I0034889

TISSUE ENGINEERING
Applications and Advancements

TISSUE ENGINEERING

Applications and Advancements

Edited by
Rajesh K. Kesharwani, PhD, MTech
Raj K. Keservani, MPharm
Anil K. Sharma, PhD, MPharm

AAP APPLE
ACADEMIC
PRESS

First edition published 2022

Apple Academic Press Inc.
1265 Goldenrod Circle, NE,
Palm Bay, FL 32905 USA

4164 Lakeshore Road, Burlington,
ON, L7L 1A4 Canada

CRC Press
6000 Broken Sound Parkway NW,
Suite 300, Boca Raton, FL 33487-2742 USA

2 Park Square, Milton Park,
Abingdon, Oxon, OX14 4RN UK

© 2022 Apple Academic Press, Inc.

Apple Academic Press exclusively co-publishes with CRC Press, an imprint of Taylor & Francis Group, LLC

Reasonable efforts have been made to publish reliable data and information, but the authors, editors, and publisher cannot assume responsibility for the validity of all materials or the consequences of their use. The authors, editors, and publishers have attempted to trace the copyright holders of all material reproduced in this publication and apologize to copyright holders if permission to publish in this form has not been obtained. If any copyright material has not been acknowledged, please write and let us know so we may rectify in any future reprint.

Except as permitted under U.S. Copyright Law, no part of this book may be reprinted, reproduced, transmitted, or utilized in any form by any electronic, mechanical, or other means, now known or hereafter invented, including photocopying, microfilming, and recording, or in any information storage or retrieval system, without written permission from the publishers.

For permission to photocopy or use material electronically from this work, access www.copyright.com or contact the Copyright Clearance Center, Inc. (CCC), 222 Rosewood Drive, Danvers, MA 01923, 978-750-8400. For works that are not available on CCC please contact mpkbookspermissions@tandf.co.uk

Trademark notice: Product or corporate names may be trademarks or registered trademarks and are used only for identification and explanation without intent to infringe.

Library and Archives Canada Cataloguing in Publication

Title: Tissue engineering : applications and advancements / edited by Rajesh K. Kesharwani, PhD, MTech, Raj K. Keservani, MPharm, Anil K. Sharma, PhD, MPharm.

Names: Kesharwani, Rajesh Kumar, 1978- editor. | Keservani, Raj K., 1981- editor. | Sharma, Anil K., 1980- editor.

Description: First edition. | Includes bibliographical references and index.

Identifiers: Canadiana (print) 2021034444X | Canadiana (ebook) 20210344482 | ISBN 9781774630204 (hardcover) | ISBN 9781774638774 (softcover) | ISBN 9781003180531 (ebook)

Subjects: LCSH: Tissue engineering.

Classification: LCC R857.T55 T57 2022 | DDC 610.28—dc23

Library of Congress Cataloging-in-Publication Data

Names: Kesharwani, Rajesh Kumar, 1978- editor. | Keservani, Raj K., 1981- editor. | Sharma, Anil K., 1980- editor.

Title: Tissue engineering : applications and advancements / edited by Rajesh K. Kesharwani, Raj K. Keservani, Anil K. Sharma.

Other titles: Tissue engineering (Kesharwani)

Description: First edition. | Palm Bay, FL : Apple Academic Press, 2022. | Includes bibliographical references and index. | Summary: "This new volume on applications and advances in tissue engineering presents significant, state-of-the-art developments in this exciting area of research. It highlights some of the most important applied research on the applications of tissue engineering along with its different components, specifically different types of biomaterials. It looks at the various issues involved in tissue engineering, including smart polymeric biomaterials, gene therapy, tissue engineering in reconstruction and regeneration of visceral organs, skin tissue engineering, bone and muscle regeneration, and applications in tropical medicines. Covering a wide range of issues in tissue engineering, the volume Provides an overview of the efficacy of the different biomaterials employed in tissue engineering (such as skin regeneration, nerve regeneration, artificial blood vessels, bone regeneration). Looks at smart polymeric biomaterials in tissue engineering Discusses the hybrid approach of tissue engineering in conjunction with gene therapy Explores using tissue engineering in the management of tropical diseases Considers various skin tissue engineering applications, including wound healing methods, skin substitutes and other materials Reports on the use of various biomaterials in bone and muscle regeneration Describes the use of tissue engineering in reconstruction and regeneration of visceral organs Covers polysaccharides and proteins-based hydrogels for tissue engineering applications Providing an abundance of advanced research and information, Tissue Engineering: Applications and Advancements will be a valuable resource for medical researchers, pharmaceutical manufacturers, healthcare personnel, and academicians"-- Provided by publisher.

Identifiers: LCCN 2021049654 (print) | LCCN 2021049655 (ebook) | ISBN 9781774630204 (hardback) | ISBN 9781774638774 (paperback) | ISBN 9781003180531 (ebook)

Subjects: MESH: Tissue Engineering--methods | Biocompatible Materials--therapeutic use

Classification: LCC R857.T55 (print) | LCC R857.T55 (ebook) | NLM QS 525 | DDC 612/.028--dc23/eng/20211101

LC record available at https://lccn.loc.gov/2021049654

LC ebook record available at https://lccn.loc.gov/2021049655

ISBN: 978-1-77463-020-4 (hbk)
ISBN: 978-1-77463-877-4 (pbk)
ISBN: 978-1-00318-053-1 (ebk)

About the Editors

Rajesh K. Kesharwani, PhD, MTech
Nehru Gram Bharati (Deemed to be University),
Prayagraj, Uttar Pradesh, India

Rajesh K. Kesharwani, PhD, has more than 10 years of research and eight years of teaching experience at various institutes of India, imparting bioinformatics and biotechnology education. He has received several awards, including the NASI-Swarna Jayanti Puruskar from The National Academy of Sciences of India. He has supervised one PhD and more than 20 undergraduate and postgraduate students for their research work, and has authored over 40 peer-reviewed articles, 20 book chapters, and 11 edited books with international publishers. He has been a member of many scientific communities as well as a reviewer for many international journals. He has presented many papers at various national and international conferences. Dr. Kesharwani received his PhD from the Indian Institute of Information Technology, Allahabad, and worked at NIT Warangal for two semesters. He has been a recipient of a Ministry of Human Resource Development (India) Fellowship and a Senior Research Fellowship from the Indian Council of Medical Research, India. His research fields of interest are medical informatics, protein structure and function prediction, computer-aided drug design, structural biology, drug delivery, cancer biology, nanobiotechnology, and biomedical sciences.

Raj K. Keservani, MPharm
Faculty of B. Pharmacy, CSM Group of Institutions, Allahabad, India

Raj K. Keservani, MPharm, is a member of the Faculty of B. Pharmacy, CSM Group of Institutions, Allahabad, India. He has more than 10 years of academic experience from various institutes of India in pharmaceutical education. He has published 30 peer-reviewed papers in the field of pharmaceutical sciences in national and international journals, 30 book chapters, two co-authored books, and 15 edited books. He is also active as a reviewer for several international scientific journals. Mr. Keservani graduated with a pharmacy degree from the Department of Pharmacy, Kumaun University, Nainital (Uttarakhand), India. He received his Master of Pharmacy (MPharm) (specialization in pharmaceutics) from the School of Pharmaceutical Sciences, Rajiv Gandhi Proudyogiki Vishwavidyalaya, Bhopal, India. His research interests include nutraceutical and functional foods, novel drug delivery systems (NDDS), transdermal drug delivery/ drug delivery, health science, cancer biology, and neurobiology.

Anil K. Sharma, PhD, MPharm
School of Medical and Allied Sciences, G. D. Goenka University, Sohna, Haryana, India

Anil Kumar Sharma, PhD, MPharm, is an expert in the area of pharmaceutics with a background in drug delivery. He has taught these subjects for nearly 10 years at universities such as the Delhi Institute of Pharmaceutical Sciences and Research, University of Delhi, and School of Medical and Allied Sciences, G D Goenka University, India. Prior to taking up his current role in 2018, Dr. Sharma served in academic positions such as Lecturer (Pharmaceutics) at Delhi Institute of Pharmaceutical Sciences and Research, University of Delhi. Dr. Sharma holds a PhD (Pharmaceutical Sciences) from the University of Delhi; MPharm (Pharmaceutics) from the Rajiv Gandhi Proudyogiki Vishwavidyalaya; and BPharm from the University of Rajasthan, India.

Contents

Contributors

Blessing Atim Aderibigbe
Department of Chemistry, University of Fort Hare, Alice Campus, Eastern Cape 5700, South Africa

Roberta Cassano
Department of Pharmacy, Health and Nutritional Sciences, University of Calabria, Arcavacata di Rende, Cosenza, Italy

Federica Curcio
Department of Pharmacy, Health and Nutritional Sciences, University of Calabria, Arcavacata di Rende, Cosenza, Italy

Eric G Ayom
Department of Chemistry, University of Zululand, KwaDlangezwa, KwaZulu-Natal, South Africa, 3886

Soma Mondal Ghorai
Department of Zoology, Hindu College, University of Delhi, Delhi-110007, India

Maria Luisa Di Gioia
Department of Pharmacy, Health and Nutritional Sciences, University of Calabria, Arcavacata di Rende, Cosenza, Italy

Merve Erginer Hasköylü
IBSB, Department of Bioengineering, Marmara University, 34722, İstanbul, Turkey

Hardeep Kaur
Department of Zoology, Ramjas College, University of Delhi, Delhi 110007, India

Akhilesh Kumar Maurya
Chemistry Laboratory Department of Applied Sciences, Indian Institute of Information Technology, Allahabad, India

Nidhi Mishra
Chemistry Laboratory Department of Applied Sciences, Indian Institute of Information Technology, Allahabad, India

Sudhanshu Mishra
Department of Advanced Science & Technology, Nims University Rajasthan, Jaipur-303121, India

Ebru Toksoy Öner
IBSB, Department of Bioengineering, Marmara University, 34722, İstanbul, Turkey

Shesan John Owonubi
Department of Chemistry, University of Zululand, KwaDlangezwa, KwaZulu-Natal 3886, South Africa

Debora Procopio
Department of Pharmacy, Health and Nutritional Sciences, University of Calabria, Arcavacata di Rende, Cosenza, Italy

Neerish Revaprasadu
Department of Chemistry, University of Zululand, KwaDlangezwa, KwaZulu-Natal, South Africa, 3886

Sinem Selvin Selvi
IBSB, Department of Bioengineering, Marmara University, 34722, İstanbul, Turkey

Sonia Trombino
Department of Pharmacy, Health and Nutritional Sciences, University of Calabria, Arcavacata di Rende, Cosenza, Italy

Viroj Wiwanitkit
Department of Community Medicine, Dr DY Patil University, Pune, India

Sora Yasri
Private Academic Practice, Bangkok, Thailand

Abbreviations

AAV	adeno-associated virus
ADA	adenosine deaminase
ALL	acute lymphoblastic leukemia
ASC	adipose-derived stem cells
ASCs	adipose stem cells
BC	bacterial cellulose
BCP	biphasic calcium phosphate
CA	cellulose acetate
CAP	cellulose acetate phthalate
CEAs	cultured epithelial autografts
CMC	carboxymethyl cellulose
CMCS	carboxymethyl chitosan
CNC	cellulose nanocrystals
CNTs	carbon nanotubes
CPBs	calcium phosphate biomaterials
CPCs	calcium phosphate cements
CPTi	commercially pure titanium
CS	chondroitin sulfate
CSA	chondroitin sulfate A
CSGT	cancer suicide gene therapy
CT	computed tomography
DBCO	dibenzyl cyclooctyne
DEAE	diethylaminoethyl
dECM	decellularized ECM
DMAc	dimethylacetamide
DSM	decellularized skeletal muscle
EBs	embryoid bodies
EC	ethyl cellulose
ECM	extracellular matrix
ECs	endothelial cells
EGF	epidermal growth factor
ELRs	elastin-like recombinamers
EPCs	endothelial progenitor cells
ESC	embryonic stem cells

EXOs   exosomes
FGF   fibroblast growth factor
FNS   fibronectins
GAGs   glycosaminoglycans
GAM   gene-activated matrix
GGT   germline gene therapy
GI   gastrointestinal
HA   hydroxyapatite
HAC   human artificial chromosomes
HCF   heparin-conjugated fibrin
hKCs   human keratinocytes
HPMC   hydroxypropyl methylcellulose
HSV   herpes simplex virus
IDD   insulin-dependent diabetes
IEPs   isoelectric points
IHC   immunohistochemistry
IM   intermediate mesoderm
INH   isoniazid
IPNs   interpenetrating networks
LCA   Leber congenital amaurosis
LIF   leukemia inhibitory factor
MC   methyl cellulose
MeHA   methacrylated HA
MM   metanephric mesenchyme
MPS   microphysiological system
MRI   magnetic resonance imaging
MSCs   mesenchymal stem cells
NaCMC   sodium carboxymethyl cellulose
NAG N-acetyl-D-glucosamine
NGF   nerve growth factor
NK   natural killer
NMMO N-methylmorpholine-N-oxide
pDNA   plasmid DNA
PEDOT   poly(3,4-ethylendioxythiophene)
PEEk   polyetheretherketone
PEG   polyethylene glycol
PEO   polyethylene oxide
PGA   polyglycolic acid
PHAs   polyhydroxyalkanoates

PLA	polylactic acid
PLGA	poly(lactide-*co*-glycolide)
PLL	poly-L-lysine
PMMA	polymethyl methacrylate
PIGS	polyimmunoglobulin G scaffold
PRP	platelet-rich plasma
PTMC	poly(trimethylene carbonate)
PUs	polyurethanes
PVA	polyvinyl alcohol
PVP	polyvinylpyrrolidone
PVPI	povidone-iodine
RGD	arginine-glycine-asparagine
RWM	restrata wound matrix
SA	sodium alginate
SCGT	somatic cell gene therapy
SCID	severe combined immunodeficiency
SDS	sodium dodecyl sulfate
SF	silk fibroin
SIS	small intestinal submucosa
STZ	streptozotocin
SVF	stromal vascular fraction
TA	tibialis anterior
TE	tissue engineering
TEPS	tissue-engineered pancreatic substitute
TK	thymidine kinase
TNF	tumor necrosis factor
TTCP	tetracalcium phosphate
UCST	upper critical solution temperature
VEGF	vascular endothelial growth factor

Foreword

It is a matter of great pleasure for me to write foreword for this book, *Tissue Engineering: Applications and Advancements*. Tissue engineering is a specialized branch under biomedical engineering (bioengineering). Owing to its outstanding advantages, tissue engineering is considered as an ultimately ideal medical treatment to regenerate a patient's own tissues and organs that are entirely free of low bio-functionality and severe immune rejection.

Tissue engineering evolved from the field of biomaterials development and refers to the practice of combining scaffolds, cells, and biologically active molecules into functional tissues. It involves medical devices, tissue replacement, repair, and regeneration. This book covers different applied aspects in tissue engineering, such as for example, smart polymeric biomaterials, gene therapy, tissue engineering application in tropical medicines, skin tissue engineering, bone and muscle regeneration, and tissue engineering in reconstruction and regeneration of visceral organs.

The volume also provides an overview of the efficacy of different biomaterials employed in tissue engineering (such as skin regeneration, nerve regeneration, artificial blood vessels, and bone regeneration) and varied aspects of tissue engineering and gene therapy, their advantages and future prospects as well as the challenges pertaining to the combination of the two. This book also describe the bioengineering of visceral organs and the various challenges that are faced in the field of tissue engineering and reconstructive surgery.

All the contributing authors have provided advanced and rich information that provide valuable insight for scientists, medical researchers, faculty, and students working in the field of material and biomedical Sciences.

I congratulate the editors for bringing together experts of *biomaterials* and *tissue engineering* and the authors for their excellent contributions.

—Prof. Krishna Misra
Honorary Professor, Indian Institute of Information Technology Allahabad,
Devghat, Jhalwa, Prayagraj 211015, Uttar Pradesh, India

Preface

This new book, *Tissue Engineering: Applications and Advancements* focuses on the ever-growing and very important topics that give a state-of-art picture of biomaterial and its application with the emphasis on its present, past, and future. There have been significant developments in the field of biomaterial and its advancement used in tissue engineering, and this volume highlights some of the most important developments in the field. The book covers different applied research involved in tissue engineering, biomaterial, smart polymeric biomaterials, gene therapy, tissue engineering in reconstruction and regeneration of visceral organs, skin tissue engineering, bone and muscle regeneration, and application in tropical medicines.

With high demand for organs and tissues all over world, the research on tissue engineering is of more concern, and this volume will be a valuable resource for medical researchers, pharmaceutical manufacturers, healthcare personnel, and academicians.

The present book includes eight chapters containing information about the advanced research on biomaterial, and tissue engineering with different applications for human welfare.

Chapter 1, entitled "Biomaterials in Tissue Engineering" authored by B. A. Aderibigbe and S. J. Owonubi, focuses on biomaterials and their use to replace the natural function of a defective organ/tissue, which can be classified as either synthetic (such as metals, polymers, ceramics) or biological material (such as natural polymers, carbon-based nanomaterials). This chapter gives an overview of the efficacy of different biomaterials employed in tissue engineering (such as skin regeneration, nerve regeneration, artificial blood vessels, and bone regeneration).

The role of smart polymeric biomaterials in tissue engineering is well demonstrated by Nidhi Mishra and her coauthor in Chapter 2. Polymeric biomaterials are one of the basics of tissue engineering. A wide range of materials has been used in the medical field. The advancement of synthetic and natural biomaterials has led to the development of stimuli responsive biomaterials, known as "smart biomaterials." These polymers have been used in the development of various medical devices, artificial organs and organ parts, targeted and controlled drug delivery with effect of specificity of biomaterials. More advanced and smart biomaterials will be developed in the future. This chapter is focused on development of smart biomaterials. It discuses natural and synthetic polymers used in their preparation and the most recent applications as biomaterials.

Chapter 3, "Gene Therapy in Tissue Engineering: Prospects and Challenges," written by Soma Mondal Ghorai and Hardeep Kaur, emphasizes gene therapy holds great prospects for future clinical therapeutics as it can be effortlessly united with tissue engineering and can repair the damaged tissue at the cellular and molecular levels. This hybrid approach of conjunction between tissue engineering and gene therapy provides the optimum environment for therapeutic protein expression for regeneration of cells and tissues; it thereby holds immense potential in areas of skin, bone, and cartilage repair. The aim of this chapter is to provide readers with the varied aspects of tissue engineering and gene therapy, their advantages, and future prospects as well as the challenges pertaining to the combination of the two.

Chapter 4, "Tissue Engineering and Application in Tropical Medicine," is authored by Sora Yasri and Viroj Wiwanitkit, with reference to application in tropical medicine. The modeling of the natural tissue growth and development is the basic concept and process of the novel tissue engineering. Introducing the new technology such as tissue engineering for the management of tropical diseases becomes a new challenging issue in tropical medicine.

Since skin is the outermost layer of human body and protects it from external hazards, any damage of this tissue, like wounds and burns may result in serious health problems. Chapter 5, "Skin Tissue Engineering: Past, Present, Future Perspectives" is written by Sinem Selvin Selvi and his colleague. Skin tissue engineering applications are found to be one of the first ones in history because of their importance and urgency. Here in this chapter, the authors discuss the history of tissue engineering, wound healing methods, skin substitutes, materials used with the current and promising applications.

The details about regeneration or repair of skeletal muscle tissue or bone are well described in Chapter 6, "Biomaterial in Bone and Muscle Regeneration," by Shesan John Owonubi and his associates. Biomaterials have been employed over the years in the regeneration of bones and muscles. The regeneration or repair of skeletal muscle tissue or muscles is necessary when innate muscle or bones cannot on initiate their own repair. This chapter introduces biomaterials and the advancement of biomaterials, is it indicates exactly what both bone and muscle regeneration involves, and with numerous research findings reported, it dwells on biomaterials in bone regeneration.

Chapter 7, "Tissue Engineering in Reconstruction and Regeneration of Visceral Organs," by Soma Mondal Ghorai and Sudhanshu Mishra, well describes reconstruction and regeneration of visceral organs and limitations due to imperding shortage of donor tissues/organs and low rates of successful surgeries, mainly in pediatric patients. Tissue engineering is an innovative field that combines engineering with biology and is the answer to the above mentioned limitation. This strategy helps to reconstruct and regenerate damaged and diseased tissues/organs. This chapter discusses bioengineering of visceral organs and the various challenges that are faced in the field of tissue engineering and reconstructive surgery.

Chapter 8, "Polysaccharides and Proteins Based Hydrogels for Tissue Engineering Applications," is written by Sonia Trombino and her colleagues, in very precise manner with scientific fact. The authors describe specifically the natural biomaterials based on polysaccharides and proteins used in tissue engineering and their most important applications.

The present volume, *Tissue Engineering: Applications and Advancements,* provides detailed information on application of tissue engineering and its different components especially different types of biomaterials, and their applications in various types of tissue/organ regeneration. This book provides advanced research and a wealth of information that will be valuable to medical scientists, researchers, academicians, and students.

CHAPTER 1

Biomaterials in Tissue Engineering

BLESSING ATIM ADERIBIGBE[1*] and SHESAN JOHN OWONUBI[2]

[1]Department of Chemistry, University of Fort Hare, Alice Campus, Eastern Cape 5700, South Africa

[2]Department of Chemistry, University of Zululand, KwaDlangezwa, KwaZulu-Natal 3886, South Africa

*Corresponding author. E-mail: blessingaderibigbe@gmail.com

ABSTRACT

Biomaterials used to replace the natural function of a defective organ/tissue can be classified as either synthetic (such as metals, polymers, and ceramics) or biological materials (such as natural polymers and carbon-based nano-materials). These materials interact with the biological system. They can be modified to enhance their biostability, biocompatibility, physicochemical properties, mechanical properties, and their interaction with the biological system. Biomaterials have been employed in tissue engineering as regenerative scaffolds, for bone regeneration, as implants, etc. In the selection of biomaterials for tissue engineering, several factors are taken into consideration such as the nature and properties of the biomaterial, etc. This chapter gives an overview and efficacy of the different biomaterials employed in tissue engineering (such as skin regeneration, nerve regeneration, artificial blood vessels, and bone regeneration).

1.1 INTRODUCTION

Tissue engineering is an interdisciplinary field, which is focused on the regeneration of functional human tissues/organs (Keane and Badylak, 2014; Tur, 2009; O'brien, 2011). These materials are developed for the regeneration of tissues/organs and are in continuous contact with the body tissue cells (Keane and Badylak, 2014). These biomaterials are combined with cells and bioactive molecules (Keane and Badylak, 2014; Tur, 2009). Biomaterials are classified as biological and synthetic depending on their sources. A biomaterial scaffold provides shape, mechanical and structural support with a tailored surface suitable for cell attachment, cell–cell interaction, and cell proliferation and differentiation (Khan and Tanaka, 2017). Biomaterials are placed within the body and as such, they must be biocompatible, nontoxic, and have adequate physicochemical and mechanical properties (Tur, 2009). They have been used in various biomedical applications such as skin regeneration, bone regeneration, tissue/organ regeneration, dental applications, etc. The success of a biomaterial developed for implantation is determined by the host response to the scaffold material after years of implantation. There are advantages and disadvantages for each biomaterial used in tissue engineering. This chapter will give an overview of biomaterials used in tissue/organ regeneration.

1.2   CLASSES OF BIOMATERIALS

Biomaterials used in tissue engineering are classified as synthetic biomaterials and biological/natural biomaterials (Figure 1.1) (He and Lu, 2016). Synthetic biomaterials are further classified as polymers, composites, metals, ceramics, and glasses (He and Lu, 2016; Nigam and Mahanta, 2014). The biological/natural biomaterials are further classified as carbon-based materials, cell, tissue, protein, peptides, etc. (Bhat and Kumar, 2012; Ha et al., 2013). Some biomedical-based scaffolds are prepared from the combination of synthetic and natural biomaterials resulting in scaffolds with excellent physicochemical properties (Mengyan et al., 2005; Galler et al., 2018). The biomedical applications of biomaterials include dental, orthopedic, skin regeneration, etc. (Galler et al., 2018).

1.2.1   SYNTHETIC-BASED BIOMATERIALS USED IN TISSUE ENGINEERING

1.2.1.1   METALS

Metals are used in the design of scaffolds for implantation due to their unique feature such as excellent strength. However, they are prone to corrosion resulting in the release of metal ions that cause toxic reactions and their poor biocompatibility limits their use as implants (Saini et al., 2015). Metal-based biomaterials are used for the development of biomedical devices for orthopedic, artificial organs, dental, bone applications, etc. (Bose et al., 2012; Xiao et al., 2012). Some of the metals used are Ti- and Co-based alloys, stainless steel, magnesium, and iron and the metal-based nanoparticles used are Ag, Cu, Au, or Co nanoparticles (Prasad et al., 2017; Yoo et al., 2008).

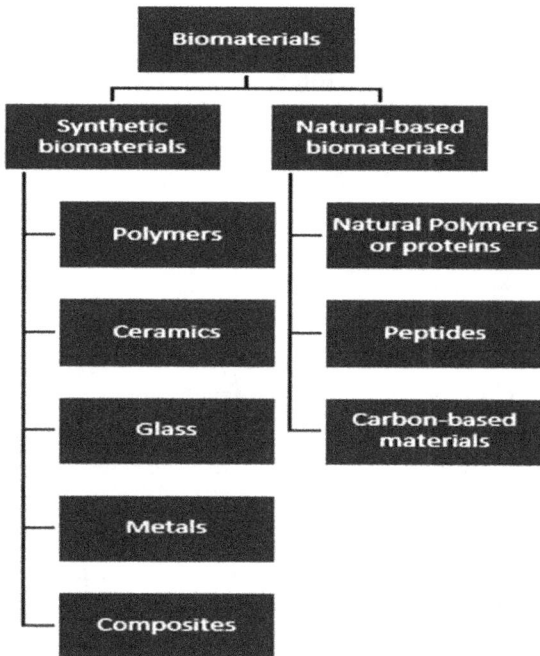

FIGURE 1.1   Classification of synthetic biomaterials and biological/natural biomaterials.

1.2.1.1.1   Metal-based Biomaterials for Bone and Joint Replacement

Selected metals such as surgical cobalt–chromium (Co–Cr) alloys, stainless steel (316L), and titanium (Ti) alloys are commonly used metals for fracture fixation and bone remodeling (Prasad et al., 2017). They exhibit long-term stability resulting from their low corrosion, excellent mechanical properties, and friction. Surgical stainless-steel alloys (316L) made with varying amounts of nickel, iron, and chromium have been used in the manufacture of prostheses (Yoo et al., 2008). The low carbon content in surgical stainless steel reduces corrosion and metal allergic reactions (Yoo et al., 2008). However, it is prone to stress corrosion and cracking. Its use is often limited in biomedical application where strength is not required for a prolonged period (Pruitt and Chakravartula, 2012). Stainless steels are less expensive when compared to other alloys. However, some metals lack a biologically active surface that can induce osteointegration or prevent infections resulting in more research which involves the coating of implants. In the selection of coatings for metal implants used for bone replacement, factors such as biocompatibility, the capability to induce osteoblasts, good mechanical stability, and antimicrobial activity must be considered (Godbole et al., 2016; Kiel et al., 2008). Metal implants are used for artificial hip joints, bone plates, spinal fixation devices, and artificial dental roots. The mechanical biocompatibility of metals used for implants is measured by Young's modulus, which describes the response of a material to stress and strain (Niinomi and Nakai, 2014). Metals with Young's modulus, equal to that of the bone, are ideal for metallic implants, thereby reducing the stress shielding effect (Niinomi and Nakai, 2014).

Titanium alloys have been developed for bone replacement by several researchers. They are employed in the development of orthopedic devices such as knee and hip implants because of their excellent mechanical properties and resistance to infections. However, there have been concerns about their long-term effect on human health. Powderized titanium–tantalum alloy, which is highly biocompatible for bone replacements, was prepared using selective laser melting by blending jagged tantalum powder with titanium microspheres powder. The stress shielding effect, which is common in metal-based implants, when they are too elastic, thereby transferring insufficient loads to the neighboring bones, was not observed in the powderized titanium-tantalum alloy indicating their potential to improve patient care (Nikels, 2016). Sumitomo et al. investigated the biocompatibility of low rigidity titanium alloy (Ti-29Nb-13Ta-4.6Zr) in bone plate fixation *in vivo* using rabbit (Sumitomo et al., 2008). Experimental fractures were made in rabbit tibiae and fixed using the titanium alloy. It was compared to the conventional bone plates of SUS316L and Ti-6Al-4V. The diameter of the tibia bone was increased in the titanium alloy indicating bone remodeling when compared to SUS316L and Ti-6Al-4V. The elastic modulus of the bone plate influenced bone tissue reaction to the bone plate fixation. The elastic modulus of the titanium alloy was 58 GPa when compared to SUS316L and Ti-6Al-4V which was 161 GPa and 108 GPa, respectively. The low rigidity of the titanium alloy delayed the bone atrophy and enhanced bone reorganization due to the mechanical stress, which is clinically useful for long-term implantation in aged patients and high-risk patients with severe complications (Sumitomo et al., 2008). Nakai et al. (2011) also investigated titanium alloys by self-adjustment of Young's modulus.

Young's modulus of titanium alloys via deformation-induced phase transformation was investigated. β-type titanium alloys exhibiting deformation-induced ω-phase transformation in which only Young's modulus of the deformed part was increased while the nondeformed part remains low was developed making them useful for spinal fixation devices (Nakai et al., 2011). In the development of spinal fixation implants, implants with high rigidity result in the stress shielding effect. Materials with low Young's modulus are often preferred for healthy spine formation (Shi et al., 2012; Wang et al., 2013; Nakai et al., 2015). Implants are usually subjected to bending during surgery in order to obtain the curvature of the spine indicating that the implant must have a high Young's modulus (Nakai et al., 2011, 2015; Noshchenko et al., 2011). The degree of spring back of the implant is influenced by the strength and the Young's modulus of the spinal fixation implant. Higher Young's modulus will exhibit a smaller spring back (Niinomi and Nakai, 2011). The aforementioned factor has resulted in the development of deformation-induced ω-phase transformation in β-type Ti alloys in which the deformed material exhibits high Young's modulus, while the nondeformed part exhibits low Young's modulus thereby satisfying the conflicting requirement of Young's modulus (Nakai et al., 2015; Zhao et al., 2011a, 2011b, 2012a, 2012b; Liu et al., 2014).

In magnetic resonance imaging used for the diagnosis of various diseases, metallic orthopedic devices implanted in the human body cause distortions of the images of the organs and tissues around the implant thereby hindering correct diagnosis. The distortion of the images formed is due to the difference in magnetic susceptibilities between living tissues and metallic materials (Nakai et al., 2015). This magnetic susceptibility of Ti is lower when compared to ferromagnetic iron and Co. However, it is higher than water. Zirconium, Zr, exhibits a smaller magnetic susceptibility of 1.3×10^{-6} cm^3 g^{-1} and some of its alloys have been employed for implants (Nakai et al., 2015; Kondo et al., 2011; Suyalatu et al., 2010, 2011).

Cobalt-chromium-based alloys have been used for prosthetic arthroplasty. Their unique mechanical properties make them suitable for total hip and knee joint arthroplasty (Bal et al., 2007). Cobalt is not a biocompatible biomaterial. However, the addition of 15–30% chromium creates a passivating oxide film which is stable in the body (Haynes et al., 2000; Rabiei, 2010). CoCr alloys exhibit good corrosion resistance. However, they are difficult to fabricate due to their brittle nature (Haynes et al., 2000; Rabiei, 2010). Ogawa et al. seeded CoCr-based alloy implant surface with rabbit marrow mesenchymal cells and left the other side unseeded (Ogawa et al., 2012). The CoCr implants were then implanted in rabbit bone defects. After 3 weeks, the implantation revealed new bone formation. However, no bone formation was detected on the unseeded side indicating that early fixation of CoCr-based alloy can result in cementless fixation in various joint arthroplasties (Ogawa et al., 2012). The wear resistance of Co alloys is higher when compared to Ti alloys and stainless steel alloys (Niinomi, 2002). The head of the joint in artificial hip joints is subjected to wear. To increase the resistance of Co alloy to wear, it has been overcome by dispersing carbide in Co alloys and by transforming the metastable γ phase to the ε martensitic phase (Niinomi, 2008). Grandfield et al. studied *in vivo* response to the free-form fabricated CoCr implants with and without hydroxyapatite (HA) plasma-sprayed coatings in the tibial metaphysis of New Zealand white rabbits. After 6 weeks, the plasma-sprayed coating of HA to implants enhanced *in vivo* interaction suggesting resorption and increased interface strength (Grandfield et al., 2011). The coating of the implants also has the potential to prevent the release of metallic ions at the implant surface, which can induce periprosthetic bone loss resulting in implant failure (Haynes et al., 2000). The addition of a biocompatible layer, such as HA, may act as a buffer to prevent the release of biologically harmful metallic ions. There have been reports of high concentration of chromium and cobalt in blood after implants resulting in neurological problems (Clark et al., 2014; Bradberry et al., 2014; Campbell and Estey, 2013). Cobalt from implants is found in two forms inside the body. The divalent (Co^{II}) state is more toxic when compared to the metallic ($Co0$) state. Chromium has three states which are metallic (Cr^{o}), trivalent (Cr^{III}), and hexavalent (Cr^{VI}). Trivalent chromium is mildly toxic, while the hexavalent chromium compounds are strongly carcinogenic and can cause kidney damage (Swiatkowska et al., 2018).

The most commonly used steel alloys are 316 and 316L grades. 316L steel alloy is preferred for implant fabrications because of its reduced carbon content which decreases the possibility of chromium carbide formation which can result in intergranular corrosion, thereby making it resistant to corrosion by physiological saline. However, it is prone to corrosion by chloride ions and reduced sulfur compounds (Manivasagam et al., 2010; Xu et al., 2006). Microorganism on the metal surface can affect the concentration of the electrolytic constituents, pH, and oxygen levels negatively (Maniva-sagam et al., 2010; Xu et al., 2006). Furthermore, studies have revealed that over 90% of the failure of 316L stainless steel implants result from pitting and crevice corrosion attack (Sivakumar et al., 1995). Ti alloy implants have been reported to suppress the development of inflammation when compared to stainless-steel alloy implants (Akyol et al., 2017).

1.2.1.1.2 Metal-based Biomaterials for Dental Application

Metal-based biomaterials have been used as dental implants such as artificial tooth root which is inserted in the jaw for tooth replacement (Duraccio et al., 2015). The implant is surgically inserted and the shape of the implant varies. The formation of a strong bond between the implant and jawbone is known as osseointegration, which anchors the implant by the development of bone tissue around the implant. However, it is important to mention that an absolute bone-to-implant contact does not occur (Duraccio et al., 2015). There are several factors that influence osseointegration such as the medical state of the patient, habits, for example, smoking, the properties and the design of the implant, quality of the bone, radiation therapy, and bacterial contamination, etc. (Duraccio et al., 2015; Goutam et al., 2013; Park et al., 2006). The common metals, which are used for dental implants, are pure titanium and the alloy of titanium and zirconium dioxide. The unique properties of titanium, which include its nontoxicity, biocompatibility, resistance to corrosion, good fatigue strength, controlled degradability, and modulus of elasticity, are useful for dental applications (Duraccio et al., 2015). Titanium implant surfaces are usually modified by roughening and coating in order to enhance the rate of osseointegration (Duraccio et al., 2015).

Methods used for creating a rough surface of titanium implant include titanium plasma spraying, anodization, blasting with ceramic particles, and acid etching (Bauer et al., 2013). In titanium plasma-spraying method, titanium powder is injected onto the implant resulting in the formation of a film with enhanced surface area and tensile strength (Jemat et al., 2015). Knabe et al. investigated a titanium surface having a porous titanium plasma-sprayed coating on rat bone marrow cells. The titanium surface enhanced facilitated rat bone marrow cells growth with high cell density which indicates that it is suitable for dental implants (Knabe et al., 2002). Hung et al. developed dental implants by plasma-sprayed HA coating on titanium (Ti-6Al-4V ELI) surfaces with a coating thickness of approximately 120 μm. The implants were uniformly covered by the HA coating and exhibited high biocompatibility (Hung et al., 2013). Eom et al. also showed that the HA coating of implants shortens the time of bone healing at poor bone quality sites and they are useful for early loading after the placement of the implant (Eom et al., 2012). Huang et al. reported the antibacterial effect of surface treatment of titanium. ZrO_2–silver (Ag) and ZrO_2–copper (Cu) coatings were sprayed onto titanium surface resulting in an improved antibacterial performance of the coated titanium implant when compared to the pure titanium implants (Huang et al., 2013). Titanium surface is also roughened by blasting with hard ceramic particles. However, particles must be stable, biocompatible, and should not interfere or hinder the osseointegration of the implants (Duraccio et al., 2015). Alumina has been used for blasting of titanium surfaces due to its insolubility in acid.

Gehrke et al. evaluated the effects of aluminum and titanium dioxide (TiO_2) microparticles for blasting during the sandblasting acid surface treatment in titanium dental implants using a rabbit tibia model (Gehrke et al., 2016). The residual blasting titanium particles on the surface of dental implants did not affect the osseointegration of the titanium dental implants but resulted in high osteoconductivity and good bone formation (Gehrke et al., 2016). Diniz et al. characterized titanium surfaces blasted with aluminum oxide particles followed by the treatment with a hydrofluoric acid-based solution. The treatment resulted in depressions up to 10 μm on the homogeneous surfaces (Diniz et al., 2005). After the chemical treatment, the surfaces were smooth, homogeneous with a regular microtopography when compared to surfaces without chemical treatment which exhibited irregular morphology and depressions (Diniz et al., 2005). In another report by Gehrke et al., *in vivo* host response of a surface sandblasted with particles of titanium oxide followed by acid etching was studied. The implants were placed in the tibia of six rabbits. The surface of the implants was homogeneous with uniform irregularities and small residues of the metal oxides. Reduced risk of contamination by the residual metal oxide from the blasting procedure was observed. The titanium oxide blasting produced an enhanced effect on the osseointegration and on the biomechanical features of the implants. The residual blasting titanium particles on the surface of dental implants did not affect the osseointegration of titanium dental implants (Gehrke et al., 2015). Etching with strong acids is another approach for the roughening of titanium dental implants, which creates micropits on the surface of the implant (Duraccio et al., 2015). It also enhances osseointegration (Herrero-Climent et al., 2013; Okazaki et al., 2017). The use of dual acid etching produces a microrough surface and enhances the osteoconductive process resulting in bone formation directly on the surface of the implant (Al-Radha and Sahib, 2016; Giner et al., 2017). The titanium anodized surface results in micro- and nanosurfaces, which increases blood clot retention and favors osseointegration (Traini et al., 2018). The anodization process is complex and is influenced by factors such as the concentration of acid used, the density of the current, the composition, and the temperature of the electrolyte (Traini et al., 2018; Shayganpour et al., 2015).

In titanium surface coating, different methods have been developed such as sol–gel coating, plasma spraying, sputter deposition, etc. Hyun-Pil et al. evaluated coated TiO_2 nanotube with HA by the sol–gel process on osteoblast-like cell and bone formation in rat tibia. Cell viability was studied after 1, 3, and 7 days of incubation *in vitro*. Implants were inserted into the tibia of rats. After 7 days of implantation, there was high cell viability on the coated TiO_2 nanotube with enhanced hydrophilicity and improved osseointegration. The findings suggest that HA-coated TiO_2 nanotube can be used as dental implants (Lim et al., 2018). Catauro et al. coated commercially pure titanium (CPTi) grade 4 substrates by a sol–gel process with poly(ε-caprolactone) (PCL) and silica.

Significant HA nucleation was observed on the surface of the coated substrates after soaking in a fluid simulating human blood plasma. The coating improved the bioactivity and biocompatibility of the implants (Catauro et al., 2018). The coating with PCL produced a crack-free surface (Catauro et al., 2018; Teng et al., 2014). Harle et al. developed sol–gel coatings on titanium substrates with various compositions under controlled processing conditions and evaluated the biological efficacy of the coatings. *In vitro* studies on primary human osteoblast cells revealed significant proliferation and attachment on the sol–gel-coated surfaces when compared to the uncoated titanium (Harle et al., 2006).

Zirconia has also been used to fabricate dental implants because of its properties such as tooth-like color, excellent mechanical properties, and biocompatibility. The use of zirconia prevents complication such as gingival recession (Depprich et al., 2008; Piconi and Maccauro, 1999). Despite its excellent mechanical properties, its long-term durability is uncertain. There have been reports of its failure *in vivo* caused by low-temperature degradation or aging (Lughi and Sergo, 2010). In the presence of water, there is a slow transformation from the tetragonal into the monoclinic phase resulting in its progressive deterioration. The results of the aging process are surface and strength degradation with grain pullout and microcracking (Lughi and Sergo,

2010). Some of its physical and mechanical properties include low thermal conductivity, favorable fracture resistance, wear and corrosion resistance, and high flexural strength (900–1200 MPa) (Cionca et al., 2016). Thoma et al. placed zirconia dental implants (BPI, VC, ZD) in six dogs. The implant systems demonstrated significant loss of marginal bone between the baseline and the crown insertion ranging between 0. 29 and 0.80 mm. The zirconia implants were prone to fracture prior to and after loading with one-piece zirconia implants when compared to the two-piece zirconia implants and titanium implants (Thoma et al., 2015). The fracture was influenced by the implant design. Gahlert et al. reported that zirconia implants with a diameter of 3. 25 and 4 mm are prone to fracture. The fractured implants were located at the anterior side of the maxilla and the mandibular. The fracture was caused by strong bruxism. Mechanical overloading also caused the fracture of the implants. The proper handling of the material, the surface modification, and the design had an impact on the strength of zirconia (Gahlert et al., 2011).

Bormann et al. compared zirconia implants with sandblasted and acid-etched titanium implants. All implants had a diameter of 4.1 mm and a length of 10 mm. The zirconia implants properties were similar to the roughened titanium surface. There were no statistically significant differences between the two materials after a healing period of 4 and 12 weeks (Bormann et al., 2011). Hempel et al. evaluated Saos-2 cells on either a sandblasted or a sandblasted/etched zirconia and compared with a sandblasted/etched titanium. A high adherent of cells after 24-h incubation on zirconia when compared with titanium was observed. The rate of cell proliferation after 48 h was high with zirconia when compared with titanium. The result indicated that zirconia has a significant effect on cell adhesion, proliferation, and differentiation when compared with titanium (Hempel et al., 2010). Chung et al. evaluated and compared the osseointegration in rabbit tibiae of smooth and roughened powder injection-molded zirconia implants with or without (Ti, Zr)O$_2$ surface coatings. The coatings changed the surface topography and chemical composition of the zirconia implants. The smooth and roughly coated zirconia implants revealed enhanced bone to implant contact when compared to the uncoated implants. The roughly coated and uncoated implants exhibited high mechanical anchorage (Chung et al., 2013). Montero et al. evaluated titanium and zirconia implants placed into fresh extraction sockets in beagles without oral hygiene attention or a soft diet during postoperative healing. The implant failure rate for the zirconia implants was 3.5 times higher when compared to the titanium implants. The zirconia implants were characterized by a less favorable topography, a significantly lower roughness (Ra = 0.85 ± 0.04 pm), negative skewness of the surface profile (−1.56 ± 0. 27), and higher kurtosis (7.88 ± 1.99) (Montero et al., 2015). Schliephake et al. reported that after 4 weeks, the mean bone to implant contact of sandblasted and sandblasted/etched zirconia surfaces was comparable to sandblasted/etched titanium surfaces *in vivo*. After 13 weeks, there was a continuous increase in the mean bone to implant contact in the titanium group. However, the mechanical anchorage was significantly lower in the zirconia implant when compared to the titanium implants after 4 weeks (Schliephake et al., 2010). However, it is important to mention that most of the clinical studies on zirconia implants are short term indicting that there is a need for substantial results from long-term clinical trials. More research to prevent the aging, improve the structure, surface properties, and osseointegration of zirconia implant is needed.

1.2.1.1.3 *Metal-based Biomaterials for Facial Reconstruction*

The application of metal-based biomaterials for the restoration of the shape and function of the maxillofacial region has been reported. Metals used for maxillofacial surgery require specific mechanical properties such as good tensile strength, shear stress, elasticity, and yield strength (Pacifici, 2016). The commonly used metals for maxillofacial surgery are titanium, gold, stainless steel, and vitallium. 3D-printed titanium TRUMATCH® maxillofacial implants have been designed for jaw and facial reconstruction (Goble, 2017). Clinical studies reported that the reconstruction of maxillectomy defects and through cheek defects using a titanium mesh in combination with folded-free anterolateral thigh flap are a feasible approach with high success rate and a low incidence of complications (Wu et al., 2016). Titanium is chemically inert with little hypersensitive reaction, it is easily trimmed, it resists mechanical strains, and it maintains a proper shape (Wu et al., 2016). However, there is a risk of infection after reconstruction. The use of titanium mesh implantation for skeletal reconstruction after maxillectomy is beneficial for fragile and aged patients (Wu et al., 2016). Costan et al. studied the efficacy of titanium mesh panels for reconstructing the craniofacial skeleton between January 2015 and December 2017. The study on 26 patients in 20 trauma-related cases and six cases of postablative defects when titanium mesh was covered using locoregional flaps revealed restoration of facial dimensions (Costan et al., 2018). The use of titanium mesh resulted in a proper reconstruction of the orbital floor, without complaints of postoperative diplopia. The mesh was not exposed postoperatively (Costan et al., 2018). There are other reports on the application of titanium implant for facial reconstruction (Crainiceanu et al., 2016; Yi et al., 2012; Gear et al., 2002; Schön et al., 2006). The titanium mesh is a malleable system that provides good support where there is a lack of bone support (Sixto et al., 2016). Nasal reconstruction can be performed using titanium mesh and external skin reconstruction without the repair of the intranasal lining, thereby decreasing operation time. However, titanium mesh is not suitable for patients who had prior postoperative radiotherapy (Kao et al., 2017).

Vitallium mesh has also been used for facial reconstruction as a replacement for the bony skeleton without complications or morbidity (Sengezer and Sadove, 1992). However, its use is dependent on its rigid fixation (Sengezer and Sadove, 1992). Study on animal models showed that it is less biocompatible when compared to titanium which is characterized by an increase in the accumulation of metal ions in the implant surrounding area (Pacifici, 2016; Jakobsen et al., 2010).

1.2.1.2   POLYMERS

Polymers used in regenerative medicine can be classified as natural or synthetic polymers. They represent the most significant biomaterials resulting from their inert nature. Their physicochemical properties are easily tailored based on their applications. Synthetic polymers are characterized by good mechanical properties. However, their biocompatibility is poor when compared to natural polymers. Polymers have been used for the regeneration of bone, cartilage, skin, etc.

1.2.1.2.1   Polymers Application for Skin Regeneration

Polymer-based materials such as hydrogels, films, composites, fibers, etc., have been developed for skin regeneration. Severe skin damage resulting from injury can be life-threatening. Skin regeneration involves a combination of complex biological processes such as inflammation, proliferation, and remodeling. Despite the availability of a wide range of wound dressings, wound healing still remains a clinical challenge globally among the aged people, people with chronic conditions, burn patients, etc. (Han and Ceilley, 2017).

Polymers have been designed for skin regeneration in chronic and acute wounds. Synthetic polymers such as polyethylene glycol (PEG), poloxamer, pluronic, polylactic acid (PLA), polyacrylic acid, PCL, polyvinylpyrrolidone, and polyvinyl alcohol (PVA) have been used as biomaterials to develop hydrogels for skin regeneration (Mogoşanu and Grumezescu, 2014; Sell et al., 2010). Synthetic polymers have good mechanical properties but some of them are not biocompatible. PEG-based materials have been designed for skin regeneration and they are characterized by rapid wound closure and bleeding control, tissue adhesion, controlled degradability, and elastomeric mechanical properties suitable for skin regeneration (Chen et al., 2018b).

They are also characterized by good biocompatibility, which provide adequate moisture to the wound bed with gradual resorption and replacement by structured skin tissue suitable for the management of complicated wounds (Venzin and Jacot, 2016). Incorporating chemokines onto PEG-based wound dressing materials is useful for skin regeneration in chronic wounds resulting in the reduction of inflammation, increased granulation tissue formation, vascularization, and wound closure (Lohmann et al., 2017). PEG-based wound dressings have been designed as injectable gels with excellent pH response, rapid gelation time, excellent deformability, and good mechanical strength with the capability to stop bleeding in severe traumatic injuries (Zhang et al., 2018). PEG-based scaffold has also been designed as bilayered microenvironment, which supports fibroblasts on the top and keratinocytes at the bottom (Tsao et al., 2014).

The combination of polycaprolactone with poloxamer to develop nano-fibers resulted in materials with excellent mechanical strength and good biocompatibility. The nanofiber acted as a protective barrier and integrated with the host skin tissue. The tensile strength and the hydrophilic property of the nanofibers provided good resilience and compliance to movement as a skin graft (Pan et al., 2014). Polycaprolactone scaffolds incorporated with ZnO nanoparticles can act as skin substitute materials, thereby promoting wound healing. It enhances cell adhesion and migration without the formation of a scar (Augustine et al., 2014). The combination of PEG, poly-caprolactone, and natural polymers to produce scaffolds further enhanced epithelial differentiation. *In vivo* efficacy studies on a second-degree burn wound model in Wistar rats revealed an increased rate of wound contraction (Bhowmick et al., 2018).

Polycaprolactone-based materials used to develop engineered skin substitute exhibited good cell adhesion and inhibited early shrinkage of the material after seeding with fibroblasts (Bhowmick et al., 2018). Nanofibers prepared from a combination of chitosan and PCL were evaluated *in vivo* on a mouse cutaneous excisional skin defect model. An increased wound healing rate and complete wound closure were observed when compared to the commercially available occlusive dressing (Levengood et al., 2017).

Other synthetic polymers have also been used to develop materials for skin regeneration. However, due to the poor biocompatibility of synthetic polymers, they are combined with natural polymers for enhanced biocompatibility. Polyvinylpyrrolidone has been combined with gelatin for skin grafts applications.

The skin grafts were biocompatible and biodegradable resulting from gelatin, while polyvinylpyrrolidone is an inert component with good water affinity (Kenawy et al., 2014). PVA is one of the oldest synthetic polymers used to develop materials for wound dressing due to its good biocompatibility (Kenawy et al., 2014). However, materials developed from PVA do not have sufficient elasticity and exhibit poor hydrophilicity properties when used as a wound dressing polymeric material (Yang et al., 2010). PLA-based nanofibers have been found to be effective in wound healing by protecting the wound, preventing the loss of moisture, enhancing the proliferation of cells, and the closure of large wounds (Sundaramurthi et al., 2014).

1.2.1.2.2 Polymers Application for Bone and Cartilage Regeneration

The design of polymer-based scaffolds for bone and cartilage regeneration is a potential approach, which can eliminate the problems of supply scarcity, potential pathogen transfer, and immunogenicity (Pina et al., 2015). In the design of scaffolds for bone and cartilage regeneration, the physicochemical, structural, and biological properties of the scaffolds should mimic the natural extracellular matrix (ECM) thereby providing desired environment for cell proliferation, differentiation, and bone or cartilage regeneration (Chan and Leong, 2008). The porosity of the scaffolds also plays a major role in maintaining the diffusion of nutrients and metabolites (Loh and Choong, 2013). Among the materials used for the preparation of scaffolds for bone and cartilage regeneration, polymers and their composites are the most promising candidates due to their good biocompatibility and biodegradability (Puppi et al., 2010).

Synthetic polymers such as PLA, polyglycolic acid, and polycaprolactone have been used for the development of scaffolds for bone tissue regeneration.

However, synthetic polymers are combined with inorganic materials and bioactive molecules for optimized osteogenic outcomes (Puppi et al., 2010). The synthesis of synthetic polymers is via controlled conditions resulting in good mechanical properties, controlled rate of degradation, and microstructure, which are reproducible by the incorporation of selected functional groups (Ma et al., 2016). Aliphatic polyesters such as PLA, polyglycolic acid, etc., degrade *in vivo* by hydrolysis, which are nonenzymatic resulting in products which are not toxic (Shi et al., 2016). PLA scaffolds prepared by the interface of the Ti3C2Tz nanosheets with the hydrophobic matrix of PLA exhibited a tensile strength of 72 MPa which is over 33% higher than the pure PLA membrane.

The scaffolds exhibited excellent biocompatibility, increased cell adhesion, proliferation, and osteogenic differentiation indicating their potential application for bone regeneration (Chen et al., 2018a). PLA-based scaffold, prepared from the combination of high concentration solvent casting, particulate leaching, and room temperature compression molding, exhibited good pore size and mechanical properties. The concentration of HA in the scaffold influenced its mechanical properties and porous structure. The scaffold with 20% HA exhibited porosity, contact angle, compressive yield strength, and weight loss of 84. 28 ± 7.04%, 45.13 ± 2.40, 1.57 ± 0.09 MPa, and 4.77 ± 0.32%, respectively, after 56 days (Mao et al., 2018). The aforementioned properties revealed the effect of combining synthetic polymers with ceramics. Poly(lactic-*co*-glycolic acid)-based scaffolds exhibited an interconnected porous architecture with pore sizes of 200–400 µm. SBA-15 modification provided the desired environment for the cell attachment, spreading, and proliferation on the scaffolds. The scaffolds exhibited excellent biocompatibility and biodegradability with effective osteogenesis *in vivo* (Wu et al., 2017).

Polycaprolactone-based scaffolds have also been used in bone regeneration. The design of a 3D polycaprolactone scaffold with properties such as porosity and biocompatibility with mechanical strength suitable for the proliferation and regeneration of tissues has been reported. The pore size was in a range of 200–400 µm and Young's modulus (E) was in the range of 0.121–0.171 GPa, which are compatible with the modulus of natural bone. The scaffolds cell proliferation capability revealed their ability to enhance osseous tissue formation, which is suitable for bone tissue regeneration (Gómez-Lizárraga et al., 2017). Polycaprolactone scaffolds seeded with bone morphogenetic protein-7-transduced human gingival fibroblasts and implanted subcutaneously in immunocompromised mice for a period of 4 and

8 weeks indicated good bone penetration into high permeability scaffolds, with visible blood vessel infiltration at 4 weeks. The results indicate that polycaprolactone scaffold with regular architecture and good permeability is suitable *in vivo* for bone regeneration (Mitsak et al., 2011). Polycaprolactone scaffolds have been utilized for the delivery of mesenchymal stem cells. The scaffolds were not enriched with biologically active agents. The scaffold provided a suitable environment for osteogenic differentiation of the mesenchymal stem cells illustrating the potential capability of polycaprolactone-based scaffolds as bone grafts (Rumiński et al., 2017).

Other synthetic polymers such as PVA, polyphosphoester (PPE), poly(trimethylene carbonate) (PTMC), polyurethanes (PUs), and poly-γ-glutamic acid (γ-PGA) have also been used for scaffolds for bone regeneration. PVA-based scaffolds exhibit good water uptake indicating a good hydrophilic property. They also possess uniform pore size with diameters ranged between 142 and 519 μm and are nontoxic in nature which is suitable for bone tissue regeneration (Pineda-Castillo et al., 2018). Scaffolds prepared from a combination of modified cellulose and PVA exhibit an average diameter in the range of 117–500 nm; decreased degree of crystallinity and the presence of glycosidic linkage further enhanced the biocompatibility of the scaffolds (Chahal et al., 2013).

Combining biphasic calcium phosphate (BCP) and PVA resulted in porous scaffold with interconnected pore structure, good mechanical strength, good biodegradation rate, and cytocompatibility essential for bone tissue regeneration (Nie et al., 2012). Coating scaffolds prepared from the combination of PVA and hydroxyethyl cellulose with nano-HA enhanced the tensile strength and decreased the elongation at breakage of the scaffolds. The coating influenced cell proliferation and differentiation (Chahal et al., 2016). The release mechanism of recombinant human bone morphogenetic protein-2 (rhBMP-2) from scaffolds of PPE loaded with rhBMP-2 was a combination of burst and sustained release. The cytotoxic effect of the scaffolds was reduced and the scaffolds were biocompatible. The bioactivity of rhBMP-2 was retained after the polymerization process of the scaffolds (Tian et al., 2012). PPE is a biodegradable polymer with excellent biocompatibility (Qiu et al., 2006).

Polyurethane-based scaffolds exhibit homogeneous morphology and a regular pore size of 407 μm. Biomineralization of the scaffolds enhanced the mechanical properties of scaffolds and made the surface of the scaffolds suitable for cell attachment and proliferation suggesting that it promotes osteoconductivity and bone bonding (Meskinfam et al., 2018). PU scaffolds with dense shell and a porous core have been reported for the treatment of oromaxillary bone defects. The scaffolds were biocompatible and suitable for guided bone regeneration applications (Giannitelli et al., 2015).

Polyurethane scaffolds loaded with lovastatin exhibited porous structure with interconnected pores suitable for cell attachment and proliferation. *In vivo* studies revealed their good osteoconductive potential and biocompatibility (Yoshii et al., 2010). γ-PGA-based scaffolds prepared from covalent cross-linking using an organosilane promoted cell attachment and were not cytotoxic (Poologasundarampillai et al., 2010). γ-PGA is biodegradable with carboxylic acid functional groups useful for modification. It degrades enzymatically from the surface and the degradation rate is influenced by its environment, the concentration of enzymes present, and the surface area exposed to enzyme activity (Poologasundarampillai et al., 2010). γ-PGA-silica hybrid scaffolds exhibit tailorable physiochemical properties useful for bone tissue regeneration (Gao et al., 2016).

Synthetic polymers, used for the design of scaffolds for cartilage regeneration, are easily molded with microstructure, mechanical properties, and degradation suitable for bone regeneration. PEG-based scaffolds have been demonstrated to be a potential platform for cartilage regeneration. PEG-based hydrogels prepared by Michael addition reaction were reported to be biocompatible. Collagen type II and chondroitin sulfate accumulated over time in the gels (Jin et al., 2010). PEG-based cross-linked hydrogels prepared by Diels–Alder click reaction from hyaluronic acid and PEG exhibited good mechanical properties and short gelation time suitable for cartilage tissue engineering (Yu et al., 2014). Encapsulation of rabbit chondrocytes into the injectable hydrogels prepared from a combination of γ-PGA and alginate revealed the viability of the entrapped cells. The gel exhibited good mechanical stability, cell ingrowth, and ectopic cartilage formation (Yan et al., 2014). In another report in which hydrogels were fabricated for cartilage regeneration by click reaction, the hydrogels exhibited fast gelation with antifatigue properties, a storage modulus of 27 kPa, breakage strength of 109.4 kPa, and compressive strain of 81.9% with high metabolic cell viability and proliferation *in vitro* suitable for cartilage tissue engineering (Yu et al., 2018). An electrospun scaffold of gelatin-incorporated poly(L-lactide-*co*-ε-caprolactone) exhibited mechanical properties similar to natural cartilage.

In vivo studies on the scaffolds indicated good cartilage formation in partial-thickness defects of rabbit knees (Kim et al., 2012b). PU-based scaffold prepared for cartilage regeneration exhibited excellent water uptake similar to natural cartilage with compressive modulus in the range of 1.9–14.4 MPa similar to the articular cartilage. The cell viability using human chondrocytes showed 14% and 33% increase in cell viability (Bonakdar et al., 2010). Poly(L-glutamic acid)-based scaffolds encapsulation with rabbit chondrocytes revealed the viability of the entrapped cells with a rapid *in vivo* gel formation and significant mechanical stability and ectopic cartilage formation (Yan et al., 2016). Swine auricular chondrocytes were photoencapsulated into PEG dimethacrylate copolymer scaffolds with either a degradable or nondegradable macromers. The photoencapsulated chondrocytes survived with significant cell proliferation. Scaffold with a 100% nondegradable PEG dimethacrylate inhibited cell–cell interactions of the chondrocytes and the formation of contiguous cartilage. Scaffolds with ratios of degradable and nondegradable macromers of 60:40 and 70:30 were suitable for engineering auricular cartilage. The scaffolds supported *in vivo* chondrogenesis by photoencapsulating auricular chondrocytes (Papadopoulos et al., 2011). Degradable polymers are preferred for articular cartilage repair because they form a temporary scaffold for mechanical support and when new cartilage starts forming within the defect site, these polymer materials degrade leaving behind the regenerated tissue (Seal, 2001).

1.2.1.2.3 *Polymers Application for Tissue/Organ Regeneration*

Synthetic polymers have also been employed for the design of scaffolds for organ regeneration such as nerve, liver, and cardiovascular system (heart, arteries, lungs, veins, and capillaries). The human nervous system lacks the capability to regenerate its components when damaged (Maiti and Díaz Díaz, 2018). Nerve injuries can cause partial or total loss of autonomic, sensory, and motor functions (Navarro et al., 2007). Nerve injuries are treated by autograft method, which involves transplanting tissue from one part of the body to another.

However, autograft method suffers from several limitations such as it is expensive, time-consuming, there is a need for a secondary surgical site, immunogenic rejection, the risk of transference of disease, a diameter mismatch between defected nerves, and newly grafted nerves (Maiti and Díaz Díaz, 2018; Pi et al., 2015). Polymers, which are biodegradable, have been used to construct nerve guide channels, which avoid the need of a second surgery to remove the nerve guide channels from the body, thereby preventing chronic tissue responses or nerve compression (Maiti and Díaz Díaz, 2018).

Polyphosphoester has been used for nerve regeneration. Polymer-based microspheres loaded with nerve growth factors prepared from biodegradable

PPE and loaded into PPE conduits provided prolonged and site-specific delivery of nerve growth factors (NGFs). *In vivo* studies in rat sciatic nerve model, 3 months after implantation, revealed higher values of fiber diameter, population, and density when compared to the control conduits loaded confirming a long-term promoting effect of exogenous NGF on the regeneration of peripheral nerves. This finding confirmed the potential of polymers in enhancing the functional recovery in patients with injured nerves (Xu et al., 2003). Poly(L-lactide-*co*-glycolide) has also been used for nerve regeneration. Poly(L-lactide-*co*-glycolide)-based fibers were used for the fabrication of the conduits. The degradation of the conduit was via fiber breakage revealing the bulk hydrolysis of the polymer. *In vivo* studies in rat sciatic nerve model with a 12-mm gap revealed the absence of inflammatory response after implantation, good biological response of the conduit which was characterized by the formation of a fibrin matrix cable.

After 4 weeks of implantation, nerve regeneration was observed in the rats. The implants were flexible and permeable revealing their efficacy in nerve regeneration and repair (Bini et al., 2003). Poly(lactic-*co*-glycolic acid) (PLGA) conduits have been reported to have good plasticity, intensity, and elasticity indicating that they are useful for the repair of sciatic nerve injury (Yu et al., 2013). Poly(L-lactide-*co*-glycolide) biodegradable polymer nanofibers fabricated to conduits functioned as nerve guidance channels. *In vivo* studies on rat sciatic nerve model with a 10-mm gap length revealed successful nerve regeneration and the absence of tube breakage and inflammatory response. The nanofiber nerve guidance conduits were also flexible and permeable with no sign of swelling (Bini et al., 2004). Stem cells from human exfoliated deciduous teeth seeded in poly(L-lactide-*co*-glycolide) scaffolds and implanted in sciatic nerve transection rat model with a 7-mm nerve gap bridge revealed an improved function in sciatic functional index, significant functional recovery, and nerve regeneration.

Scaffolds with stem cells accelerated nerve recovery (dos Santos et al., 2019). The scaffold enhanced cells attachment, migration, and growth as conditioning for axonal outgrowths, which is essential for nerve regeneration (dos Santos et al., 2019). NGF-loaded poly(L-lactide-*co*-glycolide) microspheres have been reported to be useful for nerve regeneration in peripheral nerve injury with a significant effect on functional recovery in the long term. The release of NGF-loaded microspheres in small gap tubulization facilitated nerve regeneration (Kaka et al., 2017; Wang et al., 2014b; de Boer et al., 2012). Biodegradable synthetic polymers such as PLA and PCL have also been used as scaffolds for nerve regeneration.

Poly(ε-caprolactone) scaffold loaded with NGF in a nerve conduit used in repairing the transected rat sciatic nerve by implantation into the 10-mm right sciatic nerve defects revealed motor and sensory functional recovery and significant motor distal latency The scaffold mechanical properties and biocompatibility improved sciatic nerve regeneration in rats (Mohamadi et al., 2018). Nanocomposites prepared from a mixture of PCL and carbon-based nanoparticles exhibited improved cell adhesion, facilitated a twofold increased in the number of myelinated axons in the repaired nerves suggesting their potential in nerve tubulization repair (Assaf et al., 2017). PCL films with modified surfaces with selected functional groups influenced their cellular response, hydrophilicity, hydrophobicity, and mechanical properties. Hydrolyzed films exhibited significant hydrophilicity and the aminolysis of the films decreased their mechanical properties. Improved cell attachment was significant on the modified films with amino groups on the material surface (de Luca et al., 2012). PCL scaffold prepared possessed good hydrophilicity and flexibility. *In vitro* study revealed that the scaffold promoted Schwann cell adhesion, elongation, and proliferation. *In vivo* test revealed that the porous nerve conduits supported nerve regeneration through an 8-mm sciatic nerve gap in adult rats successfully.

The implanted polymer scaffold nerve conduits facilitated significant axons regeneration via the conduit lumen and gradually degraded which is essential for longer nerve defect (Yu et al., 2011). PLA, an aliphatic polyester, has low allergenic potential, low toxicity, and is biocompatible with predictable kinetics of degradation. PLA microporous hollow fiber application as a conduit to bridge a nerve gap in a mouse sciatic nerve injury model revealed a significant increase in the number of myelinated fibers and blood vessels in animals, good overall tissue organization, and a significant improvement in functional recovery indicating that PLA conduits are potential alternative to autograft (Goulart et al., 2016). PLA is used in nerve conduit due to its biocompatibility, easily shaped properties, and degradation to low toxic lactic acid. However, its use is restricted by its hydrophobicity and lack of binding sites for cellular activities. Incorporation of graphene oxide into PLA nanofibers enhanced its mechanical properties and hydrophilicity, thereby making it suitable for peripheral nerve regeneration application (Öztatlı and Ege, 2016).

Polymers have also been used for liver tissue regeneration. A nanofibrous scaffold was fabricated from polycaprolactone. The nanofibers were characterized by few diameters, better pore, size, and good orientation (Semnani et al., 2016). Polymers have also been employed for the regeneration of cardiovascular system. Their biocompatibility makes them to be used for cardiovascular application such as prosthetic heart valves, vascular grafts to stents, catheters, hemodialyzer, heart assist devices, etc. (Jaganathan et al., 2014). Some of the polymers used are polytetrafluorethylene, polyethylene terephthalate, PU, PVA, and polyamide (Helmus and Snyder, 2009). The cardiovascular system is composed of the heart and the blood vessels. Polymers used for the regeneration of cardiovascular system may have contact with blood and a number of other cells. They interact with the heart, blood, and blood vessels. However, they are susceptible to failure resulting from thrombosis resulting in heart attacks, strokes, damage of blood cells, reduce oxygen carrying capability of the blood, paralysis, and organ failure (Helmus and Snyder, 2009).

Polyamides are used for the development of catheters and hemodialysis membranes. Polytetrafluorethylene is a monofilament plastic polymer, which is durable with good flexibility, biostability, and breaking strength with negative charge-like native endothelium (El Khoury and Vohra, 2012). It exhibits good hemodynamic properties but its use in the development of prosthetic heart valves and vascular grafts is limited by calcification, thrombosis, and stiffening of leaflets (Hayabuchi et al., 2007; Saha et al., 2011; Mehta et al., 2011). Polyethylene terephthalate has been used for the sewing cuffs of prosthetic heart valves *in vitro*. The pretreatment of prosthetic heart valves with antibiotics reduced the risk of bacterial adhesion and infections. The soaking of prosthetic heart valves in antibiotic solutions before implantation and combination with fibrin glue can prevent the development of early prosthetic valve endocarditis (Mashaqi et al., 2011).

A fibrous composite prepared from polyethylene terephthalate polyethylene exhibited physical and mechanical properties revealing its potential application for the valve leaflet function (Amri et al., 2018). Woven polyethylene terephthalate polyethylene has been reported to exhibit small pores with the capability to reduce leakage of blood and good efficiency as vascular grafts when compared to knit one (Jaganathan et al., 2014). Polyethylene terephthalate polyethylene grafts are also coated with protein such as collagen or albumin resulting in reduced loss of blood and good biocompatibility (Kudo et al., 2002). Textile polyester provides unique folding and strength properties with good biocompatibility. Its mechanical and hemodynamic properties were compared with biological tissue. The textile valves elasticity and mechanical strength were superior when compared to the biological tissue.

The flexibility of polyester textile valve leaflets was similar to the biological leaflets. The regurgitation and turbulent patterns of the polyester textile valves were significant resulting from its increased porosity and rapid tissue ingrowth postimplantation when compared to the biological tissue revealing the efficacy of polyester for the development of heart valve leaflet material (Yousefi et al., 2016). PCL has long degradation time, good flexibility, and biocompatibility and its small-diameter grafts are promising alternatives to polyethylene terephthalate polyethylene grafts resulting from its healing characteristics. Tubular PCL reinforced with different polyethylene terephthalate-knitted fabric structures to form multilayer composites was reported to mimic human blood vessels with good mechanical properties, suture retention, water permeability, and elastic recovery. The loop density influenced the compressive strength, suture retention strength, and elastic recovery. The mechanical properties were better than the commercially expanded polytetrafluoroethylene (Wang et al., 2014a). After an average implantation of 6 years, the expanded polytetrafluoroethylene/Gore exhibits stronger resistance against dilatation when compared to polyester/Braun and polyester/Vascutek tube grafts. No graft failure or rupture occurred with a graft patency of 100% (Stollwerck et al., 2011).

Some of the commercially available vascular grafts are Vascutek®-knitted polyester grafts, GORE-TEX® vascular grafts, CoreoGraft™, etc. PU-based grafts have also been reported to significantly increase endothelial cell proliferation *in vitro* with 100% patency after implant with no signs of aneurysmal dilatation. The thin-walled grafts were found to be desirable form of a biodegradable vascular implant with the potential of long-term performance characteristics (Bergmeister et al., 2015). PU-based grafts have been designed with good cytocompatibility, porous architecture, average fiber range of 1.5–2.0 µm, good tensile strength, and significant biostability suitable for vascular grafts (Arjun and Ramesh, 2012; Styan et al., 2012). PVA-based cryogels coated with lyophilized decellularized vascular matrix resulted in enhanced adhesion of human umbilical vein endothelial cells. However, the implantation of the coated scaffold into the abdominal aorta of Sprague Dawley rats resulted in the mortality of all the animals' 3–4 days after surgery indicating that the coating produced a thrombogenic surface. The rat implanted with PVA without coating survived 12 months after implantation suggesting the potential of PVA for the fabrication of artificial vessels (Conconi et al., 2014). PVA hydrogel has excellent potential as a vascular graft because of its unique properties such as mechanical properties that are tunable, bioinert, high water content, and low thrombogenicity. PVA hydrogel grafts, with submillimeter diameter and the mechanical properties, are similar to the rabbit femoral artery that was reported. *The graft exhibited low thrombogenicity, improved perfusion of the distal limb, and was* patent over 2 weeks after implant without the use of anticoagulant or antithrombotics.

On the luminal surface of the grafts, endothelial cells were visible indicating their potential application as a vascular replacement in microvascular surgery (Cutiongco et al., 2016). Moreover, vascular grafts composed of weft knits have high porous connectivity and compliance similar to native vessels (Lin et al., 2017). PVA tubes have also been reported to exhibit thickness of 344 ± 13 μm almost similar to a human artery, which is in a range of 350–710 μm. Its suture retention was 140 ± 11 g, which was also close to that of human vessels and the burst pressure was 507 ± 25 mm Hg which is more than three times higher than the human healthy systolic arterial pressure. No leakage was observed at arterial pressure, which was contrary to vascular expanded polytetrafluoroethylene prostheses. Implantation in rats did not result in thrombotic complications. These findings indicate that cross-linking method of PVA results in mechanical properties, which are compliance and compatible with the circulatory blood flow with no thrombotic complications (Chaouat et al., 2008).

1.2.1.2.4 Polymers Application for Cosmetic Surgery

Polymers have been designed for cosmetic surgery, which includes breast implant and facial reconstruction. Hydrogels prepared from 2.5% polyacrylamide have been reported to be useful for the reconstruction of facial lipoatrophy resulting from combination of antiretroviral therapy. Clinical studies in 110 patients, who received two to six injections every 4 weeks, resulted in average cheek skin thickness of 9.7 mm at baseline increased by an average of 4.4 mm at month 12 and a further increased by an average of 0.87 mm at month 24. No severe adverse effects related to the polyacrylamide hydrogel were observed (Mole et al., 2012). Polyacrylamide hydrogel injections significantly improved the quality of life of HIV-infected patients with facial lipoatrophy. However, polyacrylamide hydrogel injections suffer from limitations such as infections (Kalantarhormozi et al., 2008). Porous polymethylmethacrylate implants filled with a gel that releases antibiotics to protect the tissue from infection have been designed. The thermogel is composed of block copolymer for the controlled release of colistin, an antibiotics and turns into a gel at body temperature followed by a slow degradation over the period of implantation up to 28 days (Mountziaris et al., 2016). Cranial implants have been developed from a biocompatible polymer, ultrahigh molecular weight polyethylene, by computerized tomographies of the patient, converting them into a 3D model using the software InVesalius.

The use of polymer based for cranial implants has advantages such as lightweight, low heat conductivity with mechanical properties similar to bone, and low cost (Bagudanch et al., 2018). Resorbable polymer implants prepared from polylactide and polyglycolide polymers are potential devices for the treatment of acquired and congenital cranio-facial deformities (Cohen et al., 2004). A porous shape memory-polymer foam prepared from PCL had interconnected pores which promoted bone cells to migrate in and grow. It is potentially useful for craniomaxillofacial bone grafting. The foam coated with polydopamine locks the polymer into place by inducing the formation of a mineral found in bone. It induces osteoblasts to adhere and spread throughout the polymer. The biodegrad-able nature of the foam results in its biodegradation leaving behind only the new bone tissue (Mann, 2014).

Computed tomographic biomodeled, heat cured, and prefabricated polymethyl methacrylate implants are well tolerated in patient in long term. Their advantages are long-term biocompatibility, customized design, and distinct esthetic results (Groth et al., 2006). Polymethyl methacrylate produces minimal thermal, electrical, and magnetic conductivity making it useful for orbital implantation (Chiarini et al., 2004). High-density polyethylene has been used for dorsum nasi augmentation due to its long-term structural stability and lack of resorption (Dresner and Hilger, 2008). It is also used for chin and malar augmentation. The histopathological results indicated soft-tissue ingrowth and collagen deposition with signifi-cant vascularization. Complications were few and 91% of the implants remained unchanged (Niechajev, 2012). Polyethylene terephthalate is used for correction in nasal reconstruction (Rai et al., 2013). However, it cannot be used for structural support. It is a good alloplastic implant for facial skeleton augmentation, if autogenous grafts cannot be harvested. However, it can be rigid and infection is a complication which has been reported (Ionita et al., 2015).

Polymers have also been designed for breast implants. Polymeric fillers synthesized from acrylamide by redox polymerization are biocompatible and are permanent injectable filler material for breast reconstruction (Kim et al., 2018). Polymers are also alternative to the use of acellular dermal matrices and are used as temporary reinforcement in patients undergoing breast reconstruction (Becker and Lind, 2013). An arborescent block copolymer prepared and investigated as breast implant did not exhibit leakage that can provoke inflammatory responses in patients (Becker and Lind, 2013). It is biocompatible when compared to silicone in the long term (Becker and Lind, 2013). Silicone gel-filled breast implants with a silicone outer shell are filled with silicone gel. They are approved by FDA for breast augmentation and reconstruction in women age 22 years or older. However, complications associated with silicone breast implants are capsular contracture, implant rupture, wrinkling, asymmetry, scarring, pain, infection, and anaplastic large cell lymphoma (FDA, 2017). A branched arborescent polyisobutylene core was reported to be an alternative biomaterial to silicone rubber. Implantation in a rabbit model revealed that the material exhibited excellent tissue–material interactions resulting from the lower surface energy of polyisobutylene that forms a thin layer on the surface of the material. No acute inflammation was observed and the material was highly biostable (Teck Lim et al., 2013).

1.2.1.3   CERAMICS

Ceramics have been used widely in bone regeneration. They are designed for a strong bonding to bone and are an alternative to metallic implants. They are characterized by excellent corrosion resistance, biocompatibility, hard brittle surface, and osteoconductivity. However, they are limited by poor brittleness, fracture toughness, elasticity, and high stiffness (Salinas and Vallet-Regí, 2013). Some examples of ceramics used in tissue regeneration are calcium phosphate (CaP), HA, $CaCO_3$ (argonite), $CaSO_4 \cdot 2H_2O$ (plaster of Paris), $Ca_3(PO_4)_2$ [tricalcium phosphate (TCP)], etc.

A 3D-fabricated ceramic scaffold prepared from HA/TCP exhibited pore sizes smaller than scaffolds prepared from HA. The release of calcium ions from the scaffolds was higher in TCP scaffold. The HA/TCP scaffolds had a greater capacity to enhance bone regeneration when compared to HA scaffolds. The calcium ion releasing effect of the scaffolds and the rough surface morphology induced bone regeneration indicating their potential in complex bone defects (Seol et al., 2014). (BCP ceramics are biocompatible, osteoconductive, bioactive, and can induce differentiation of stem cells. Ceramics are easily tailored into matrix for bone regeneration (Lobo and Livingston Arinzeh, 2010). Scaffolds composed of different concentrations of HA and β-tricalcium phosphate (β-TCP) exhibit controlled bioactivity with a balance between resorption/solubilization, which influences their stability and also promotes bone growth (Daculsi et al., 1990).

The high release of calcium from ceramic scaffolds to the microenvironment induces an inflammatory response, resulting in a change of the pH and it promotes fibrous tissue formation (Hing et al., 2007). High calcium ion levels influence osteoclastic activity and the controlled levels of calcium ions promote the formation of an apatite layer useful for HA/β-TCP ceramics bioactivity (Daculsi and LeGeros, 2008). Ceramic scaffolds can cause the transformation of macrophages into an M2c phenotype, genes associated with remodeling. These findings indicate that macrophages must be in direct contact with the scaffold for tissue regeneration (Graney et al., 2016). The use of dielectric barrier discharge plasma with oxygen can enhance the hydrophilicity of nonporous HA surfaces. *In vivo* implantation of plasma-treated interconnected porous calcium HA exhibited significant bone ingrowth. Plasma-treated interconnected porous calcium HA promoted osteogenic differentiation of seeded marrow mesenchymal stem cells indicating the osteoconductive potential of interconnected porous calcium HA when used as bone substitutes (Moriguchi et al., 2018). Some physical properties of ceramics when compared with the human natural bone include mechanical properties. CaP ceramics promote bone repair, but have limited lifetime and cannot adapt to skeletal changes (Oryan and Alidadi, 2017). Synthetic HA exhibits a strong affinity to the host bone tissue resulting from its chemical similarity with mineralized human bone tissue (Oryan and Alidadi, 2017). It resorbs slowly and undergoes little transforming into a bone-like material after implantation when compared to β-TCP. β-TCP scaffolds often possess lower strength when compared to the HA scaffolds (Oryan and Alidadi, 2017).

Several researchers have investigated the potential of ceramic-based scaffolds in bone regeneration. HA scaffolds seeded with rabbit mesenchymal stem cells (rMSCs) with 54%–81% porosity exhibited significant bone regeneration in rabbit mandible defects (Guo et al., 2009). HA scaffolds induced bone formation after implantation into immunodeficient male mice (Teixeira et al., 2009). β-TCP scaffolds loaded with BMP-2 placed in rabbit femoral defects induced bone formation significantly (Sohier et al., 2009). β-TCP scaffolds cocultured with rMSCs and rMSC-derived endothelial cells followed by implantation into rabbit large segmental defects resulted in bone regeneration at week 16 revealing enhanced osteogenesis and vascularization (Zhou et al., 2010). Scaffolds composed of 60:4 HA:β-TCP ratio and interconnected pores of 300–800 μm with 75%–85% porosity were cultured in mouse mesenchymal stem cells. The scaffolds differentiate into osteoblast-like cells and implantation in rat lower jaw bones and tibias resulted in bone formation (Kim et al., 2012a).

1.3 BIOLOGICAL-BASED BIOMATERIAL IN TISSUE ENGINEERING

Biological-based biomaterials are used in tissue engineering due to their unique properties such as excellent biocompatibility, nontoxic nature, biodegradability, and they are readily available. Some examples of biological-based biomaterials are natural polymers, peptides, carbon-based materials, etc. They have been used in the design of scaffolds for bone and cartilage regeneration, skin regeneration, cosmetic surgery, soft-tissue regeneration, etc.

1.3.1 NATURAL POLYMERS

Natural polymers such as silk, keratin, chitosan, alginate, fibronectin, collagen, fibrin, hyaluronic acid, and amylose are used in tissue engineering. They are biodegradable and can be replaced upon the generation of new tissues. However, they are limited by their immunological integrity and poor mechanical properties (Sproul et al., 2018). They can be further classified based on their sources such as animal-based and plant-based polymers. They are used for bone and cartilage regeneration, skin regeneration, cosmetic surgery, and soft-tissue regeneration.

1.3.2 FIBRIN

Fibrin plays an important role in blood clotting. It is the primary component in clots and is useful in hemostasis and tissue repair (Sproul et al., 2018). It is used as a tissue sealant, biodegradable, and biocompatible with a high cell binding and good signaling capacity (Sproul et al., 2018). The precursors of fibrin, fibrinogen and thrombin, can be isolated from patients' blood which limits immunogenicity (Janmey et al., 2008; Huang and Fu, 2010). Its network exhibits properties useful for the development of skin substitutes and the rate of polymerization, architecture, the pore size of the scaffolds, and the thickness can be easily tailored (Huang and Fu, 2010; Bencherif et al., 2017). Its cost of isolation is affordable when compared to other natural polymers (Bencherif et al., 2017; Ahmed et al., 2008). Fibrin-based scaffolds provide adequate time suitable for neomatrix formation with slow resorption influenced by the action of proteases (Bencherif et al., 2017).

The aforementioned factors make it useful in wound healing and skin regeneration. Heparin-conjugated fibrin (HCF) scaffold was loaded with fibroblast growth factor 2 (FGF2). It was used as a vehicle for long-term delivery of FGF2. It was implanted into full-thickness skin defects of mice and the formation of neoepidermis was significantly thick indicating the efficacy of fibrin in skin regeneration mediated by FGF2 (Bhang et al., 2010). Fibrin-based interpenetrating polymer networks prepared by photochemistry provided good mechanical support for cellular growth. It was cultured in human dermal equivalent cells and the surface of the network supported cell growth revealing excellent biocompatibility. *In vivo* studies after subcutaneous implantation in an animal model did not induce inflammation indicating that it is a potential scaffold for human skin substitute (Gsib et al., 2018).

The application of engineered 3D PEGylated fibrin scaffold loaded with adipose-derived stem cells (ADSCs) in burn injury model showed the presence of stem cells at the wound site 2 weeks after application. Enhanced vascularization and granulation tissue formation were significant (Chung et al., 2016). A PVA hydrogel loaded with granule-lyophilized platelet-rich fibrin exhibited good mechanical strength and degradation rate, which was influenced by the concentration of the granule-lyophilized platelet-rich fibrin. However, the excellent elastic properties and biocompatibility of the hydrogel were not influenced by the concentration of granule-lyophilized platelet-rich fibrin. Application of the scaffold to an acute full-thickness dorsal skin wounds enhanced wound closure at days 7 and 9. The scaffold enhanced the formation of granulation tissue, collagen deposition, and new vessel (Xu et al., 2018). Scaffold prepared from a combination of synthetic polymers, fibrin and loaded with platelet lysate exhibited sustained release of the platelet lysate *in vitro*. The application of the scaffold on genetically diabetic mouse full-thickness skin wound enhanced wound closure at day 15. Re-epithelialization, granulation tissue formation, and collagen deposition were increased indicating their potential use for the treatment of diabetic foot ulcers (Losi et al., 2015). Fibrin scaffold has been developed into a three-layered skin substitute by embedding ADSCs and mature adipocytes in the hydrogel with fibroblasts for the construction of the dermal layer. On top of the two layers was loaded keratinocytes to mimic the epidermal layer. After 3 weeks, the loaded stem cells and the fibroblasts were viable and proliferated and differentiated into matured adipocytes with morphology similar to native adipose tissue. The keratinocytes formed an epithelial-like layer (Kober et al., 2015). Fibrin scaffolds cultured in human fibroblasts and seeded with human keratinocytes on the top of the scaffold healing potential was assessed in deep partial and full-thickness burns *in vivo*. Good cell attachment and colony spreading of keratinocytes and fibroblasts on the scaffold were visible. The appearance of the skin did not differ from the areas of transplanted skin indicating good healing (Kljenak, 2016). Fibrin glue has been applied for the closure of a meshed skin graft with reduced scarring and decreased infection. Addition of angiogenic growth factor further enhanced the growth of blood vessels from the wound bed into the graft (Feldman and Osborne, 2018).

Fibrin has also been used in cosmetic surgery for facelift surgery. Aerosolized fibrin glue used in facelifts surgery resulted in less bruising, reduced swelling, and a rapid healing response. The risk of hematoma was also reduced with shortened operating times by 13.3 minutes when compared to facelift surgery with the use of glue (Fezza et al., 2002). Autologous platelet-rich fibrin matrix enhances patient's natural wound healing ability. It induces the formation of viable blood vessels, fat cells, and collagen deposits. It is used with minimal invasive and for open surgical procedures (Sclafani and Saman, 2012). In facial implant and uplift, it promotes rapid integration of the implant into the surrounding tissues. Fibrin scaffolds have also been loaded with fibroblasts for regeneration of new facial nerve in pigs indicating the potential application of fibrin for facial nerve regeneration (Lasso et al., 2015).

Fibrin-based scaffolds have also been used in bone regeneration by several researchers. Platelet-rich fibrin enhanced osteoblast proliferation and differentiation indicating their effect on bone regeneration with low risk of complications (Kim et al., 2017). A comparison study on the effects of fibrin and collagen on proliferation and differentiation of osteoblasts and protein adsorption revealed that fibrin adsorbed approximately 6.7 times more when compared to serum fibronectin. Fibrin stimulated the proliferation of larger MC3T3-E1 preosteoblasts at a low cell density and promoted enhanced osteoblast differentiation when compared to collagen revealing the superiority of fibrin to collagen in bone regeneration (Oh et al., 2014). Leukocyte-platelet-rich fibrin has been used in the reconstruction of surgical bone defect. The closure of the bony defect by neo-osteogenesis was observed by CT scan. However, the density of the new bone was less when compared to the surrounding normal bone showing its capability to induce bone healing and regeneration at the surgical site defect (Fredes et al., 2017). Platelet-rich fibrin stimulated bone regeneration in diabetic rabbits with a mean percent of 16.87 and 29.59 at weeks 4 and 8, respectively (Durmuşlar et al., 2016). Platelet-rich fibrin application in two bicortical skull defects in 20 New Zealand white rabbits showed that it induced bone formation when used alone or when combined with autogenous bone (Pripatnanont et al., 2013).

1.3.3 COLLAGEN

Collagen is used as tissue fillers, as support matrices for matrix-rich tissues, as skin substitutes, and dermal fillers because of its natural high composition. It is the main component of cartilage, bone, skin, tendons, and ligaments (Wang et al., 2009). It exhibits excellent biocompatibility, insignificant immunogenicity, and high bioabsorbability. Collagen, obtained from fish scales and used to prepare patches, stimulated blood and lymphatic vessel formation, thus revealing its potential use for tissue repair and regeneration. Collagen enhances wound healing and acts as a drug carrier such as growth factors, etc., which activates wound healing process (Wang et al., 2016, 2017a). PLGA-collagen scaffold prepared by electrospinning method induced cell adhesion on the scaffold when cultured in human dermal fibroblast and human keratinocyte, which was influenced by the porosity of the scaffold.

The porosity of the scaffold was in the range of 4–30 μm. The hydrophilic nature of collagen also influenced the interaction of cells with the scaffold, thereby inducing biological signals that promote cell adhesion and proliferation (Sadeghi-Avalshahr et al., 2017). Tilapia skin collagen electrospun nanofibers were developed for wound dressing. The tensile strength of collagen nanofibers was 6.72 ± 0.44 MPa. The nanofibers induced the viability of human keratinocytes, human dermal fibroblasts, and enhanced epidermal differentiation. The nanofibers promoted effective rapid skin regeneration *in vivo* resulting from the biomimic extracellular cell matrix structure, hydrophilicity, and the multiple amino acids of the collagen nanofibers (Zhou et al., 2015). Collagen sponge transplanted directly to the wound areas of diabetic mice promoted wound healing and enhanced regeneration of capillary 14 days after cotransplantation of collagen sponge and skin-derived precursors. Superior proangiogenic effects were attributed to skin-derived precursors by paracrine secretion of proangiogenic and neurotrophic factors and direct transdifferentiating into vascular and neural components (Ke et al., 2015).

Two layers of the skin were mimicked by constructing two different porous polymeric scaffolds (sodium carboxymethyl cellulose loaded with fibroblasts as the dermis layer and chondroitin sulfate-incorporated collagen loaded with keratinocytes as the epidermis layer). The mimicked skin was characterized by interconnected porosity, excellent water content, and adequate stability. The attachment and proliferation of cells on both layers of the construct were induced by the expression of vascular endothelial growth factor (VEGF), basic FGF, and interleukin-8 (IL-8) and the production of collagen I, collagen III, laminin, and transglutaminase. Attachment and proliferation of fibroblasts on the dermal layer were reduced when compared with the keratinocyte on epidermis layer which was characterized by a dense and a stratified layer similar to the epidermis. The constructed skin is a potential graft for the treatment of deep wounds (Kilic Bektas et al., 2018).

Collagen has also been used for bone regeneration. Collagen type I was phosphorylated with alendronate sodium that accelerates mineralization in simulated body fluid *in vitro*. It was biocompatible with bone marrow mesenchymal stem cells and enhanced cell adhesion and osteogenic differentiation of the stem cells. The implantation of the scaffold into a critical-sized rat cranial defect for over 4–8 weeks revealed degradation of the scaffold and the stimulation of bone growth in the defect. The stem cells were able to attach and undergo osteogenic differentiation without the use of external osteogenic factors signifying that the presence of phosphate on a bone cell attachment surface is an important factor in the cells adhesion onto that surface of the scaffold (He et al., 2018). Collagen scaffolds have been combined with ceramics such as HA for bone regeneration in order to enhance its mechanical properties. Collagen scaffold containing varied amount of HA and loaded with doxycycline to prevent infection mimicked bone structure with compact structure and low water uptake capacity. The low water uptake was influenced by the high content of HA (Mederle et al., 2016). Scaffolds prepared from the combination of collagen and HA exhibit excellent biocompatibility, osteoconductivity, and bone-bonding ability (Cunniffe et al., 2009; Andronescu et al., 2011). The mechanical properties of collagen scaffold are improved by incorporating HA (Calabrese et al., 2016). The surface area of the collagen scaffolds can also be increased by combining it with HA resulting in good cellular adhesion (Sionkowska and Kozłowska, 2013).

The use of nano-sized HA particles increased the surface area, porosity, and induced deep and even distribution of cells effectively (Lickorish et al., 2003). HA particles can interact with the host bone tissue resulting in rapid and good bone bonding between the scaffolds and the host bone tissue. The use of micron-sized HA particles results in scaffolds with poor resorbability and brittle constructs (Kunzler et al., 2007). A rough surface area of the scaffold enhanced cell proliferation (Pasqui et al., 2013) and scaffolds containing HA exhibit enhanced cellular proliferation when compared to scaffolds without HA (Sionkowska and Kozłowska, 2013).

β-tricalcium phosphate rate of degradation is faster when compared to HA. It is used in combination with collagen composite for bone regeneration and it can be replaced by newly formed bone tissues (Arahira and Todo, 2016). Composite with a weight ratio of 9:1 collagen solution to the β-TCP powder exhibited high compressive module when compared to collagen composite indicating enhanced structural stability. It supported cell permeation and proliferation. The osteoconductive capabilities of β-TCP have also been reported to be high when compared to pure collagen composites (Cao and Kuboyama, 2010). β-TCP-collagen composites used as bone void filler in critical size defects of rabbit distal femoral condyle model showed resorption of the void filler and good bone formation without immunological response and rejection. Combining β-TCP with collagen in composite resulted in a synergistic effect on the bone healing process and provided good contact to the surrounding bone tissue (Arahira and Todo, 2014).

1.3.4 ELASTIN

Elastin is useful for soft-tissue replacement due to its biocompatibility and biostability. Elastin hydrogel loaded with endothelial cell and mesenchymal stem cells followed by the addition of fibronectin to the surface of the hydrogel resulted in cell adhesion, proliferation, and migration, which was enhanced by the addition of fibronectin. High-cell viability further indicated the potential application of elastin for artificial blood vessels (Ravi et al., 2012). A 3D tubular-shaped composite-layered scaffold with high surface roughness due to the nanofibrous layer and the good biophysical properties resulting from the microfibrous layer was sprayed with elastin proteins. The composite exhibited antithrombogenic surface with the potential to overcome thrombosis and intimal hyperplasia (Jang et al., 2014).

A 3D collagen-elastin scaffold was encapsulated with valve interstitial cells and cultured with valve endothelial cells onto the surface. The valve interstitial cells proliferated with a stable expression level of integrin $\hat{I}^2 1$ and the expression of integrin $\hat{I}^2 1$ was low in valve endothelial cells. Over a period of 7 days, 20% valve endothelial cells were transformed to mesenchymal phenotype with a high expression of integrin $\hat{I}^2 1$. These results demonstrate that the scaffold is a potential tool for heart valve regeneration (Lacerda et al., 2018). Biodegradable photopolymer scaffolds coated with elastin exhibited good cell adhesion and proliferation. The adhesion of endothelial cells to functionalized substrates demonstrates the possibility to bioactivate the polymeric graft for vascular applications (Barenghi et al., 2014; Wang et al., 2018; Waterhouse et al., 2011).

1.3.5   SILK

Silk is isolated from mulberry and nonmulberry and silkworms are obtained from cocoons. Silk has been used for the regeneration of bone. Composite hybrid prepared from silk and HA followed by implantation in a critical-sized, $7 \times 4 \times 1.5$ mm alveolar defect created in Sprague-Dawley rats resulted in the formation of 85% new bone at 12 weeks. Osteoid tissues were surrounded by osteoblasts, which were visible in the center of the scaffold implanted at week 8 with no immunological reaction (Koh et al., 2018). Silk composite with a compressive strength of 13 MPa exhibited high surface roughness and porosity, which enhanced human bone marrow-derived mesenchymal stem cell differentiation toward bone-like tissue *in vitro* (Mandal et al., 2012). Porous silk scaffolds with pore size in the range of 400–500 μm loaded with stem cells were used for the repair of rat critical-sized calvarial defects. The loaded cells promoted angiogenesis and osteogenesis with the stimulation of VEGF and BMP-2. The porous nature of the scaffolds was suitable for the delivery of seed cells for bone regeneration (Zhang et al., 2014). Silk fibroin impregnated with poly(3-hydroxybutyrate-*co*-3-hydroxyvalerate) nanofibrous scaffolds with HA exhibited average fiber diameter and porosity of 450–850 nm and 80–85%, respectively. *In vitro* cell culture of the scaffolds in MG-63 osteosarcoma human cells for 10 days indicated enhanced cell viability, alkaline phosphatase activity, and total cellular protein. The scaffolds induced cell penetration and the production of type I collagen revealing that they are promising bone-filling material for tissue regeneration (Colpankan Gunes et al., 2018). Increasing the content of silk nanofiber content in the composite scaffolds decreased the pore size.

The small pores in nanofibers influenced cell growth such as proliferation, adhesion, and differentiation into osteoblasts *in vitro*. The scaffold stimulated the formation of new bone formation in rabbit calvarial defect model *in vivo* (Park et al., 2015). Silk scaffolds have also been used to deliver stem cells into a bone defect area with prolonged viability of the cells after implantation. The scaffold with 1.0×10^7/mL concentration of the stem cells exhibited the best osteogenic effect *in vivo* with the formation of new bone at 8 weeks after implantation (Ding et al., 2017).

Silk scaffolds have also been used in eye regeneration. The grafts for keratoplasty are obtained for replacement of corneal tissue. However, there is a risk of transmission of infectious diseases such as HIV, hepatitis B and C virus, syphilis, etc. (Liu et al., 2012). Silk-based transparent films with a thickness of 5 μm coated with collagen and a chondroitin sulfate laminin mixture promoted cell adhesion and proliferation making it a potential substratum for the transplantation of tissue constructs for keratoplasty (Madden et al., 2011). Silk film with 0.5–5.0 mm diameter pores was suitable for cell alignment and translamellar diffusion of nutrients. The silk film constructs resemble the physiological characteristics of a normal cornea (Lawrence et al., 2009).

The capability of silk-based films to continuously support cornea cells can prevent the destruction of collagenase and promote corneal tissue regeneration (Madden et al., 2011). The preparation of films from the combination of silk and synthetic polymers for corneal regeneration can enhance the attachment and proliferation of corneal epithelial cells. Films prepared from silk and PEG exhibited increased permeability and topographic surface roughness. An increase in the rigidity resulted in an increase in cell proliferation in the long term. The films exhibited a high nuclear-to-cytoplasmic ratio indicating a more proliferative phenotype (Suzuki et al., 2015). Functionalization of arginine-glycine-aspartic acid (RGD)-containing peptide onto silk scaffolds induced cell attachment significantly. However, the ratio of RGD-containing peptide with silk influenced human corneal limbal epithelial cells attachment (Bray et al., 2013). Silk scaffolds support epithelial cells and keratocytes in rabbit eyes after implantation (Hazra et al., 2016).

Silk is also used for nerve regeneration. Silk-based films cultured with dorsal root ganglion neurons showed that the films supported the growth and neurite extension of neurons revealing it can promote the repair of the peripheral nervous system (Benfenati et al., 2012). Functionalization of the films with NGF promoted the adhesion, migration, and proliferation of neurites (Benfenati et al., 2012). Scaffolds prepared from the combination of silk and chitosan bridged a 10-mm long sciatic nerve gap in rats. The scaffold was similar to an acellular nerve graft, a nerve tissue-derived ECM scaffold, but superior to the plain chitosan/SF scaffold (Gu et al., 2014). Fabrication of a nanofiber composite from silk and NGF with the core coated with PLA preserved and sustained the release of NGF. The scaffold enhanced attachment and differentiation of PC12 cells resulting in elongated neurites outgrowth of 95 mm after 11 days and increased surface hydrophilicity (Tian et al., 2015).

Silk is also used for skin regeneration due to its unique properties such as biocompatibility, slow rate degradation, and its capability to stimulate the collagen synthesis of fibroblasts and rapid tissue reconstruction (Jao et al., 2016). Skin substitute construct was reported with a trilayer skin equivalent with silk sponge as the hypodermis, collagen as the dermis, and keratinocytes as the overlaying of the epidermis seeded with endothelial and ADSCs onto the silk sponge and fibroblasts in the collagen layer. The construct showed expression of keratin 10 and collagens I and IV with the production of glycerol and leptin, which are markers of adipose metabolism. These constructs are potential skin substitutes for deep burn and incision wounds (Bellas et al., 2012). Silk-based nanofiber material blended poly(ethylene oxide) and functionalized with fibronectin-induced cellular adhesion, proliferation, and migration of normal human dermal fibroblasts (Chutipakdeevong et al., 2013). Silk-elastin scaffolds accelerated re-epithelialization of wound sites. Cross-linking of genipin reduced the pore size of the scaffold and mimicked natural dermal constructs suitable for burn wounds (Vasconcelos et al., 2012). Fabricated porous 3D silk-keratin scaffolds enhanced fibroblast growth, attachment, and proliferation (Bhardwaj et al., 2015).

1.4   CARBON-BASED MATERIALS

Carbon-based materials such as graphene, carbon nanotubes (CNTs), and fullerenes are used for the development of scaffolds for tissue regeneration. Their physicochemical properties such as their high surface area-to-volume ratio, their hollow structure, electrical conductance, good thermal conductivity, mechanical properties, and their tunable properties via functionalization. They can be conjugated with specific biomolecules such as polymers, peptides, proteins, nucleic acids, and other therapeutic agents to target specific types of tissue/organs (Yun, 2012).

Fullerenes C_{60} is a stable cage-like molecule with a diameter of ~0.7 nm which facilitates its passive diffusion into cells and nuclei. It is available as a pure compound when compared to graphene and CNT. It is biocompatible and does not induce cellular apoptosis/death (Raoof et al., 2012). It has used in bone regeneration application. A pretreatment of fullerol for 7 days promoted osteogenic differentiation in a dose-dependent manner when combined with osteogenic medium. It was nontoxic toward human ADSCs even at a dose up to 10 μM and it was a reactive oxygen species scavenger for human ADSCs indicating that it can be used as alternative to growth factors for the tissue engineering-based repair of bone fractures and defects (Yang et al., 2014).

Carbon nanotubes can be classified as single-walled, double-walled, and multiwalled CNTs. They have been used in tissue regeneration (Bosi et al., 2013). Seeding dissociated embryonic rat hippocampal neurons on a mat of multi-walled CNTs deposited onto polyethylenimine (PEI)-induced neurites. However, the neurites did not form branches on the CNT (Mattson et al., 2000). CNTs noncovalent functionalization with 4-hydroxynonenal increased the number of neurons and the length of their neurites significantly when compared to the unfunctionalized CNTs. The surface charge of CNTs influenced the neurite growth with significant neurite branching in neurons grown on positively charged multi-walled CNTs when compared to the neutral or negatively charged multiwalled CNTs (Hu et al., 2005). Similar reports showed that positively charged CNT surface grafted with PEI enhanced neuronal growth *in vitro* (Hu et al., 2005). CNT roughness and the large surface area played an important role in their capability to promote neuronal adhesion (Sorkin et al., 2008).

Polyethylene glycol-functionalized CNT derivatives without neurotrophins *in vitro* resulted in an extended neurite length and a reduced number of neurites (Ni et al., 2005). The aforementioned finding is attributed to the inhibition of endocytic processes and not the exocytotic ones (Bosi et al., 2013; Malarkey et al., 2008). The long length of the nanotubes inhibited the vesicle from closing and pinching off, thereby preventing endocytosis. The physical configuration of nanotubes sticking in vesicles did not hinder exocytosis (Bosi et al., 2013; Malarkey et al., 2008). Hybridization of CNTs with biopolymers of PLGA and poly(L-lactic acid-*co*-ε-caprolactone) (PLCL) promoted neurite outgrowth *in vitro* in neural cells (Lee et al., 2010; Jin et al., 2011). CNT is also used in bone regeneration.

Chitosan scaffolds containing functionalized multi-walled CNTs exhibited porosity in the range of 93.6%–94.5%. The mechanical characteristics of the scaffolds were increased by the functionalized-MWCNTs. The pore size of the scaffolds was decreased after introducing the functionalized MWCNTs. The scaffolds were nontoxic and biocompatible with the capability to be used in bone regeneration (Zadeh et al., 2018). MWCNT 3D blocks loaded with rhBMP-2 followed by implantation in mouse muscle resulted in the formation of ectopic bone.

The bone marrow densities of the blocks were similar to PET-reinforced collagen sheets loaded with rhBMP-2. MC3T3-E1 preosteoblasts were attached to the scaffold surface of blocks when compared to PET-reinforced collagen sheets. The blocks also exhibited maximum compression strength similar to the cortical bone. The blocks served as bone defect filler (Tanaka et al., 2017). Single-walled CNTs-PLGA composites fabricated with varied amounts of SWCNT followed by cell seeding with MC3T3-E1 and hBMSCs revealed biocompatibility. Composites with 10 mg of SWCNT exhibited significant cell proliferation. Gene expressions of alkaline phosphatase, collagen I, osteocalcin, osteopontin, Runx2, and bone sialoprotein were visible in all the composites indicating their potential use for musculoskeletal regeneration and bone tissue engineering (Gupta et al., 2013). Furthermore, *in vivo* studies on the composites indicated biocompatibility over a period of 12 weeks with a high mechanical strength which mimicked the microstructure of human trabecular bone (Gupta et al., 2015).

Graphene is a crystalline form of carbon. It is composed of a single monolayer of sp2 hybridized orbitals in a tightly packed two-dimensional honeycomb lattice. Its sheets can be transformed into graphene materials such as graphene oxide (GO) and reduced GO (rGO) with unique properties which can be tailored (Shin et al., 2016). It has been used in neural regeneration due to its electrical properties. Graphene-based substrates promoted neuronal adhesion and growth of mammalian differentiated postmitotic neurons *in vitro*. The substrate did not alter the cell differentiation, synaptogenesis, and spontaneous synaptic activity. It retained neuronal signaling properties suggesting that carbon-based substrates have the capability to preserve neuronal activity (Fabbro et al., 2016). Graphene substrate promoted human neural stem cell adhesion and differentiation into neurons (Park et al., 2011). *In vitro* studies of mouse hippocampal culture model on graphene-based substrates revealed excellent biocompatibility. The neurite numbers and average length were enhanced at day 2–7. On day 2, neurite sprouting and outgrowth was maximum. The expression of growth-associate protein-43 was also enhanced which might have influenced the neurite sprouting and growth (Li et al., 2011). rGO microfibers are characterized by good flexibility, excellent mechanical strength, nanoporous surface, biodegradability, and cytocompatibility that supported neural stem cells adhesion, proliferation, and differentiation into neurons forming a dense neural network around the microfiber (Guo et al., 2017). GO-decellularized scaffold applied to the injury of a sciatic nerve in rats repaired the injury of the sciatic nerve and facilitated the regeneration of injured nerve which was characterized by a thickness of myelin sheath, the diameter of axon, and dominant muscle rehabilitation level (Wang et al., 2017b). Graphene-based scaffolds have also been used in bone regeneration.

Scaffolds prepared from graphene-based material and collagen-induced significant osteogenic differentiation of human mesenchymal stem cells (Kang et al., 2015; Dinescu et al., 2014). 3D-printed scaffolds prepared from chitosan and GO promoted bone regeneration *in vivo* in calvarial defects of a mouse with an increase in alkaline phosphatase activity, expression of

BMP, and Runx2 factor (Hermenean et al., 2017). Factors that contribute to the cell attachment ability of the scaffolds are the polarity and the hydroxyl functional group of the GO (Ruan et al., 2015). GO/gelatin/HA scaffolds enhanced osteogenic differentiation of human mesenchymal stem cells. The cell proliferation on day 1 was higher than on day 7 and 14 but reduced on day 21. The scaffolds enhanced cell proliferation and osteogenic differentiation of human mesenchymal stem cells without the addition of osteogenic supplements (Nair et al., 2015). GO-silk fiber scaffolds enhanced the proliferation of MC3T3-E1 osteoblast cells. The addition of GO to the scaffold reduced the pore diameter and influenced the pore morphology of the scaffolds (Wang et al., 2015). Graphene-based substrate has been used in combination with synthetic polymers to develop scaffolds for bone regeneration.

Polycaprolactone-GO scaffolds induced mesenchymal stem cells and PC12 cells growth. The scaffolds with 1.0 wt % GO exhibited reduced cell proliferation and scaffolds with 0.3% and 0.5% concentration of GO displayed significant differentiation of mesenchymal stem cells into osteogenic cells (Song et al., 2015). PCL-graphene nanosheet scaffolds displayed regular and reproducible architecture. The scaffold was coated with P1-latex protein obtained from the *Hevea brasiliensis* rubber tree. *In vitro* evaluation of the scaffold with human ADSCs did not reveal severe toxic effects. Graphene nanosheet and P1-latex protein in the scaffolds increased their cell proliferation capability (Caetano et al., 2018). Graphene-based scaffolds have also been designed for cartilage regeneration.

Methacrylated chondroitin sulfate-PEG methyl ether-ε-caprolactone-acryloyl chloride-GO scaffold exhibited good pore size. Cartilage cells interacted with the scaffold and remained viable resulting from its biocompatibility and favorable degradation rate. The use of the scaffold with cellular supplementation *in vivo* enhanced the morphology of the chondrocyte with the formation of thick cartilage indicating its potential application in articular cartilage tissue engineering (Liao et al., 2015). A 3D graphene foam with good biocompatibility promoted cell proliferation and differentiation into osteogenic or chondrogenic cell lines useful for cartilage repair and regeneration (Yocham et al., 2018). Graphene-based scaffolds have also been developed for nerve regeneration.

Nanofibers of RGD peptide-GO cofunctionalized PLGA fabricated via electrospinning exhibited random-oriented electrospun nanofibers with an average diameter of 558 nm. The surface hydrophilicity of the nanofiber mats was increased significantly by cofunctionalizing with RGD peptide and GO. Cell attachment of cultured vascular smooth muscle cells on the nanofibers was significant indicating that they are promising scaffolds for the regeneration of vascular smooth muscle (Shin et al., 2017).

1.5 CONCLUSION

Synthetic and biological-based materials have been used in regenerative medicine. Metals used in the design of scaffolds for implants exhibit excellent mechanical properties. However, their use is limited resulting from their poor compatibility and their ability to release metal ions that can cause toxic reactions. Some metals lack a biologically active surface that can induce osteointegration or prevent infections resulting in the coatings of implants. The coating of the implants has the potential to prevent the release of metallic ions. High concentration of metals in the blood from implant causes neurological problems and is also carcinogenic. The surface of some of the metals implants such as titanium is usually modified by roughening and coating for enhanced rate of osseointegration. Synthetic polymers such as PEG have been used in skin regeneration resulting in wound closure and bleeding control, tissue adhesion, controlled degradability, and elastomeric mechanical properties suitable for skin regeneration. However, due to the poor biocompatibility of synthetic polymers, they are combined with natural polymers resulting in scaffolds with improved biocompatibility.

Polymers have also been used in facial reconstruction, and bone and cartilage regeneration. Polymers can be tailored into scaffolds with unique properties depending on their applications. Ceramics are characterized by excellent corrosion resistance, biocompatibility, hard brittle surface, and good osteoconductivity. However, their application is limited by poor brittleness, fracture toughness, elasticity, and high stiffness. To overcome the aforementioned limitations, they are combined with polymers resulting in excellent biocompatibility, good osteoconductivity, and bone-bonding ability. Natural polymers-based films prepared from the silk have been reported to enhance the attachment and proliferation of corneal epithelial cells.

Carbon-based materials have been conjugated with specific biomolecules such as polymers, peptides, and proteins for regenerative medicine applications. Their roughness, large surface area, and electrical properties influence their capability to promote neuronal adhesion. Their biocompatibility also promoted osteogenic differentiation of human mesenchymal stem cells *in vitro* and promoted bone regeneration *in vivo*. Despite the potential of carbon-based materials in regenerative medicine, their safety in long-term use must be investigated thoroughly.

Despite the several research reports on biomaterials used in regenerative medicine, factors such as unforeseen technical challenges for manufacturing of scaffolds/implants, limited commercialization expertise, and inadequate preclinical safety and risk assessment have reduced the successful translation of biomaterials to clinical applications.

ACKNOWLEDGMENT

The financial support of National Research Foundation (NRF), South Africa and South Africa Medical Research Council (MRC) (Self-Initiated Research) toward this research is hereby acknowledged. The views and opinions expressed in this manuscript are those of the authors and not of MRC or NRF. SJO specially thanks the NRF for SARChI Postdoctoral Research Fellowship.

KEYWORDS

- **biomaterials**
- **polymers**
- **ceramics**
- **metals**
- **carbon nanotubes**
- **graphene**
- **tissue engineering**

REFERENCES

Ahmed, T. A. E., Dare, E. V. & Hincke, M. Fibrin: a versatile scaffold for tissue engineering applications. *Tissue Eng Part B Rev.* **2008,** 14(2): 199–215.

Akyol, S., Bozkus, H., Adin Cinar, S. & Hanci, M. M. Which is better stainless steel or titanium alloy? *Turk Neurosurg.* **2017.**

Al-Radha, D. & Sahib, A. The influence of different acids etch on dental implants titanium surface. *IOSR J Dent Med Sci.* **2016,** 15(8): 87–91.

Amri, A., Laroche, G., Chakfe, N. & Heim, F. Fibrous composite material for textile heart valve design: *in vitro* assessment. *Biomed Eng Biomed.* **2018,** 63(3): 221–230.

Andronescu, E., Voicu, G., Ficai, M., Mohora, I. A., Trusca, R. & Ficai, A. Collagen/ hydroxyapatite composite materials with desired ceramic properties. *J Electron Microsc (Tokyo).* **2011,** 60(3): 253–259.

Arahira, T. & Todo, M. Effects of Proliferation and differentiation of mesenchymal stem cells on compressive mechanical behavior of collagen/β-TCP composite scaffold. *J Mech Behav Biomed.* **2014,** 39: 218–230.

Arahira, T. & Todo, M. Variation of mechanical behavior of β-TCP/collagen two phase composite scaffold with mesenchymal stem cell *in vitro*. *J Mech Behav Biomed.* **2016,** 61: 464–474.

Arjun, G. N. & Ramesh, P. Structural characterization, mechanical properties, and *in vitro* cytocompatibility evaluation of fibrous polycarbonate urethane membranes for biomedical applications. *J Biomed Mater Res A.***2012,** 100A(11): 3042–3050.

Assaf, K., Leal, C. V., Derami, M. S., de Rezende Duek, E. A., Ceragioli, H. J. & de Oliveira, A. L. R. Sciatic nerve repair using poly(ε-caprolactone) tubular prosthesis associated with nanoparticles of carbon and graphene. *Brain Behav.* **2017,** 7(8): e00755.

Augustine, R., Dominic, E. A., Reju, I., Kaimal, B., Kalarikkal, N. & Thomas, S. Electrospun polycaprolactone membranes incorporated with ZnO nanoparticles as skin substitutes with enhanced fibroblast proliferation and wound healing. *RSC Advances.* **2014,** 4(47): 24777.

Bagudanch, I., García-Romeu, M. L., Ferrer, I. & Ciurana, J. Customized cranial implant manufactured by incremental sheet forming using a biocompatible polymer. *Rapid Prototyp J.* **2018,** 24(1): 120–129.

Bal, B. S., Garino, J., Ries, M. & Rahaman, M. N. A review of ceramic bearing materials in total joint arthroplasty. *Hip Int.* **2007,** 17(1): 21–30.

Barenghi, R., Beke, S., Romano, I., Gavazzo, P., Farkas, B., Vassalli, M. et al. Elastin-coated biodegradable photopolymer scaffolds for tissue engineering applications. *Bio Med Res Int.* **2014,** 2014: 1–9.

Bauer, S., Schmuki, P., von der Mark, K. & Park, J. Engineering biocompatible implant surfaces. *Prog Mater Sci.* **2013,** 58(3): 261–326.

Becker, H. & Lind, J. G. The use of synthetic mesh in reconstructive, revision, and cosmetic breast surgery. *Aesthetic Plast Surg.* **2013,** 37(5): 914–921.

Bellas, E., Seiberg, M., Garlick, J. & Kaplan, D. L. *In vitro* 3D full-thickness skin-equivalent tissue model using silk and collagen biomaterials. *Macromol Biosci.* **2012,** 12(12): 1627–1636.

Bencherif, S., Gsib, O. & Egles, C. Fibrin: an underrated biopolymer for skin tissue engineering. *J Mol Biol Biotech.* **2017,** 2: 1–4.

Benfenati, V., Stahl, K., Gomis-Perez, C., Toffanin, S., Sagnella, A., Torp, R. et al. Biofunctional silk/neuron interfaces. *Adv Funct Mater.* **2012,** 22(9): 1871–1884.

Bergmeister, H., Seyidova, N., Schreiber, C., Strobl, M., Grasl, C., Walter, I. et al. Biodegradable, thermoplastic polyurethane grafts for small diameter vascular replacements. *Acta Biomater.* **2015,** 11: 104–113.

Bhang, S. H., Sun, A. Y., Yang, H. S., Rhim, T., Kim, D. I. & Kim, B. S. Skin regeneration with fibroblast growth factor 2 released from heparin-conjugated fibrin. *Biotechnol Lett.* **2010,** 33(4): 845–851.

Bhardwaj, N., Sow, W. T., Devi, D., Ng, K. W., Mandal, B. B. & Cho, N. J. Silk fibroin–keratin-based 3D scaffolds as a dermal substitute for skin tissue engineering. *Integr Biol.* **2015,** 7(1): 53–63.

Bhat, S. & Kumar, A. Biomaterials in regenerative medicine. *J Postgrad Med Edu Res.* **2012,** 46(2): 81–89.

Bhowmick, S., Thanusha, A. V., Kumar, A., Scharnweber, D., Rother, S. & Koul, V. Nanofibrous artificial skin substitute composed of mPEG–PCL grafted gelatin/hyaluronan/chondroitin sulfate/sericin for 2nd degree burn care: *in vitro* and *in vivo* study. *RSC Advances.* **2018,** 8(30): 16420–16432.

Bini, T. B., Gao, S., Tan, T. C., Wang, S., Lim, A., Hai, L. B. et al. Electrospun poly(L-lactide-co-glycolide) biodegradable polymer nanofibre tubes for peripheral nerve regeneration. *Nanotechnol.* **2004,** 15(11): 1459–1464.

Bini, T. B., Gao, S., Xu, X., Wang, S., Ramakrishna, S. & Leong, K. W. Peripheral nerve regeneration by microbraided poly(L-lactide-co-glycolide) biodegradable polymer fibers. *J. Biomed Mater Res.* **2003,** 68A(2): 286–295.

Bonakdar, S., Emami, S. H., Shokrgozar, M. A., Farhadi, A., Ahmadi, S. A. H. & Amanzadeh, A. Preparation and characterization of polyvinyl alcohol hydrogels crosslinked by biodegradable polyurethane for tissue engineering of cartilage. *Mater Sci Eng C.* **2010,** 30(4): 636–643.

Bormann, K. H., Gellrich, N. C., Kniha, H., Dard, M., Wieland, M. & Gahlert, M. Biomechanical evaluation of a microstructured zirconia implant by a removal torque comparison with a standard Ti-SLA implant. *Clin Oral Implants Res.* **2011,** 23(10): 1210–1216.

Bose, S., Roy, M. & Bandyopadhyay, A. Recent advances in bone tissue engineering scaffolds. *Trends Biotechnol.* **2012,** 30(10): 546–554.

Bosi, S., Fabbro, A., Ballerini, L. & Prato, M. Carbon nanotubes: a promise for nerve tissue engineering? *Nanotechnol Rev.* **2013,** 2(1).

Bradberry, S. M., Wilkinson, J. M. & Ferner, R. E. Systemic toxicity related to metal hip prostheses. *Clin Toxicol.* **2014,** 52(8): 837–847.

Bray, L., Suzuki, S., Harkin, D. & Chirila, T. Incorporation of exogenous RGD peptide and inter-species blending as strategies for enhancing human corneal limbal epithelial cell growth on bombyx mori silk fibroin membranes. *J Funct Biomater.* **2013,** 4(2): 74–88.

Caetano, G. F., Wang, W., Chiang, W. H., Cooper, G., Diver, C., Blaker, J. J. et al. 3D-printed poly(ε-caprolactone)/graphene scaffolds activated with P1-latex protein for bone regeneration. *3D Print Add Manufactur.* **2018,** 5(2): 127–137.

Calabrese, G., Giuffrida, R., Fabbi, C., Figallo, E., Lo Furno, D., Gulino, R. et al. Collagen-Hydroxyapatite scaffolds induce human adipose derived stem cells osteogenic differentiation *in vitro*. *PLoS One.* **2016,** 11(3): e0151181.

Campbell, J. R. & Estey, M. P. Metal release from hip prostheses: cobalt and chromium toxicity and the role of the clinical laboratory. *Clin Chem Lab Med.* **2013,** 51(1).

Cao, H. & Kuboyama, N. A biodegradable porous composite scaffold of PGA/β-TCP for bone tissue engineering. *Bone.* **2010,** 46(2): 386–395.

Catauro, M., Bollino, F. & Papale, F. Surface modifications of titanium implants by coating with bioactive and biocompatible poly(ε-caprolactone)/SiO_2 hybrids synthesized via sol–gel. *Arab J Chem.* **2018,** 11(7): 1126–1133.

Chahal, S., Hussain, F. S. J. & Yusoff, M. B. M. Characterization of modified cellulose (MC)/poly(vinyl alcohol) electrospun nanofibers for bone tissue engineering. *Proced Eng.* **2013,** 53: 683–688.

Chahal, S., Hussain, F. S. J., Yusoff, M. M., Abdull Rasad, M. S. B. & Kumar, A. Nano-hydroxyapatite-coated hydroxyethyl cellulose/poly(vinyl) alcohol electrospun scaffolds and their cellular response. *Int J Polymer Mater Polymer Biomater.* **2016,** 66(3): 115–122.

Chan, B. P. & Leong, K. W. Scaffolding in tissue engineering: general approaches and tissue-specific considerations. *Eur Spine J.* **2008,** 17(S4): 467–479.

Chaouat, M., Le Visage, C., Baille, W. E., Escoubet, B., Chaubet, F., Mateescu, M. A. et al. A novel cross-linked poly(vinyl alcohol) (PVA) for vascular grafts. *Adv Funct Mater.* **2008,** 18(19): 2855–2861.

Chen, K., Chen, Y., Deng, Q., Jeong, S. H., Jang, T. S., Du, S. et al. Strong and biocompatible poly(lactic acid) membrane enhanced by Ti 3 C 2 T z (MXene) nanosheets for guided bone regeneration. *Mater Lett.* **2018a,** 229: 114–117.

Chen, S. L., Fu, R. H., Liao, S. F., Liu, S. P., Lin, S. Z. & Wang, Y. C. A PEG-based hydrogel for effective wound care management. *Cell Transplant.* **2018b,** 27(2): 275–284.

Chiarini, L., Figurelli, S., Pollastri, G., Torcia, E., Ferrari, F., Albanese, M. et al. Cranioplasty using acrylic material: a new technical procedure. *J Craniomaxillofac Surg.* **2004,** 32(1): 5–9.

Chung, E., Rybalko, V. Y., Hsieh, P. L., Leal, S. L., Samano, M. A., Willauer, A. N. et al. Fibrin-based stem cell containing scaffold improves the dynamics of burn wound healing. *Wound Repair Regen.* **2016,** 24(5): 810–819.

Chung, S. H., Kim, H. K., Shon, W. J. & Park, Y. S. Peri-implant bone formations around (Ti, Zr)O$_2$-coated zirconia implants with different surface roughness. *J Clin Periodontol.* **2013,** 40(4): 404–411.

Chutipakdeevong, J., Ruktanonchai, U. R. & Supaphol, P. Process optimization of electrospun silk fibroin fiber mat for accelerated wound healing. *J Appl Polym Sci.* **2013,** 130(5): 3634–3644.

Cionca, N., Hashim, D. & Mombelli, A. Zirconia dental implants: where are we now, and where are we heading? *Periodontol 2000.* **2016,** 73(1): 241–258.

Clark, M. J., Prentice, J. R., Hoggard, N., Paley, M. N., Hadjivassiliou, M. & Wilkinson, J. M. Brain structure and function in patients after metal-on-metal hip resurfacing. *Am J Neuroradiol.* **2014,** 35(9): 1753–1758.

Cohen, S. R., Holmes, R. E., Meltzer, H. S., Levy, M. L. & Beckett, M. Z. Craniofacial reconstruction with a fast resorbing polymer: a 6- to 12-month clinical follow-up review. *Neurosurg Focus.* **2004,** 16(3): 1–3.

Colpankan Gunes, O., Unalan, I., Cecen, B., Ziylan Albayrak, A., Havitcioglu, H., Ustun, O. et al. Three-dimensional silk impregnated HAp/PHBV nanofibrous scaffolds for bone regeneration. *Int J Polymer Mater Polymer Biomater.* **2018,** 68(5): 217–228.

Conconi, M. T., Borgio, L., Di Liddo, R., Sartore, L., Dalzoppo, D., Amist À, P. et al. Evaluation of vascular grafts based on polyvinyl alcohol cryogels. *Mol Med Rep.* **2014,** 10(3): 1329–1334.

Costan, V., Sulea, D., Nicolau, A., Drochioi, C., Luchian, S. & Boisteanu, O. The use of titanium mesh in facial contour reconstruction. *Med Surg J Rev Med Chir.* **2018,** 122(1): 167–175.

Crainiceanu, Z., Ianes, E., Matusz, P., Bloanca, V., Seleacu, E., Narad, V. et al. Innovative method of titanium plate use for morphological and functional human face recontruction. *Mat Plast.* **2016,** 53: 518–521.

Cunniffe, G. M., Dickson, G. R., Partap, S., Stanton, K. T. & O'Brien, F. J. Development and characterisation of a collagen nano-hydroxyapatite composite scaffold for bone tissue engineering. *J Mater Sci Mater Med.* **2009**, 21(8): 2293–2298.

Cutiongco, M. F. A., Kukumberg, M., Peneyra, J. L., Yeo, M. S., Yao, J. Y., Rufaihah, A. J., Le et al. Submillimeter diameter poly(vinyl alcohol) vascular graft patency in rabbit model. *Front Bioeng Biotechnol.* **2016**, 4.

Daculsi, G. & LeGeros, R. (**2008**). Biphasic calcium phosphate (bcp) bioceramics: chemical, physical, and biological properties. In *Encyclopedia of Biomaterials and Biomedical Engineering, Second Edition—Four Volume Set*, 359–366: CRC Press.

Daculsi, G., LeGeros, R. Z., Heughebaert, M. & Barbieux, I. Formation of carbonate-apatite crystals after implantation of calcium phosphate ceramics. *Calcif Tissue Int.* **1990**, 46(1): 20–27.

de Boer, R., Borntraeger, A., Knight, A. M., Hébert-Blouin, M. N., Spinner, R. J., Malessy et al. Short- and long-term peripheral nerve regeneration using a poly-lactic-co-glycolic-acid scaffold containing nerve growth factor and glial cell line-derived neurotrophic factor releasing microspheres. *J Biomed Mater Res Part A.* **2012**, 100A(8): 2139–2146.

de Luca, A. C., Terenghi, G. & Downes, S. Chemical surface modification of poly-ε-caprolactone improves Schwann cell proliferation for peripheral nerve repair. *J Tissue Eng Regen Med.* **2012**, 8(2): 153–163.

Depprich, R., Zipprich, H., Ommerborn, M., Naujoks, C., Wiesmann, H. P., Kiattavorncharoen, S. et al. Osseointegration of zirconia implants compared with titanium: an *in vivo* study. *Head Face Med.* **2008**, 4(1).

Dinescu, S., Ionita, M., Pandele, A. M., Galateanu, B., Iovu, H., Ardelean, A., Costache, M. et al. *In vitro* cytocompatibility evaluation of chitosan/graphene oxide 3D scaffold composites designed for bone tissue engineering. *Biomed Mater Eng.* **2014**, 24(6): 2249–2256.

Ding, X., Yang, G., Zhang, W., Li, G., Lin, S., Kaplan, D. L. et al. Increased stem cells delivered using a silk gel/scaffold complex for enhanced bone regeneration. *Sci Rep.* **2017**, 7(1).

Diniz, M. G., Pinheiro, M. A. S., Andrade Junior, A. C. C. & Fischer, R. G. Characterization of titanium surfaces for dental implants with inorganic contaminant. *Braz Oral Res.* **2005**, 19(2): 106–111.

dos Santos, F. P., Peruch, T., Katami, S. J. V., Martini, A. P. R., Crestani, T. A., Quintiliano, K. et al. Poly(lactide-co-glycolide) (PLGA) scaffold induces short-term nerve regeneration and functional recovery following sciatic nerve transection in rats. *Neuroscience.* **2019**, 396: 94–107.

Dresner, H. & Hilger, P. An overview of nasal dorsal augmentation. *Semin Plast Surg.* **2008**, 22(2): 65–73.

Duraccio, D., Mussano, F. & Faga, M. G. Biomaterials for dental implants: current and future trends. *J Mater Sci.* **2015**, 50(14): 4779–4812.

Durmuşlar, M. C., Ballı, U., Öngöz Dede, F., Bozkurt Doğan, Ş., Mısır, A. F., Barış, E. et al. Evaluation of the effects of platelet-rich fibrin on bone regeneration in diabetic rabbits. *J Craniomaxillofac Surg.* **2016**, 44(2): 126–133.

El-Khoury, G. & Vohra, H. A. Polytetrafluoroethylene leaflet extensions for aortic valve repair. *Eur J Cardiothorac Surg.* **2012**, 41(6): 1258–1259.

Eom, T. G., Jeon, G. R., Jeong, C. M., Kim, Y. K., Kim, S. G., Cho, I. H. et al. Experimental study of bone response to hydroxyapatite coating implants: bone-implant contact and removal torque test. *Oral Surg Oral Med Oral Pathol Oral Radiol.* **2012**, 114(4): 411–418.

Fabbro, A., Scaini, D., León, V., Vázquez, E., Cellot, G., Privitera, G. et al. Graphene-based interfaces do not alter target nerve cells. *ACS Nano.* **2016**, 10(1): 615–623.

FDA, U. (**2017**). Update on the Safety of Silicone Gel-Filled Breast Implants (2011)—Executive Summary.

Feldman, D. & Osborne, S. Fibrin as a tissue adhesive and scaffold with an angiogenic agent (FGF-1) to enhance burn graft healing *in vivo* and clinically. *J Funct Biomater.* **2018**, 9(4): 68.

Fezza, J. P., Cartwright, M., Mack, W. & Flaharty, P. The Use of Aerosolized Fibrin Glue in Face-Lift Surgery. *Plast Reconstr Surg.* **2002**, 110(2): 658–664.

Fredes, F., Pinto, J., Pinto, N., Rojas, P., Prevedello, D. M., Carrau, R. L. et al. Potential effect of leukocyte-platelet-rich fibrin in bone healing of skull base: a pilot study. *Int J Otolaryngol.* **2017**, 2017: 1–7.

Gahlert, M., Burtscher, D., Grunert, I., Kniha, H. & Steinhauser, E. Failure analysis of fractured dental zirconia implants. *Clin Oral Implants Res.* **2011**, 23(3): 287–293.

Galler, K. M., Brandl, F. P., Kirchhof, S., Widbiller, M., Eidt, A., Buchalla, W. et al. Suitability of different natural and synthetic biomaterials for dental pulp tissue engineering. *Tissue Eng Part A.* **2018**, 24(3–4): 234–244.

Gao, C., Ito, S., Obata, A., Mizuno, T., Jones, J. R. & Kasuga, T. Fabrication and *in vitro* characterization of electrospun poly(γ-glutamic acid)-silica hybrid scaffolds for bone regeneration. *Polymer.* **2016**, 91: 106–117.

Gear, A. J. L., Lokeh, A., Aldridge, J. H., Migliori, M. R., Benjamin, C. I. & Schubert, W. Safety of titanium mesh for orbital reconstruction. *Ann Plast Surg.* **2002**, 48(1): 1–9.

Gehrke, S. A., Ramírez-Fernandez, M. P., Granero Marín, J. M., Barbosa Salles, M., Del Fabbro, M. & Calvo Guirado, J. L. A comparative evaluation between aluminium and titanium dioxide microparticles for blasting the surface titanium dental implants: an experimental study in rabbits. *Clin Oral Implants Res.* **2016**, 29(7): 802–807.

Gehrke, S. A., Taschieri, S., Del Fabbro, M. & Coelho, P. G. Positive Biomechanical Effects of Titanium Oxide for Sandblasting Implant Surface as an Alternative to Aluminium Oxide. *J Oral Implantol.* **2015**, 41(5): 515–522.

Giannitelli, S. M., Basoli, F., Mozetic, P., Piva, P., Bartuli, F. N., Luciani, F. et al. Graded porous polyurethane foam: a potential scaffold for oro-maxillary bone regeneration. *Mater Sci Eng C Mater Biol Appl.* **2015**, 51: 329–335.

Giner, L., Mercadé, M., Torrent, S., Punset, M., Pérez, R. A., Delgado, L. M. et al. Double acid etching treatment of dental implants for enhanced biological properties. *J Appl Biomater Funct Mater.* **2018**, 16(2): 83–89.

Goble, V. (**2017**). MATERIALISE's 3D-Printed Maxillofacial Implants in Titanium Are First to Get Green Light for U.S. Market.

Godbole, N., Yadav, S., Ramachandran, M. & Belemkar, S. A review on surface treatment of stainless steel orthopedic implants. *Int J Pharm Sci Rev Res.* **2016**, 36(1): 190–194.

Gómez-Lizárraga, K. K., Flores-Morales, C., Del Prado-Audelo, M. L., Álvarez-Pérez, M. A., Piña-Barba, M. C. & Escobedo, C. Polycaprolactone- and polycaprolactone/ceramic-based 3D-bioplotted porous scaffolds for bone regeneration: a comparative study. *Mater Sci Eng C.* **2017**, 79: 326–335.

Goulart, C. O., Pereira Lopes, F. R., Monte, Z. O., Dantas, S. V., Souto, A., Oliveira, J. T. et al. Evaluation of biodegradable polymer conduits—poly(l-lactic acid)—for guiding sciatic nerve regeneration in mice. *Methods.* **2016**, 99: 28–36.

Goutam, M., Chandu, G., Mishra, S. K., Singh, M. & Tomar, B. S. Factors affecting osseointegration: a literature review. *J Orofacial Res.* **2013,** 3(3): 197–201.

Grandfield, K., Palmquist, A., Gonçalves, S., Taylor, A., Taylor, M., Emanuelsson, L. et al. Free form fabricated features on CoCr implants with and without hydroxyapatite coating *in vivo*: a comparative study of bone contact and bone growth induction. *J Mater Sci Mater Med.* **2011,** 22(4): 899–906.

Graney, P. L., Roohani-Esfahani, S. I., Zreiqat, H. & Spiller, K. L. *In vitro* response of macrophages to ceramic scaffolds used for bone regeneration. *J R Soc Interface.* **2016,** 13(120): 20160346.

Groth, M. J., Bhatnagar, A., Clearihue, W. J., Goldberg, R. A. & Douglas, R. S. Long-term efficacy of biomodeled polymethyl methacrylate implants for orbitofacial defects. *Arch Facial Plast Surg.* **2006,** 8(6).

Gsib, O., Deneufchatel, M., Goczkowski, M., Trouillas, M., Resche-Guigon, M., Bencherif, S. et al. FibriDerm: interpenetrated fibrin scaffolds for the construction of human skin equivalents for full thickness burns. *IRBM.* **2018,** 39(2): 103–108.

Gu, Y., Zhu, J., Xue, C., Li, Z., Ding, F., Yang, Y. et al. Chitosan/silk fibroin-based, Schwann cell-derived extracellular matrix-modified scaffolds for bridging rat sciatic nerve gaps. *Biomaterials.* **2014,** 35(7): 2253–2263.

Guo, H., Su, J., Wei, J., Kong, H. & Liu, C. Biocompatibility and osteogenicity of degradable Ca-deficient hydroxyapatite scaffolds from calcium phosphate cement for bone tissue engineering. *Acta Biomater.* **2009,** 5(1): 268–278.

Guo, W., Qiu, J., Liu, J. & Liu, H. Graphene microfiber as a scaffold for regulation of neural stem cells differentiation. *Sci Rep.* **2017,** 7(1).

Gupta, A., Liberati, T. A., Verhulst, S. J., Main, B. J., Roberts, M. H., Potty, A. G. R. et al. Biocompatibility of single-walled carbon nanotube composites for bone regeneration. *Bone Joint Res.* **2015,** 4(5): 70–77.

Gupta, A., Woods, M. D., Illingworth, K. D., Niemeier, R., Schafer, I., Cady, C. et al. Single walled carbon nanotube composites for bone tissue engineering. *J Orthop Res.* **2013,** 31(9): 1374–1381.

Ha, T. L. B., Quan, T. M. & Vu, D. N. **(2013).** Naturally derived biomaterials: preparation and application. In *Regenerative medicine and tissue engineering*: IntechOpen.

Han, G. & Ceilley, R. Chronic wound healing: a review of current management and treatments. *Adv Ther.* **2017,** 34(3): 599–610.

Harle, J., Kim, H. W., Mordan, N., Knowles, J. C. & Salih, V. Initial responses of human osteoblasts to sol–gel modified titanium with hydroxyapatite and titania composition. *Acta Biomater.* **2006,** 2(5): 547–556.

Hayabuchi, Y., Mori, K., Kitagawa, T., Sakata, M. & Kagami, S. Polytetrafluoroethylene graft calcification in patients with surgically repaired congenital heart disease: evaluation using multidetector-row computed tomography. *Am Heart J.* **2007,** 153(5): 806.e1–8.

Haynes, D. R., Crotti, T. N. & Haywood, M. R. Corrosion of and changes in biological effects of cobalt chrome alloy and 316L stainless steel prosthetic particles with age. *J Biomed Mater Res.* **2000,** 49(2): 167–175.

Hazra, S., Nandi, S., Naskar, D., Guha, R., Chowdhury, S., Pradhan, N. et al. Non-mulberry silk fibroin biomaterial for corneal regeneration. *Sci. Rep.* **2016,** 6(1).

He, Y. & Lu, F. Development of synthetic and natural materials for tissue engineering applications using adipose stem cells. *Stem Cells Int.* **2016,** 2016: 1–12.

He, Y., Zhu, T., Liu, L., Shi, X. & Lin, Z. Modifying collagen with alendronate sodium for bone regeneration applications. *RSC Advances.* **2018,** 8(30): 16762–16772.

Helmus, M. N. & Snyder, R. W. (**2009**). Biomedical engineering and design handbook. Vol. 1, 383 (Ed M. Kutz). New York.

Hempel, U., Hefti, T., Kalbacova, M., Wolf-Brandstetter, C., Dieter, P. & Schlottig, F. Response of osteoblast-like SAOS-2 cells to zirconia ceramics with different surface topographies. *Clin Oral Implants Res.* **2010,** 21(2): 174–181.

Hermenean, A., Codreanu, A., Herman, H., Balta, C., Rosu, M., Mihali, C. V. et al. Chitosan-graphene oxide 3D scaffolds as promising tools for bone regeneration in critical-size mouse calvarial defects. *Sci. Rep.* **2017,** 7(1).

Herrero-Climent, M., Lázaro, P., Vicente Rios, J., Lluch, S., Marqués, M., Guillem-Martí, J. et al. Influence of acid-etching after grit-blasted on osseointegration of titanium dental implants: *in vitro* and *in vivo* studies. *J Mater Sci Mater Med.* **2013,** 24(8): 2047–2055.

Hing, K. A., Wilson, L. F. & Buckland, T. Comparative performance of three ceramic bone graft substitutes. *Spine J.* **2007,** 7(4): 475–490.

Hu, H., Ni, Y., Mandal, S. K., Montana, V., Zhao, B., Haddon, R. C. et al. Polyethyleneimine functionalized single-walled carbon nanotubes as a substrate for neuronal growth. *J Phys Chem B.* **2005,** 109(10): 4285–4289.

Huang, H. L., Chang, Y. Y., Weng, J. C., Chen, Y. C., Lai, C. H. & Shieh, T. M. Anti-bacterial performance of zirconia coatings on titanium implants. *Thin Solid Films.* **2013,** 528: 151–156.

Huang, S. & Fu, X. Naturally derived materials-based cell and drug delivery systems in skin regeneration. *J Control Release.* **2010,** 142(2): 149–159.

Hung, K. Y., Lo, S. C., Shih, C. S., Yang, Y. C., Feng, H. P. & Lin, Y. C. Titanium surface modified by hydroxyapatite coating for dental implants. *Surf Coat Technol.* **2013,** 231: 337–345.

Ionita, S., Popescu, S. & Lascar, I. Polypropylene meshes and other alloplastic implants for soft tissue and cartilage nasal reconstructive surgery—a literature review. *Roman J Rhinol.* **2015,** 5(18): 87–94.

Jaganathan, S. K., Supriyanto, E., Murugesan, S., Balaji, A. & Asokan, M. K. Biomaterials in cardiovascular research: applications and clinical implications. *Biomed Res Int.* **2014,** 2014: 1–11.

Jakobsen, S. S., Baas, J., Jakobsen, T. & Soballe, K. Biomechanical implant fixation of CoCrMo coating inferior to titanium coating in a canine implant model. *J Biomed Mater Res Part A.* **2010,** 94A(1): 180–186.

Jang, J., Ko, J., Cho, D. W., Jun, M. B. & Kim, D. H. (**2014**). Elastin-sprayed tubular scaffolds with microstructures and nanotextures for vascular tissue engineering. In *ASME 2013 Summer Bioengineering Conference*: American Society of Mechanical Engineers Digital Collection.

Janmey, P. A., Winer, J. P. & Weisel, J. W. Fibrin gels and their clinical and bioengineering applications. *J R Soc Interface.* **2008,** 6(30): 1–10.

Jao, D., Mou, X. & Hu, X. Tissue regeneration: a silk road. *J Funct Biomater.* **2016,** 7(3): 22.

Jemat, A., Ghazali, M. J., Razali, M. & Otsuka, Y. Surface modifications and their effects on titanium dental implants. *Biomed Res Int.* **2015,** 2015: 1–11.

Jin, G. Z., Kim, M., Shin, U. S. & Kim, H. W. Neurite outgrowth of dorsal root ganglia neurons is enhanced on aligned nanofibrous biopolymer scaffold with carbon nanotube coating. *Neurosci Lett.* **2011,** 501(1): 10–14.

Jin, R., Moreira Teixeira, L. S., Krouwels, A., Dijkstra, P. J., van Blitterswijk, C. A., Karperien, M. et al. Synthesis and characterization of hyaluronic acid–poly(ethylene glycol) hydrogels via Michael addition: an injectable biomaterial for cartilage repair. *Acta Biomater.* **2010,** 6(6): 1968–1977.

Kaka, G., Arum, J., Sadraie, S. H., Emamgholi, A. & Mohammadi, A. Bone marrow stromal cells associated with poly L-lactic-co-glycolic acid (PLGA) nanofiber scaff old improve transected sciatic nerve regeneration. *Iran J Biotechnol.* **2017,** 15(3): 149–156.

Kalantarhormozi, A., Mozafari, N. & Rasti, M. Adverse effects after use of polyacrylamide gel as a facial soft tissue filler. *Aesthet Surg J.* **2008,** 28(2): 139–142.

Kang, S., Park, J. B., Lee, T. J., Ryu, S., Bhang, S. H., La, W. G. et al. Covalent conjugation of mechanically stiff graphene oxide flakes to three-dimensional collagen scaffolds for osteogenic differentiation of human mesenchymal stem cells. *Carbon.* **2015,** 83: 162–172.

Kao, K., Chen, C., Gross, J., Hahn, S., Chi, J., Branham, G. et al. Titanium mesh nasal repair without nasal lining. *Facial Plast Surg.* **2017,** 33(1): 52–57.

Ke, T., Yang, M., Mao, D., Zhu, M., Che, Y., Kong, D. et al. Co-transplantation of skin-derived precursors and collagen sponge facilitates diabetic wound healing by promoting local vascular regeneration. *Cell Physiol Biochem.* **2015,** 37(5): 1725–1737.

Keane, T. J. & Badylak, S. F. Biomaterials for tissue engineering applications. *Semin Pediatr Surg.* **2014,** 23(3): 112–118.

Kenawy, E. R., Kamoun, E. A., Mohy Eldin, M. S. & El-Meligy, M. A. Physically crosslinked poly(vinyl alcohol)-hydroxyethyl starch blend hydrogel membranes: synthesis and characterization for biomedical applications. *Arab J Chem.* **2014,** 7(3): 372–380.

Khan, F. & Tanaka, M. Designing smart biomaterials for tissue engineering. *Int J Mol Sci.* **2017,** 19(1): 17.

Kiel, M., Krauze, A. & Marciniak, J. Corrosion resistance of metallic implants used in bone surgery. *Arch Mater Sci Eng.* **2008,** 30(2): 77–80.

Kilic Bektas, C., Kimiz, I., Sendemir, A., Hasirci, V. & Hasirci, N. A bilayer scaffold prepared from collagen and carboxymethyl cellulose for skin tissue engineering applications. *J Biomater Sci Poly Ed.* **2018,** 29(14): 1764–1784.

Kim, H. J., Park, I. K., Kim, J. H., Cho, C. S. & Kim, M. S. Gas foaming fabrication of porous biphasic calcium phosphate for bone regeneration. *Tissue Eng Reg Med.* **2012a,** 9(2): 63–68.

Kim, J., Ha, Y. & Kang, N. H. Effects of Growth Factors From Platelet-Rich Fibrin on the Bone Regeneration. *J Craniofac Surg.* **2017,** 28(4): 860–865.

Kim, M., Hong, B., Lee, J., Kim, S. E., Kang, S. S., Kim, Y. H. et al. Composite system of PLCL scaffold and heparin-based hydrogel for regeneration of partial-thickness cartilage defects. *Biomacromolecules.* **2012b,** 13(8): 2287–2298.

Kim, S., Shin, B., Yang, C., Jeong, S., Shim, J., Park, M. et al. Development of poly(HEMA-Am) polymer hydrogel filler for soft tissue reconstruction by facile polymerization. *Polymers.* **2018,** 10(7): 772.

Kljenak, A. Fibrin gel as a scaffold for skin substiture - production and clinical experience. *Acta Clin Croat.* **2016,** 55(2): 279–288.

Knabe, C., Klar, F., Fitzner, R., Radlanski, R. J. & Gross, U. *In vitro* investigation of titanium and hydroxyapatite dental implant surfaces using a rat bone marrow stromal cell culture system. *Biomaterials.* **2002,** 23(15): 3235–3245.

Kober, J., Gugerell, A., Schmid, M., Kamolz, L. P. & Keck, M. Generation of a fibrin based three-layered skin substitute. *Biomed Res Int.* **2015,** 2015: 1–8.

Koh, K. S., Choi, J. W., Park, E. J. & Oh, T. S. Bone regeneration using silk hydroxyapatite hybrid composite in a rat alveolar defect model. *Int J Med Sci.* **2018,** 15(1): 59–68.

Kondo, R., Nomura, N., Suyalatu, T. Y., Doi, H. & Hanawa, T. Microstructure and mechanical properties of as-cast Zr–Nb alloys. *Acta Biomater.* **2011,** 7(12): 4278–4284.

Kudo, F., Nishibe, T., Miyazaki, K., Flores, J. & Yasuda, K. Albumin-coated knitted Dacron aortic prostheses: study of postoperative inflammatory reactions. *Int Angiol.* **2002,** 21(3): 214–217.

Kunzler, T. P., Drobek, T., Schuler, M. & Spencer, N. D. Systematic study of osteoblast and fibroblast response to roughness by means of surface-morphology gradients. *Biomaterials.* **2007,** 28(13): 2175–2182.

Lacerda, C. M. R., Wang, X., Ali, M., Mendiola, G. & Scott, H. (**2018**). Collagen-elastin scaffolds for heart valve tissue engineering. In *18 AIChE Annual Meeting*Pittsburgh, United States.

Lasso, J. M., Prieto Montalvo, J., Deleyto, E., Castellano, M., Pérez Cano, R. & Fernández-Santos, M. E. Reconstruction of the facial nerve in pigs with facial nerve allografts wrapped in a fibrin scaffold containing fibroblasts transduced with adenovirus encoding VEGF 156. *Enliven Surg Transplan.* **2015,** 2(4).

Lawrence, B. D., Marchant, J. K., Pindrus, M. A., Omenetto, F. G. & Kaplan, D. L. Silk film biomaterials for cornea tissue engineering. *Biomaterials.* **2009,** 30(7): 1299–1308.

Lee, H. J., Yoon, O. J., Kim, D. H., Jang, Y. M., Kim, H. W., Lee, W. B. et al. Neurite outgrowth on nanocomposite scaffolds synthesized from PLGA and carboxylated carbon nanotubes. *Adv Eng Mater.* **2010,** 11(12): B261-B266.

Levengood, S. L., Erickson, A. E., Chang, F. C. & Zhang, M. Chitosan–poly(caprolactone) nanofibers for skin repair. *J Mater Chem B.* **2017,** 5(9): 1822–1833.

Li, N., Zhang, X., Song, Q., Su, R., Qi, Z. & Kong, T. The promotion of neurite sprouting and outgrowth of mouse hippocampal cells in culture by graphene substrates. *Biomaterials.* **2011,** 32.

Liao, J., Qu, Y., Chu, B., Zhang, X. & Qian, Z. Biodegradable CSMA/PECA/Graphene Porous Hybrid Scaffold for Cartilage Tissue Engineering. *Sci Rep.* **2015,** 5(1).

Lickorish, D., Ramshaw, J. A. M., Werkmeister, J. A., Glattauer, V. & Howlett, C. R. Collagen-hydroxyapatite composite prepared by biomimetic process. *J Biomed Mater Res.* **2003,** 68A(1): 19–27.

Lim, H. P., Park, S. W., Yun, K. D., Park, C., Ji, M. K., Oh, G. J. et al. Hydroxyapatite coating on TiO_2 nanotube by sol–gel method for implant applications. *J Nanosci Nanotechnol.* **2018,** 18(2): 1403–1405.

Lin, J. H., Hu, J. J., Tu, C. Y., Lee, M. C., Lu, C. T., Lu, P. C. et al. Tubular polyvinyl alcohol composites used as vascular grafts: manufacturing techniques and property evaluations. *Mater Lett.* **2017,** 190: 201–204.

Liu, H., Niinomi, M., Nakai, M., Hieda, J. & Cho, K. Deformation-induced changeable Young's modulus with high strength in β-type Ti–Cr–O alloys for spinal fixture. *J Mech Behav Biomed Mater.* **2014,** 30: 205–213.

Liu, J., Lawrence, B. D., Liu, A., Schwab, I. R., Oliveira, L. A. & Rosenblatt, M. I. Silk fibroin as a biomaterial substrate for corneal epithelial cell sheet generation. *Investig Opthalmol Vis Sci.* **2012,** 53(7): 4130.

Lobo, S. E. & Livingston Arinzeh, T. Biphasic calcium phosphate ceramics for bone regeneration and tissue engineering applications. *Materials.* **2010,** 3(2): 815–826.

Loh, Q. L. & Choong, C. Three-dimensional scaffolds for tissue engineering applications: role of porosity and pore size. *Tissue Eng Part B Rev.* **2013**, 19(6): 485–502.

Lohmann, N., Schirmer, L., Atallah, P., Wandel, E., Ferrer, R. A., Werner, C. et al. Glycosaminoglycan-based hydrogels capture inflammatory chemokines and rescue defective wound healing in mice. *Sci Transl Med.* **2017**, 9(386): eaai9044.

Losi, P., Briganti, E., Sanguinetti, E., Burchielli, S., Al Kayal, T. & Soldani, G. Healing effect of a fibrin-based scaffold loaded with platelet lysate in full-thickness skin wounds. *J Bioact Compat Polym.* **2015**, 30(2): 222–237.

Lughi, V. & Sergo, V. Low temperature degradation-aging-of zirconia: a critical review of the relevant aspects in dentistry. *Dent Mater.* **2010**, 26(8): 807–820.

Ma, X., He, Z., Han, F., Zhong, Z., Chen, L. & Li, B. Preparation of collagen/hydroxyapatite/alendronate hybrid hydrogels as potential scaffolds for bone regeneration. *Colloids Surf B Biointerfaces.* **2016**, 143: 81–87.

Madden, P. W., Lai, J. N. X., George, K. A., Giovenco, T., Harkin, D. G. & Chirila, T. V. Human corneal endothelial cell growth on a silk fibroin membrane. *Biomaterials.* **2011**, 32(17): 4076–4084.

Maiti, B. & Díaz Díaz, D. 3D Printed Polymeric Hydrogels for Nerve Regeneration. *Polymers.* **2018**, 10(9): 1041.

Malarkey, E. B., Reyes, R. C., Zhao, B., Haddon, R. C. & Parpura, V. Water soluble single-walled carbon nanotubes inhibit stimulated endocytosis in neurons. *Nano Lett.* **2008**, 8(10): 3538–3542.

Mandal, B. B., Grinberg, A., Seok Gil, E., Panilaitis, B. & Kaplan, D. L. High-strength silk protein scaffolds for bone repair. *Proceed Nat Acad Sc.* **2012**, 109(20): 7699–7704.

Manivasagam, G., Dhinasekaran, D. & Rajamanickam, A. Biomedical implants: corrosion and its prevention—A review. *Recent Pat Corros Sc.* **2010**, 2(1): 40–54.

Mann, D. (**2014**). New Moldable Polymer May Aid Facial Reconstruction. Vol. 2019.

Mao, D., Li, Q., Bai, N., Dong, H. & Li, D. Porous stable poly(lactic acid)/ethyl cellulose/hydroxyapatite composite scaffolds prepared by a combined method for bone regeneration. *Carbohydr Polym.* **2018**, 180: 104–111.

Mashaqi, B., Marsch, G., Shrestha, M., Graf, K., Stiesch, M., Chaberny, I. F. et al. Antibiotic pretreatment of heart valve prostheses to prevent early prosthetic valve endocarditis. *J Heart Valve Dis.* **2011**, 20(5): 582–586.

Mattson, M. P., Haddon, R. C. & Rao, A. M. Molecular functionalization of carbon nanotubes and use as substrates for neuronal growth. *J Mol Neurosci.* **2000**, 14(3): 175–182.

Mederle, N., Marin, S., Marin, M. M., Danila, E., Mederle, O., Albu Kaya, M. G. et al. Innovative biomaterials based on collagen-hydroxyapatite and doxycycline for bone regeneration. *Adv Mater Sci Eng.* **2016**, 2016: 1–5.

Mehta, R. I., Mukherjee, A. K., Patterson, T. D. & Fishbein, M. C. Pathology of explanted polytetrafluoroethylene vascular grafts. *Cardiovasc Pathol.* **2011**, 20(4): 213–221.

Mengyan, L., Mondrinos, M. J., Xuesi, C. & Lelkes, P. I. (**2005**). Electrospun blends of natural and synthetic polymers as scaffolds for tissue engineering. In 2*005 IEEE Engineering in Medicine and Biology 2*7*th Annual Conference*: IEEE.

Meskinfam, M., Bertoldi, S., Albanese, N., Cerri, A., Tanzi, M. C., Imani, R. et al. Polyurethane foam/nanohydroxyapatite composite as a suitable scaffold for bone tissue regeneration. *Mater Sci Eng C.* **2018**, 82: 130–140.

Mitsak, A. G., Kemppainen, J. M., Harris, M. T. & Hollister, S. J. Effect of polycaprolactone scaffold permeability on bone regeneration *in vivo. Tissue Eng Part A.* **2011**, 17(13–14): 1831–1839.

Mogoşanu, G. D. & Grumezescu, A. M. Natural and synthetic polymers for wounds and burns dressing. *Int J Pharm.* **2014,** 463(2): 127–136.

Mohamadi, F., Ebrahimi-Barough, S., Nourani, M. R., Ahmadi, A. & Ai, J. Use new poly(ε-caprolactone/collagen/NBG) nerve conduits along with NGF for promoting peripheral (sciatic) nerve regeneration in a rat. *Artif Cells Nanomed Biotechnol.* **2018,** 46(sup2): 34–45.

Mole, B., Gillaizeau, F., Carbonnel, E., Pierre, I., Brazille, P., Grataloup, C., Mercier, S. et al. Polyacrylamide hydrogel injection in the management of human immunodeficiency virus-related facial lipoatrophy: results of the LIPOPHILL open-label study. *AIDS Res Hum Retroviruses.* **2012,** 28(3): 251–258.

Montero, J., Bravo, M., Guadilla, Y., Portillo, M., Blanco, L., Rojo, R. et al. Comparison of clinical and histologic outcomes of zirconia versus titanium implants placed in fresh sockets: a 5-month study in beagles. *Int J Oral Maxillofac Implants.* **2015,** 30(4): 773–780.

Moriguchi, Y., Lee, D. S., Chijimatsu, R., Thamina, K., Masuda, K., Itsuki, D. et al. Impact of non-thermal plasma surface modification on porous calcium hydroxyapatite ceramics for bone regeneration. *PLoS One.* **2018,** 13(3): e0194303.

Mountziaris, P. M., Shah, S. R., Lam, J., Bennett, G. N. & Mikos, A. G. A rapid, flexible method for incorporating controlled antibiotic release into porous polymethylmethacrylate space maintainers for craniofacial reconstruction. *Biomater Sci.* **2016,** 4(1): 121–129.

Nair, M., Nancy, D., Krishnan, A. G., Anjusree, G. S., Vadukumpully, S. & Nair, S. V. Graphene oxide nanoflakes incorporated gelatin–hydroxyapatite scaffolds enhance osteogenic differentiation of human mesenchymal stem cells. *Nanotechnology.* **2015,** 26(16): 161001.

Nakai, M., Niinomi, M., Cho, K. & Narita, K. (**2015**). Enhancing functionalities of metallic materials by controlling phase stability for use in orthopedic implants. In *Interface Oral Health Science 2014*, 79–91: Springer Japan.

Nakai, M., Niinomi, M., Zhao, X. & Zhao, X. Self-adjustment of Young's modulus in biomedical titanium alloys during orthopaedic operation. *Mater Lett.* **2011,** 65(4): 688–690.

Navarro, X., Vivó, M. & Valero-Cabré, A. Neural plasticity after peripheral nerve injury and regeneration. *Prog Neurobiol.* **2007,** 82(4): 163–201.

Ni, Y., Hu, H., Malarkey, E. B., Zhao, B., Montana, V., Haddon, R. C. et al. Chemically functionalized water soluble single-walled carbon nanotubes modulate neurite outgrowth. *J Nanosci Nanotechnol.* **2005,** 5(10): 1707–1712.

Nie, L., Chen, D., Suo, J., Zou, P., Feng, S., Yang, Q. et al. Physicochemical characterization and biocompatibility *in vitro* of biphasic calcium phosphate/polyvinyl alcohol scaffolds prepared by freeze-drying method for bone tissue engineering applications. *Colloids Surf B Biointerfaces.* **2012,** 100: 169–176.

Niechajev, I. Facial reconstruction using porous high-density polyethylene (Medpor): long-term results. *Aesthetic Plast Surg.* **2012,** 36(4): 917–927.

Nigam, R. & Mahanta, B. An overview of various biomimetic scaffolds: challenges and applications in tissue engineering. *J Tissue Sci Eng.* **2014,** 5(2).

Niinomi, M. Recent metallic materials for biomedical applications. *Metallurg Mater Transact A.* **2002,** 33(3): 477–486.

Niinomi, M. Metallic biomaterials. *J Artif Organs.* **2008,** 11(3): 105–110.

Niinomi, M. & Nakai, M. Titanium-based biomaterials for preventing stress shielding between implant devices and bone. *Int J Biomater.* **2011,** 2011: 1–10.

Niinomi, M. & Nakai, M. Biomedical implant devices fabricated from low Young's modulus titanium alloys demonstrating high mechanical biocompatibility. *Mater Matters.* **2014,** 9: 39–46.

Nikels, L. 3D printed titanium alloy could replace bone. *Metal Powder Rep.* **2016,** 71(4): 288–289.

Noshchenko, A., Xianfeng, Y., Armour, G. A., Baldini, T., Patel, V. V., Ayers, R. et al. Evaluation of spinal instrumentation rod bending characteristics for in-situ contouring. *J Biomed Mater Res Part B Appl Biomater.* **2011,** 98B(1): 192–200.

O'Brien, F. J. Biomaterials & scaffolds for tissue engineering. *Mater Today.* **2011,** 14(3): 88–95.

Ogawa, M., Tohma, Y., Ohgushi, H., Takakura, Y. & Tanaka, Y. Early fixation of cobalt-chromium based alloy surgical implants to bone using a tissue-engineering approach. *Int J Mol Sci.* **2012,** 13(5): 5528–5541.

Oh, J. H., Kim, H. J., Kim, T. I. & Woo, K. M. Comparative evaluation of the biological properties of fibrin for bone regeneration. *BMB Rep.* **2014,** 47(2): 110–114.

Okazaki, Y., Oki, Y., Kobatake, R., Abe, Y. & Tsuga, K. Enhanced osseointegration of a modified titanium implant with bound phospho-threonine: a preliminary *in vivo* study. *J Funct Biomater.* **2017,** 8(2): 16.

Oryan, A. & Alidadi, S. (**2017**). Application of bioceramics in orthopedics and bone tissue engineering. In *Bone Regeneration,* 2–73 India: Avid Science.

Öztatlı, H. & Ege, D. Physical and chemical properties of poly(l-lactic acid)/graphene oxide nanofibers for nerve regeneration. *MRS Advances.* **2016,** 2(24): 1291–1296.

Pacifici, L. Metals used in maxillofacial surgery. *Oral Implantol.* **2016,** 9(Suppl. 1): 107.

Pan, J. F., Liu, N. H., Sun, H. & Xu, F. Preparation and characterization of electrospun PLCL/poloxamer nanofibers and dextran/gelatin hydrogels for skin tissue engineering. *PLoS One.* **2014,** 9(11): e112885.

Papadopoulos, A., Bichara, D. A., Zhao, X., Ibusuki, S., Randolph, M. A., Anseth, K. S. et al. Injectable and photopolymerizable tissue-engineered auricular cartilage using poly(ethylene glycol) dimethacrylate copolymer hydrogels. *Tissue Eng Part A.* **2011,** 17(1–2): 161–169.

Park, H. S., Jeong, S. H. & Kwon, O. W. Factors affecting the clinical success of screw implants used as orthodontic anchorage. *Am J Orthod Dentofacial Orthop.* **2006,** 130(1): 18–25.

Park, S. Y., Park, J., Sim, S. H., Sung, M. G., Kim, K. S., Hong, B. H. et al. Enhanced differentiation of human neural stem cells into neurons on graphene. *Adv Mater.* **2011,** 23(36): H263–H267.

Park, W. H., Kim, B. S., Park, K. E., You, H. K., Lee, J. & Kim, M. H. Effect of nanofiber content on bone regeneration of silk fibroin/poly(ε-caprolactone) nano/microfibrous composite scaffolds. *Int J Nanomed.* **2015**: 485.

Pasqui, D., Torricelli, P., De Cagna, M., Fini, M. & Barbucci, R. Carboxymethyl cellulose-hydroxyapatite hybrid hydrogel as a composite material for bone tissue engineering applications. *J Biomed Mater Res Part A.* **2013,** 102(5): 1568–1579.

Pi, H. Y., Gao, Y., Wang, Y. L., Kong, D., Qu, B., Su, X. J. & Li, H. Nerve autografts and tissue-engineered materials for the repair of peripheral nerve injuries: a 5-year bibliometric analysis. *Neur Reg Res.* **2015,** 10(6): 1003.

Piconi, C. & Maccauro, G. Zirconia as a ceramic biomaterial. *Biomaterials.* **1999,** 20(1): 1–25.

Pina, S., Oliveira, J. M. & Reis, R. L. Natural-based nanocomposites for bone tissue engineering and regenerative medicine: a review. *Adv Mater.* **2015,** 27(7): 1143–1169.

Pineda-Castillo, S., Bernal-Ballén, A., Bernal-López, C., Segura-Puello, H., Nieto-Mosquera, D., Villamil-Ballesteros, A., Muñoz-Forero, D. et al. Synthesis and characterization of poly(vinyl alcohol)-chitosan-hydroxyapatite scaffolds: a promising alternative for bone tissue regeneration. *Molecules.* **2018,** 23(10): 2414.

Poologasundarampillai, G., Ionescu, C., Tsigkou, O., Murugesan, M., Hill, R. G., Stevens, M. M. et al. Synthesis of bioactive class II poly(γ-glutamic acid)/silica hybrids for bone regeneration. *J Mater Chem.* **2010**, 20(40): 8952.

Prasad, K., Bazaka, O., Chua, M., Rochford, M., Fedrick, L., Spoor, J. et al. Metallic biomaterials: current challenges and opportunities. *Materials.* **2017**, 10(8): 884.

Pripatnanont, P., Nuntanaranont, T., Vongvatcharanon, S. & Phurisat, K. The primacy of platelet-rich fibrin on bone regeneration of various grafts in rabbit's calvarial defects. *J Craniomaxillofac Surg.* **2013**, 41(8): e191–e200.

Pruitt, L. A. & Chakravartula, A. M. (**2012**). Metals for medical implants. In *Mechanics of Biomaterials*, 26–69: Cambridge University Press.

Puppi, D., Chiellini, F., Piras, A. M. & Chiellini, E. Polymeric materials for bone and cartilage repair. *Prog Polym Sci.* **2010**, 35(4): 403–440.

Qiu, J. J., Liu, C. M., Hu, F., Guo, X. D. & Zheng, Q. X. Synthesis of unsaturated polyphosphoester as a potential injectable tissue engineering scaffold materials. *J Appl Polym Sci.* **2006**, 102(4): 3095–3101.

Rabiei, A. Recent developments and the future of bone mimicking: materials for use in biomedical implants. *Expert Rev Med Devices.* **2010**, 7(6): 727–729.

Rai, A., Datarkar, A., Arora, A. & Adwani, D. G. Utility of High Density Porous Polyethylene Implants in Maxillofacial Surgery. *J Maxillofac Oral Surg.* **2013**, 13(1): 42–46.

Raoof, M., Mackeyev, Y., Cheney, M. A., Wilson, L. J. & Curley, S. A. Internalization of C60 fullerenes into cancer cells with accumulation in the nucleus via the nuclear pore complex. *Biomaterials.* **2012**, 33(10): 2952–2960.

Ravi, S., Caves, J. M., Martinez, A. W., Haller, C. A. & Chaikof, E. L. Incorporation of fibronectin to enhance cytocompatibility in multilayer elastin-like protein scaffolds for tissue engineering. *J Biomed Mater Res Part A.* **2012**, 101A(7): 1915–1925.

Ruan, J., Wang, X., Yu, Z., Wang, Z., Xie, Q., Zhang, D. et al. Enhanced physiochemical and mechanical performance of chitosan-grafted graphene oxide for superior osteoinductivity. *Adv Funct Mater.* **2015**, 26(7): 1085–1097.

Rumiński, S., Ostrowska, B., Jaroszewicz, J., Skirecki, T., Włodarski, K., Święszkowski, W. et al. Three-dimensional printed polycaprolactone-based scaffolds provide an advantageous environment for osteogenic differentiation of human adipose-derived stem cells. *J Tissue Eng Regen Med.* **2017**, 12(1): e473–e485.

Sadeghi-Avalshahr, A., Nokhasteh, S., Molavi, A. M., Khorsand-Ghayeni, M. & Mahdavi-Shahri, M. Synthesis and characterization of collagen/PLGA biodegradable skin scaffold fibers. *Reg Biomater.* **2017**, 4(5): 309–314.

Saha, S. P., Muluk, S., Schenk, W., Burks, S. G., Grigorian, A., Ploder, B. et al. Use of fibrin sealant as a hemostatic agent in expanded polytetrafluoroethylene graft placement surgery. *Ann Vasc Surg.* **2011**, 25(6): 813–822.

Saini, M., Singh, Y., Arora, P., Arora, V. & Jain, K. Implant biomaterials: a comprehensive review. *World J Clin Cases.* **2015**, 3(1): 52–57.

Salinas, A. J. & Vallet-Regí, M. Bioactive ceramics: from bone grafts to tissue engineering. *RSC Advances.* **2013**, 3(28): 11116.

Schliephake, H., Hefti, T., Schlottig, F., Gédet, P. & Staedt, H. Mechanical anchorage and peri-implant bone formation of surface-modified zirconia in minipigs. *J Clin Periodontol.* **2010**, 37(9): 818–828.

Schön, R., Metzger, M. C., Zizelmann, C., Weyer, N. & Schmelzeisen, R. Individually preformed titanium mesh implants for a true-to-original repair of orbital fractures. *Int J Oral Maxillofac Surg.* **2006**, 35(11): 990–995.

Sclafani, A. P. & Saman, M. Platelet-rich fibrin matrix for facial plastic surgery. *Facial Plast Surg Clin North Am.* **2012,** 20(2): 177–186.

Seal, B. Polymeric biomaterials for tissue and organ regeneration. *Mater Sci Eng R Rep.* **2001,** 34(4–5): 147–230.

Sell, S. A., Wolfe, P. S., Garg, K., McCool, J. M., Rodriguez, I. A. & Bowlin, G. L. The use of natural polymers in tissue engineering: a focus on electrospun extracellular matrix analogues. *Polymers.* **2010,** 2(4): 522–553.

Semnani, D., Naghashzargar, E., Hadjianfar, M., Dehghan Manshadi, F., Mohammadi, S., Karbasi, S. et al.. Evaluation of PCL/chitosan electrospun nanofibers for liver tissue engineering. *Int J Polymer Mater Polymer Biomater.* **2016,** 66(3): 149–157.

Sengezer, M. & Sadove, R. C. Reconstruction of midface bone defects with vitallium micromesh. *J Craniofac Surg.* **1992,** 3(3): 125–133.

Seol, Y. J., Park, J. Y., Jung, J. W., Jang, J., Girdhari, R., Kim, S. W. et al. Improvement of bone regeneration capability of ceramic scaffolds by accelerated release of their calcium ions. *Tissue Eng Part A.* **2014,** 20(21–22): 2840–2849.

Shayganpour, A., Rebaudi, A., Cortella, P., Diaspro, A. & Salerno, M. Electrochemical coating of dental implants with anodic porous titania for enhanced osteointegration. *Beil J Nanotechnol.* **2015,** 6: 2183–2192.

Shi, C., Yuan, Z., Han, F., Zhu, C. & Li, B. Polymeric biomaterials for bone regeneration. *Ann Joint.* **2016,** 1: 27–27.

Shi, L., Wang, L., Guo, Z., Wu, Z. X., Liu, D., Gao, M. X. et al. A study of low elastic modulus expandable pedicle screws in osteoporotic sheep. *J Spinal Disord Tech.* **2012,** 25(2): 123–128.

Shin, S. R., Li, Y. C., Jang, H. L., Khoshakhlagh, P., Akbari, M., Nasajpour, A. et al. Graphene-based materials for tissue engineering. *Adv Drug Del Rev.* **2016,** 105: 255–274.

Shin, Y. C., Kim, J., Kim, S. E., Song, S. J., Hong, S. W., Oh, J. W. et al. RGD peptide and graphene oxide co-functionalized PLGA nanofiber scaffolds for vascular tissue engineering. *Reg Biomater.* **2017,** 4(3): 159–166.

Sionkowska, A. & Kozłowska, J. Properties and modification of porous 3-D collagen/hydroxyapatite composites. *Int J Biol Macromol.* **2013,** 52: 250–259.

Sivakumar, M., Kumar Dhanadurai, K. S., Rajeswari, S. & Thulasiraman, V. Failures in stainless steel orthopaedic implant devices: a survey. *J Mater Sci Lett.* **1995,** 14(5): 351–354.

Sixto, B. G., Ángel, M. & Prieto, R. Naso-orbital complex reconstruction with titanium mesh and canthopexy. *J Aesthet Reconstr Surg.* **2016,** 2(1): 2.

Sohier, J., Daculsi, G., Sourice, S., de Groot, K. & Layrolle, P. Porous beta tricalcium phosphate scaffolds used as a BMP-2 delivery system for bone tissue engineering. *J Biomed Mater Res Part A.* **2009,** 9999A: NA-NA.

Song, J., Gao, H., Zhu, G., Cao, X., Shi, X. & Wang, Y. The preparation and characterization of polycaprolactone/graphene oxide biocomposite nanofiber scaffolds and their application for directing cell behaviors. *Carbon.* **2015,** 95: 1039–1050.

Sorkin, R., Greenbaum, A., David-Pur, M., Anava, S., Ayali, A., Ben-Jacob, E. & Hanein, Y. Process entanglement as a neuronal anchorage mechanism to rough surfaces. *Nanotechnology.* **2008,** 20(1): 015101.

Sproul, E., Nandi, S. & Brown, A. (**2018**). Fibrin biomaterials for tissue regeneration and repair. In *Peptides and Proteins as Biomaterials for Tissue Regeneration and Repair,* 151–173: Elsevier.

Stollwerck, P. L., Kozlowski, B., Sandmann, W., Grabitz, K. & Pfeiffer, T. Long-term dilatation of polyester and expanded polytetrafluoroethylene tube grafts after open repair of infrarenal abdominal aortic aneurysms. *J Vasc Surg.* **2011,** 53(6): 1506–1513.

Styan, K. E., Martin, D. J., Simmons, A. & Poole-Warren, L. A. *In vivo* biostability of polyurethane–organosilicate nanocomposites. *Acta Biomater.* **2012,** 8(6): 2243–2253.

Sumitomo, N., Noritake, K., Hattori, T., Morikawa, K., Niwa, S., Sato, K. et al. Experiment study on fracture fixation with low rigidity titanium alloy. *J Mater Sci Mater Med.* **2008,** 19(4): 1581–1586.

Sundaramurthi, D., Krishnan, U. M. & Sethuraman, S. Electrospun nanofibers as scaffolds for skin tissue engineering. *Poly Rev.* **2014,** 54(2): 348–376.

Suyalatu, Kondo, R., Tsutsumi, Y., Doi, H., Nomura, N. & Hanawa, T. Effects of phase constitution on magnetic susceptibility and mechanical properties of Zr-rich Zr–Mo alloys. *Acta Biomater.* **2011,** 7(12): 4259–4266.

Suyalatu, Nomura, N., Oya, K., Tanaka, Y., Kondo, R., Doi, H., Tsutsumi, Y. et al. Microstructure and magnetic susceptibility of as-cast Zr–Mo alloys. *Acta Biomater.* **2010,** 6(3): 1033–1038.

Suzuki, S., Dawson, R., Chirila, T., Shadforth, A., Hogerheyde, T., Edwards, G. et al. Treatment of silk fibroin with poly(ethylene glycol) for the enhancement of corneal epithelial cell growth. *J Funct Biomater.* **2015,** 6(2): 345–366.

Swiatkowska, I., Mosselmans, J. F. W., Geraki, T., Wyles, C. C., Maleszewski, J. J., Henckel, J. et al. Synchrotron analysis of human organ tissue exposed to implant material. *J Trace Elem Med Biol.* **2018,** 46: 128–137.

Tanaka, M., Sato, Y., Haniu, H., Nomura, H., Kobayashi, S., Takanashi, S. et al. A three-dimensional block structure consisting exclusively of carbon nanotubes serving as bone regeneration scaffold and as bone defect filler. *PLoS One.* **2017,** 12(2): e0172601.

Teck Lim, G., Valente, S. A., Hart-Spicer, C. R., Evancho-Chapman, M. M., Puskas, J. E., Horne, W. I. et al. New biomaterial as a promising alternative to silicone breast implants. *J Mech Behav Biomed Mater.* **2013,** 21: 47–56.

Teixeira, S., Fernandes, H., Leusink, A., van Blitterswijk, C., Ferraz, M. P., Monteiro, F. J. et al. *In vivo* evaluation of highly macroporous ceramic scaffolds for bone tissue engineering. *J Biomed Mater Res Part A.* **2009,** 9999A: NA-NA.

Teng, S. H., Wang, P. & Dong, J. Q. Bioactive hybrid coatings of poly(ε-caprolactone)–silica xerogel on titanium for biomedical applications. *Mater Lett.* **2014,** 129: 209–212.

Thoma, D. S., Benic, G. I., Muñoz, F., Kohal, R., Sanz Martin, I., Cantalapiedra, A. G. et al. Marginal bone-level alterations of loaded zirconia and titanium dental implants: an experimental study in the dog mandible. *Clin Oral Implants Res.* **2015,** 27(4): 412–420.

Tian, L., Prabhakaran, M. P., Hu, J., Chen, M., Besenbacher, F. & Ramakrishna, S. Coaxial electrospun poly(lactic acid)/silk fibroin nanofibers incorporated with nerve growth factor support the differentiation of neuronal stem cells. *RSC Advances.* **2015,** 5(62): 49838–49848.

Tian, Z., Zhu, Y., Qiu, J., Guan, H., Li, L., Zheng, S. et al. Synthesis and characterization of UPPE-PLGA-rhBMP2 scaffolds for bone regeneration. *J Huazhong Univ Sci Technol Med Sci.* **2012,** 32(4): 563–570.

Traini, T., Murmura, G., Sinjari, B., Perfetti, G., Scarano, A., D'Arcangelo, C. et al. The surface anodization of titanium dental implants improves blood clot formation followed by osseointegration. *Coatings.* **2018,** 8(7): 252.

Tsao, C. T., Leung, M., Yu-Fong Chang, J. & Zhang, M. A simple material model to generate epidermal and dermal layers *in vitro* for skin regeneration. *J Mater Chem B.* **2014,** 2(32): 5256–5264.

Tur, K. Biomaterials and tissue engineering for regenerative repair of articular cartilage defects. *Turk J Rheumatol.* **2009,** 24(4): 206–217.

Vasconcelos, A., Gomes, A. C. & Cavaco-Paulo, A. Novel silk fibroin/elastin wound dressings. *Acta Biomater.* **2012,** 8(8): 3049–3060.

Venzin, C. & Jacot, V. Biocompatibility of pegylated fibrinogen and its effect on healing of full-thickness skin defects: a preliminary study in rats. *J Biotechnol Biomater.* **2016,** 6(2).

Wang, F. J., Mohammed, A., Li, C. J. & Wang, L. Promising poly(ε-caprolactone) composite reinforced with weft-knitted polyester for small-diameter vascular graft application. *Adv Mater Sci Eng.* **2014a,** 2014: 1–9.

Wang, H. J., Di, L., Ren, Q. S. & Wang, J. Y. Applications and degradation of proteins used as tissue engineering materials. *Materials.* **2009,** 2(2): 613–635.

Wang, J. K., Xiong, G. M., Luo, B., Choo, C. C., Yuan, S., Tan, N. S. et al.. Surface modification of PVDF using non-mammalian sources of collagen for enhancement of endothelial cell functionality. *J Mater Sci Mater Med.* **2016,** 27(3).

Wang, J. K., Yeo, K. P., Chun, Y. Y., Tan, T. T. Y., Tan, N. S., Angeli, V. et al. Fish scale-derived collagen patch promotes growth of blood and lymphatic vessels *in vivo*. *Acta Biomater.* **2017a,** 63: 246–260.

Wang, L., Lu, C., Li, Y., Wu, F., Zhao, B. & Dong, X. Green fabrication of porous silk fibroin/graphene oxide hybrid scaffolds for bone tissue engineering. *RSC Adv.* **2015,** 5(96): 78660–78668.

Wang, Q., Chen, J., Niu, Q., Fu, X., Sun, X. & Tong, X. The application of graphene oxidized combining with decellularized scaffold to repair of sciatic nerve injury in rats. *Saudi Pharma J.* **2017b,** 25(4): 469–476.

Wang, X., Ali, M. & Lacerda, C. A three-dimensional collagen-elastin scaffold for heart valve tissue engineering. *Bioengineering.* **2018,** 5(3): 69.

Wang, Z., Fu, S., Wu, Z. X., Zhang, Y. & Lei, W. Ti2448 pedicle screw system augmentation for posterior lumbar interbody fusion. *Spine (Phila Pa 1976).* **2013,** 38(23): 2008–2015.

Wang, Z., Han, N., Wang, J., Zheng, H., Peng, J., Kou, Y. et al. Improved peripheral nerve regeneration with sustained release nerve growth factor microspheres in small gap tubulization. *Am J Transl Research.* **2014b,** 6(4): 413–421.

Waterhouse, A., Wise, S. G., Ng, M. K. C. & Weiss, A. S. Elastin as a Nonthrombogenic Biomaterial. *Tissue Eng Part B Rev.* **2011,** 17(2): 93–99.

Wu, D., Liao, L., Liu, Z., Yan, H., Guo, Z. & Liu, X. K. Maxillary and cheek reconstruction with titanium mesh and folded free anterolateral thigh flap. *Arch Cancer Res.* **2016,** 4(3).

Wu, Z., Hu, S., Lim, T., Guo, G., Liu, J. & Li, S. Poly(lactic-co-glycolic acid) and SBA-15 composite scaffolds for bone regeneration. *J Biomater Tissue Eng.* **2017,** 7(10): 934–942.

Xiao, D. M., Yang, Y. Q., Su, X. B., Wang, D. & Luo, Z. Y. Topology optimization of microstructure and selective laser melting fabrication for metallic biomaterial scaffolds. *Transact Nonferrous Metals Soc China.* **2012,** 22(10): 2554–2561.

Xu, C., Zhang, Y., Cheng, G. & Zhu, W. Corrosion and electrochemical behavior of 316L stainless steel in sulfate-reducing and iron-oxidizing bacteria solutions. *Chin J Chem Eng.* **2006,** 14(6): 829–834.

Xu, F., Zou, D., Dai, T., Xu, H., An, R., Liu, Y. et al. Effects of incorporation of granule-lyophilised platelet-rich fibrin into polyvinyl alcohol hydrogel on wound healing. *Sci Rep.* **2018,** 8(1).

Xu, X., Yee, W. C., Hwang, P. Y. K., Yu, H., Wan, A. C. A., Gao, S. et al. Peripheral nerve regeneration with sustained release of poly(phosphoester) microencapsulated nerve growth factor within nerve guide conduits. *Biomaterials.* **2003,** 24(13): 2405–2412.

Yan, S., Wang, T., Feng, L., Zhu, J., Zhang, K., Chen, X. et al. Injectable in situ self-cross-linking hydrogels based on poly(l-glutamic acid) and alginate for cartilage tissue engineering. *Biomacromolecules.* **2014,** 15(12): 4495–4508.

Yan, S., Zhang, X., Zhang, K., Di, H., Feng, L., Li, G. et al. Injectable in situ forming poly(l-glutamic acid) hydrogels for cartilage tissue engineering. *J Mater Chem B.* **2016,** 4(5): 947–961.

Yang, X., Li, E., Wan, Y., Smith, P., Shang, G. & Cui, Q. Antioxidative fullerol promotes osteogenesis of human adipose-derived stem cells. *Int J Nanomed.* **2014:** 4023.

Yang, X., Yang, K., Wu, S., Chen, X., Yu, F., Li, J. et al. Cytotoxicity and wound healing properties of PVA/ws-chitosan/glycerol hydrogels made by irradiation followed by freeze–thawing. *Radiat Phys Chem.* **2010,** 79(5): 606–611.

Yi, W. S., Xu, X. L., Ma, J. R. & Ou, X. R. Reconstruction of complex orbital fracture with titanium implants. *Int J Ophthalmol.* **2012,** 5(4): 488–492.

Yocham, K. M., Scott, C., Fujimoto, K., Brown, R., Tanasse, E., Oxford, J. T. et al. Mechanical properties of graphene foam and graphene foam-tissue composites. *Adv Eng Mater.* **2018,** 20(9): 1800166.

Yoo, Y. R., Jang, S. G., Oh, K. T., Kim, J. G. & Kim, Y. S. Influences of passivating elements on the corrosion and biocompatibility of super stainless steels. *J Biomed Mater Res Part B Appl Biomater.* **2008,** 86B(2): 310–320.

Yoshii, T., Hafeman, A. E., Nyman, J. S., Esparza, J. M., Shinomiya, K., Spengler, D. M. et al. A sustained release of lovastatin from biodegradable, elastomeric polyurethane scaffolds for enhanced bone regeneration. *Tissue Eng Part A.* **2010,** 16(7): 2369–2379.

Yousefi, A., Vaesken, A., Amri, A., Dasi, L. P. & Heim, F. Heart valves from polyester fibers vs. biological tissue: comparative study *in vitro. Ann Biomed Eng.* **2016,** 45(2): 476–486.

Yu, F., Cao, X., Li, Y., Zeng, L., Yuan, B. & Chen, X. An injectable hyaluronic acid/PEG hydrogel for cartilage tissue engineering formed by integrating enzymatic crosslinking and Diels–Alder "click chemistry". *Polym Chem.* **2018,** 9(28): 3959–3960.

Yu, F., Cao, X., Li, Y., Zeng, L., Zhu, J., Wang, G. et al. Diels–Alder crosslinked HA/PEG hydrogels with high elasticity and fatigue resistance for cell encapsulation and articular cartilage tissue repair. *Polym Chem.* **2014,** 5(17): 5116–5123.

Yu, T., Zhao, C., Li, P., Liu, G. & Luo, M. Poly(lactic-co-glycolic acid) conduit for repair of injured sciatic nerve: a mechanical analysis. *Neur Reg Res.* **2013,** 8(21): 1966.

Yu, W., Zhao, W., Zhu, C., Zhang, X., Ye, D., Zhang, W. et al. Sciatic nerve regeneration in rats by a promising electrospun collagen/poly(ε-caprolactone) nerve conduit with tailored degradation rate. *BMC Neurosci.* **2011,** 12(1): 68.

Yun, Y. Carbon nanomaterials: from therapeutics to regenerative medicine. *J Nanomed Biother Discov.* **2012,** 2(1).

Zadeh, M. H. R., Seifi, M., Abdolrahimi, M. & Hadavi, M. A comprehensive *in vitro* study of the carbon nanotube enhanced chitosan scaffolds for cancellous bone regeneration. *Biomed Phys Eng Express.* **2018,** 4(3): 035027.

Zhang, W., Zhu, C., Ye, D., Xu, L., Zhang, X., Wu, Q. et al. Porous silk scaffolds for delivery of growth factors and stem cells to enhance bone regeneration. *PLoS One.* **2014,** 9(7): e102371.

Zhang, Z., Wang, X., Wang, Y. & Hao, J. Rapid-forming and self-healing agarose-based hydrogels for tissue adhesives and potential wound dressings. *Biomacromolecules.* **2018,** 19(3): 980–988.

Zhao, X., Niinomi, M. & Nakai, M. Relationship between various deformation-induced products and mechanical properties in metastable Ti–30Zr–Mo alloys for biomedical applications. *J Mech Behav Biomed Mater.* **2011a,** 4(8): 2009–2016.

Zhao, X., Niinomi, M., Nakai, M. & Hieda, J. Beta type Ti–Mo alloys with changeable Young's modulus for spinal fixation applications. *Acta Biomater.* **2012a,** 8(5): 1990–1997.

Zhao, X., Niinomi, M., Nakai, M., Hieda, J., Ishimoto, T. & Nakano, T. Optimization of Cr content of metastable β-type Ti–Cr alloys with changeable Young's modulus for spinal fixation applications. *Acta Biomater.* **2012b,** 8(6): 2392–2400.

Zhao, X., Niinomi, M., Nakai, M., Miyamoto, G. & Furuhara, T. Microstructures and mechanical properties of metastable Ti–30Zr–(Cr, Mo) alloys with changeable Young's modulus for spinal fixation applications. *Acta Biomater.* **2011b,** 7(8): 3230–3236.

Zhou, J., Lin, H., Fang, T., Li, X., Dai, W., Uemura, T. et al. The repair of large segmental bone defects in the rabbit with vascularized tissue engineered bone. *Biomaterials.* **2010,** 31(6): 1171–1179.

Zhou, T., Wang, N., Xue, Y., Ding, T., Liu, X., Mo, X. et al. Development of biomimetic tilapia collagen nanofibers for skin regeneration through inducing keratinocytes differentiation and collagen synthesis of dermal fibroblasts. *ACS Appl Mater Interfaces.* **2015,** 7(5): 3253–3262.

CHAPTER 2

Smart Polymeric Biomaterials in Tissue Engineering

AKHILESH KUMAR MAURYA and NIDHI MISHRA*

*Chemistry Laboratory Department of Applied Sciences,
Indian Institute of Information Technology, Allahabad, India*

Corresponding author. E-mail: nidhimishra@iiita.ac.in

ABSTRACT

Polymeric biomaterials are one of the bases of tissue engineering. A wide range of materials has been used in medical field. Biomaterials have been used from ancient civilization of human history. With the advancement of synthetic and natural biomaterials, it has led to the development of stimuli-responsive biomaterials known as "smart biomaterials." Smart polymeric biomaterials are more biocompatible, biodegradable, and similar to human body tissue. Smart polymer may be synthetic or natural. These polymers may be temperature, light, enzyme, pH, magnetic effect, etc., sensitive and stimuli specific. These polymers have been used in the development of various medical devices, artificial organs and organ parts, and targeted and controlled drug delivery with effect of specificity of biomaterials. More advanced and smart biomaterials will be developed with changing in present structure of biomaterials in future. This chapter is focused on the development of smart biomaterials. It discusses natural and synthetic polymers used in their preparation and the most recent applications as biomaterials.

2.1 INTRODUCTION

According to literature survey, affected human body parts had been repaired using materials of surrounding since antiquity, when wood was used to replace lost tissues (Huebsch and Mooney, 2009). In ancient human history, selection of materials was based on availability in particular area where they live and ingenuity of the individual making and applying the prosthetic. The first prostheses were appeared in Neolithic period. According to archeologists, Neanderthal man lived after amputation. Bone and teeth repair were most frequent surgical interventions. Ancient dentist used different animals' teeth such as dogs, calves, seals, and narwhals to replace human teeth (Hildebrand, 2013). Later, surgeons and scientists introduced metals as prosthetic such as gold, silver, copper, etc. (Hildebrand, 2013). However, early attempts at using materials in the human body for replacement were rather hit-and-miss. Interaction between materials and body systems was systematically examine in the beginning of last two century. In the beginning of 20th century, natural materials began to be replaced by synthetic materials such as metal alloys and ceramics which provided better performance than natural. On the basis of their applications, materials are used in medical devices. In early research, linking of materials chemistry to biological response provided a biologically inert substance (Ratner and Bryant, 2004; Anderson et al., 2008). Since 1960s molecular biology revolution and 1990s genomics and proteomics advancements, they significantly affected the design and use of biomaterials. Over the past few decades, our society developed biological active synthetically derived materials for tissue engineering (Ratner and Bryant, 2004). Polymeric biomaterials with various combination, natural–natural, synthetic–synthetic, and natural–synthetic have been designed by incorporation of distinct functional groups to control physiological, chemical, and biological properties. These advance biomaterials have been used in tissue engineering, organ replacement, wound healing, targeted drug delivery, controlled delivery, medical device development, etc. (Khan and Tanaka, 2018). In advancement of biomaterials, polymeric biomaterials have been developed in 3D scaffold which are excellent in organ and tissue replacement. Using various compositions of biomaterials, "smart polymeric biomaterials" have been developed with the advanced use in tissue engineering and drug delivery system.

2.2 EVOLUTION OF BIOMATERIALS

Study in the field of biomaterials starts about 70–80 years ago. Before 80 years, biomaterial term did not exist and there was no understanding about synthetic or artificial biomaterials and its wide use in medicine (Figure 2.1).

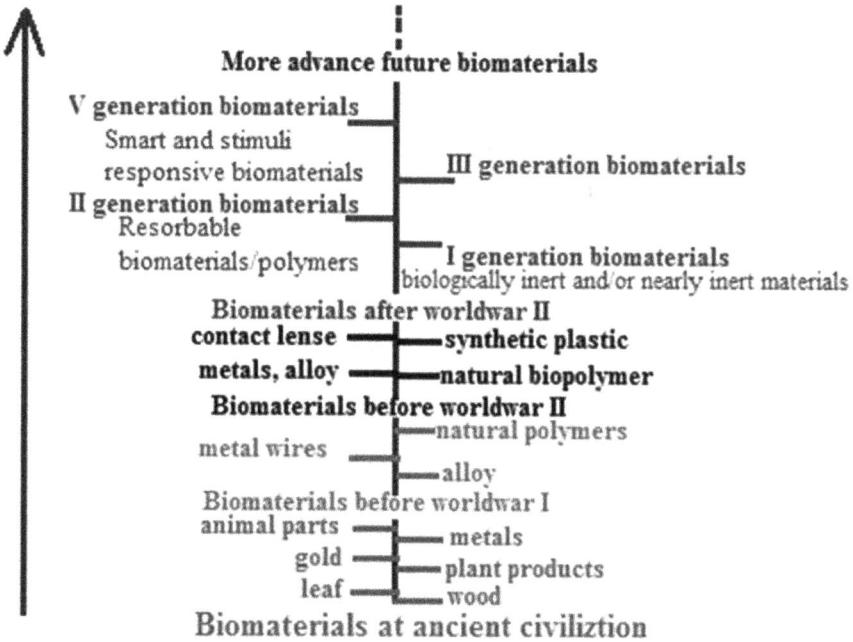

FIGURE 2.1   Evolution of biomaterial.

2.2.1   BIOMATERIALS BEFORE 1940s

Throughout the human history, nonbiological materials such as metals were used in the body. About 9000-year-old skeleton of human has been found with spear point embedded in his hip in Kennewick, Washington, USA and foreign material was embedded into skin in another example dated to about 5000 years ago (Ratner, 2004). Teeth from seashells were used by Mayan people in about 600 AD (Bobbio, 1972) and Franciscans used wrought iron dental implant in about 200 AD (Crubzy et al., 1998). The implant was described as osseointegration.

In the New Stone period, large wounds were closed by cautery or sutures. Early Egyptians used linen sutures and Europeans used catgut in middle age. Heads of large, biting ants were used in India and South Africa to clamp the wound edges together. In 1849, J Marion Sims fabricates a suture of silver wire. Those eras have no knowledge of toxicity, inflammation, sterilization, and biodegradation, yet manufacturing of sutures was very common (Ratner, 2004).

Concept of contact lenses was developed by Leonardo da Vinci in the year 1508. In about 1860, first contact lens of glass was developed by Adolf Gaston Eugen Fick. There is some controversy over who created the first pair of lenses. Some sources believe it to be German glassblower FA Muller, but others point to Swiss physician Adolf Gaston Eugen Fick and Paris optician Edouard Kalt (https://www.piedmonteye.com/history-contact-lenses). In 1948, plastic polymethyl methacrylate (PMMA) contact lenses were designed to cover only the eyes cornea. First coronary artery bypass surgery and intrathoracic transplantation by the total artificial heart in 1937 were developed by Dr Vladimir P Demikhov in a dog (Konstantinov, 2009; Critchley et al., 2011).

2.2.2   BIOMATERIALS AFTER 1940s

During and after World War II, surgeons needed high performance bioma-terial, especially biopolymeric materials to replace damaged or diseased body parts. Polyurethanes, methacrylate, silicones, stainless steel, etc., biomaterials were used. Biomaterials were commonly used as prostheses in dental, dermal, orthopedic, cardiovascular and as suture in surgery and for controlled drug delivery. Biomaterial field get accelerated after acceptance of first medical device of biomaterials on the basics of medical and scientific principles for human usage in early 1950s (Ratner et al., 2013). Research in the biomaterials field was guided and accelerated by advancement of molecular biology, material sciences, chemical sciences, and engineering. In the 20th century, development of biomaterials with medical application evolved and can be classified into four generations (Hench and Polak, 2002).

2.2.2.1   FIRST-GENERATION BIOMATERIALS

Beginning of 1960s was the period to start first-generation biomaterials. This generation was comprised of industrial materials for medical use inside the human body. Mechanical properties of tissues were recognized by Prof Bill Bonfield. His finding was pioneer for the study of interaction of biomaterials with living tissues (Hench and Thompson, 2010). First-generation biomate-rials were developed by scientist to achieve a better combination of physical properties, which match with living tissues for replacing the tissues with minimal toxic response to host (Hench, 1980).

To reduce the corrosion of metals and releasing of its ions and particles in body after implantation, biologically inert and/or nearly inert materials were used that minimize immune response in body. In the beginning of 1980s, Prof Bonfield started designing new-generation biomaterials that were "biocomposite" materials that have almost similar to mechanical properties of host tissues (Rea and Bonfield, 2004). These composite materials minimized and eliminated stress and mechanical load on the tissues. This period of time in biomaterials promoted specific response, bioactive material known as hydroxyapatite (HA) chemically similar to mineral component of human bone. HA promotes bond formation in bone tissues (Narayan, 2010). Maxillofacial implants, orthopedic implants, and dental implants are plasma sprayed with HA coatings in order to obtain fixation between the implant and the surrounding bones (Dhert, 1994).

Examples of first-generation biomaterials are metals such as stainless steel and cobalt–chrome-based alloys, Ti and Ti alloys, ceramics such as alumina (Al_2O_3), HA, calcium phosphate [$Ca_{10}(PO_4)_6(OH)_2$] and zirconia (ZrO_2), and polymers (silicone rubber, acrylic resins).

2.2.2.2 SECOND-GENERATION BIOMATERIALS

By 1980s, second-generation biomaterials had been shifted in exclusively bioinert tissue response to developed a bioactive material, which has ability to interact with micro- and macroenvironment for enhancing the biological response and materials that have the ability to biodegrade and resorbable. This generation elicited to control the reaction of implanted materials with the tissues to induce a desired therapeutic effect.

Resorbable biomaterials/polymers were most prominent in use such as drug absorbance in coronary arteries to remove drugs from body (Kukreja et al., 2008). In pharmacological agent such as drugs, antigens are released into the body fluids surrounded by the tissues; at the present time, it is the development of third-generation biomaterials (Hench et al., 2000). Various compositions of bioactive ceramics and glasses were clinically used in orthopedic and dental surgeries (Rose et al., 2001). The devices, made up of bioactive ceramics and glasses such as HeartMate®, assist patients in left ventricular for congestive heart failure. The polyurethane has integrally textured in cardiac device surface that control clotting reaction to minimize it (Yamamuro et al., 1990). The development of resorbable bioactive biomaterials, with slow release and biologically degradable with various medical applications, also include in second-generation biomaterials.

Materials with biological activity have been clinically used for orthopedics and dental surgery in 1980s. Coating on metallic prostheses has been performed to fix the bioactive and porous implant; synthetic HA ceramic has been used (Hench, 1993; Hench and Wilson, 1996). Bioactive glass ceramics, that is, bioglass have been used as ear prostheses to restore the hearing loss (Yamamuro, 1993). Replacement of vertebral column with spinal tumors has been done by tough bioactive glass ceramic, developed by Kyoto University (Hastings and Ducheyne, 1984). In second-generation biomaterials, sutures were composed of a copolymer such as polylactic acid (PLA) and polyglycolic acid (PGA) and degraded hydrolytically and resulted in CO_2 and H_2O which are easily metabolized (Freed et al., 2006).

2.2.2.3   THIRD-GENERATION BIOMATERIALS

The third-generation biomaterials are being designed to stimulate specific cellular responses, biologically active and bioresorbable, and 3D and porous, which can activate or affect the genes of regeneration of living tissues and some organs of the body. Throughout all human history, there was nonexistent of regeneration of lost tissues or organs. Now, in third-generation biomaterials with advanced tissue engineering and regenerative medicines, replacement of living tissues became possible (Critchley et al., 2011). Tissue engineering is a set of tools in the field of biomedical sciences in which biomaterials play a key role to aid tissue formation and regeneration, which produce diagnostic and/or therapeutic benefit (Mikos et al., 2006; Ingber, 2010; Jandt, 2007).

To achieve specific interactions with integrins of cells, extracellular matrix (ECM), and differentiating cells, molecular modifications are being/ have been made in resorbable polymers. Tissue engineering and in situ tissue regenerations are the routes used to repair the damaged or diseased tissues in third-generation biomaterials. Both approaches are effective in controlled tissue repairing process and can generate a specific cell response to controlled release of medicines and biochemical stimuli (Ingber, 2010). Various combinations of biomaterials have been done such as micro- and nanocellulose with glycol and many combinations of natural and synthetic polymers have been developed. Along these, polymeric biomaterials have been developed in a smart way with various combinations of polymers, now known as "smart polymer" that comes under next-generation or fourth-generation biomaterials. With smartness of biomaterials, field of nanomedicine, BioMEMS, etc., are also became more advanced (Sharma et al., 2017).

2.2.2.4   NEXT-/FOURTH-GENERATION BIOMATERIALS

The latest one is fourth-generation biomaterials that can be characterized by revolutionary development. After the implantation of fourth-generation biomaterials, biological system interacts in various ways such as degradation of materials, integration into biological system, and regulation of biological process in proper manner. These materials are "smart biomaterials," i.e., materials that can change their properties depending on external stimuli or they can mimic as biological system (Simionescu and Ivanov, 2016). Heterogeneous structures with better properties can be developed by combination of hard and soft materials with mild synthesis, withhold together by strong and weak bond association into the composite structure (Dong and Hoffman, 1987). Smart polymeric materials are environmentally sensitive and probably response in pH, temperature, pressure, light, enzyme, magnetic strength, etc., for example, poly(N-isopropylacrylamide) (PNIPAM) hydrogels are temperature sensitive (Badeau et al., 2018). Drugs and other molecules have been loaded on smart polymer and delivered at desired site. Field of smart polymeric biomaterials is evolving continuously. A recent publication (Fratzl, 2007) of new strategy of hydrogels synthesis has been introduced that degrade under user-defined environmental condition. Biocompatibility and degradability of biomaterials can be enhanced by combinatorial synthesis of naturally occurring and synthetic polymers.

Most of the polymers are made of organic components; it may be natural and/or synthetic and in this respect, their molecular properties are comparatively similar in function with lipids, proteins, and polysaccharides of biological system. Commonly used biomaterials are polyethylene (PE), polyglycolides (PGAs), polyanhydrides, PMMA, poly(lactide-co-glycolides) (PLGAs), polytetrafluoroethylene, etc., as synthetic biomaterials and fibrinogen, collagen, chitosan (CS), glycosaminoglycans (GAGs), etc., as natural biomaterials and the combination of various biomaterials develops smart polybiomaterials.

2.3   BIOMATERIALS BASED ON NATURAL POLYMER

Nature has developed few basic substances, mainly polymers and minerals, for the biological system with remarkable functional properties (Nakanishi, 1999). Natural polymers are a renewable resource that can be obtained from various sources of nature; natural polymers have variety of functional groups and can be produced by physical and/or chemical methods. These polymers can come from anywhere; generally, they originate from microbes, plants/ animal, or from abiotic sources. New biomaterial may be produced by naturally occurring biopolymers by using emerging biotechnology. Naturally occurring and modified biopolymers can be degraded into water/biological fluids and biocompatible, nontoxic, and environment friendly biomaterials. Naturally derived/modified polymeric biomaterials can be classified as proteins (elastin, keratin, fibrinogen, collagen, silk, gelatin, actin, and myosin), polysugars (cellulose, amylose, dextran, chitin, and GAGs), and polynucleotides (DNA, RNA) (Pignatello, 2011).

2.3.1 FIBRONECTIN

Fibronectins (FNs) are a multifunctional, ECM glycoprotein and are present on the surface of cell or cell organelles membrane, in plasma of blood, and other biological fluids; molecular weight of FN glycoprotein is high (~250 kDa), which interacts with other ECM molecules of body such as fibrinogen, glycosaminoglycans, and collagen (Sitterley, 2008). FNs are synthesized by various types of epithelial and mesenchymal cells such as macrophages, hepatocytes, fibroblasts, chondrocytes, myoblasts, and intestinal epithelial cells (Clark, 2013). A wide variety of cellular interactions is performed by FN with ECM and plays important roles in cell migration, adhesion, growth, proliferation, and differentiation (Sahni and Francis, 2000). FN binds with fibroblast growth factor, endothelial growth factor, and many cytokines and performs various biological functions. McManus et al. cultured neonatal rat cardiac fibroblasts onto fibrinogen electrospun scaffolds (Kozlowski, 2012).

2.3.2 CHITIN AND CHITOSAN

Chitin is a naturally occurring polysaccharide with monomer unit of N-acetyl-D-glucosamine (NAG), which is attached to each other via $\beta(1 \rightarrow 4)$ glycosidic bond (Tang et al., 2015) (Figures 2.2A and B). Chitin occurs in form of macrofibrils and it is major component of exoskeletons of arthropods and provides structural support such as the crustaceans (crabs and shrimps), insects, the radulae of molluscs, cephalopod beaks, and the scales of fish and amphibians as well as the cell walls of fungi (Azuma et al., 2015; Motiei et al., 2017).

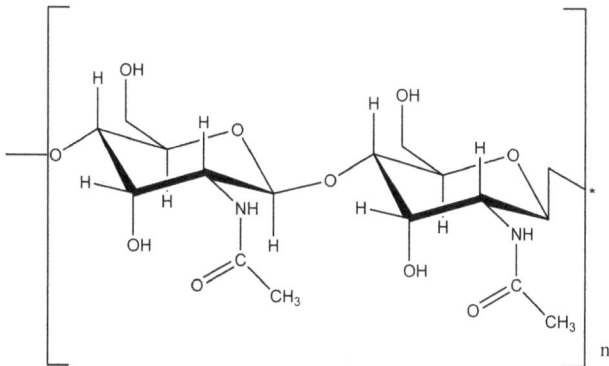

A

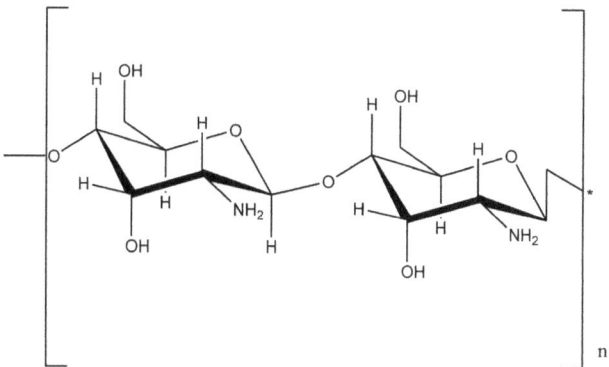

B

FIGURES 2.2 (A) Chitin (*N*-acetylglucosamine) and (B) Chitosan (D-glucosamine).

Chitosan, a biological cationic polysaccharide, can be synthesized by deacetylation of chitin. CS is one of the most abundant and distributed polybiomaterials derived from naturally occurring chitin that is commonly present in the exoskeletons of arthropods, insects, crustacean shells, and fungal cell walls (Wang et al., 2015). NAG [N-acetylglucosamine (GlcNAc)] and D-glucosamine (GlcN) make linkage of β(1→4)-linked glycosidic bond and form CS (Woraphatphadung et al., 2018). Enzymes such as lysozymes and chitosanases can break to CS bond into two monosaccharides, which can be frequently absorbed by the body (Kean and Thanou, 2010). CS is biodegradable, biocompatible, bioactive, and nontoxic biomaterial (Sahu et al., 2017). Nanogels/nanobiomaterials, having pH-sensitive properties that were prepared by using CS and coated with eucalyptus oil, are used in the controlled drug delivery (Belabassi et al., 2017), while PEGylated and fluorinated CS nanogels are used in the targeted drug delivery (Sun et al., 2017; Gupta et al., 2010). CS-based pH-sensitive polymeric micelles are used in the colon-targeted drug delivery (Kean and Thanou, 2010). Arginine-modified nanomaterial of CS is used in anticancer drug delivery (Sheikhi, 2019).

2.3.3 CELLULOSE

All green plants have structural scaffold of polysaccharide, mainly cellulose. Cellulose is found in wood (dry and living) and plant cell walls. Monomer of cellulose is D-glucose that is linked by $\beta(1\rightarrow4)$ glycosidic bonds with repeating unit of D-glucose (Figure 2.3). Different type of acid treatment produces various types of nanocellulose structures such as hairy cellulose nanofibril, CNF, bacterial CNF, and cellulose nanocrystals (CNC) (Pääkkö et al., 2007). Nanosized cellulose is used in the fabrication of hydrogels (Lin and Dufresne, 2014). Nanocelluloses in the form of nanoparticles, hydrogels, foams, electrospun fibers, nanomaterials, and polymer nanocomposite membranes have various biomedical applications including targeted drug delivery (Lee et al., 2014).

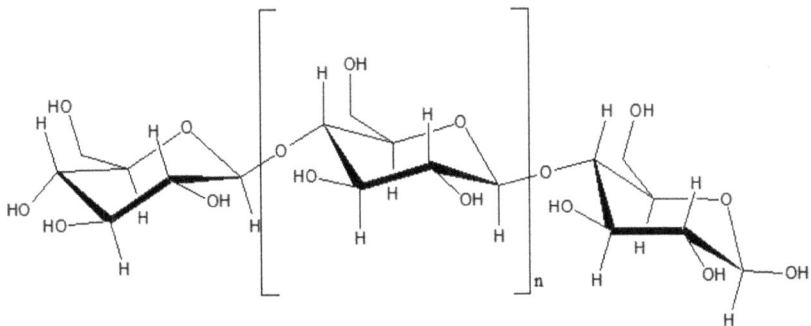

FIGURE 2.3   Cellulose repeating unit of glucose $\beta(1\rightarrow4)$ glycosidic bond.

Chemical and physical interactions between CNC, CNF or BC, and cellular matrix achieve prolonged and/or stimuli-responsive release of drugs and tissue regeneration (Herrera et al., 2016). Various types of carriers such as membranes, beads, aerogels, suspensions, hydrogels, and fibers have been developed using nanocellulose-polymer composites (Keservani et al., 2016). Nanocomposites of cellulose have tendency of swelling and shrinking uniformly, which enhance encapsulation capacity and release profile by physiochemical stimuli such as pH, ionic strength, and temperature (Kundu, 2014). The un-spoilt CNFs can use in wound healing, while oxidized CNF in the form of gels has applications in dressings for chronic wounds (Ferrari and Cappello, 1997).

2.3.4 SILK FIBROIN (SF)

Silk fibroin is a natural biopolymer produced by Bombycoidea family of insect, that is, silkworms. *Bombyx mori* (*B. mori*) is the main source of silk that is produced by the Bombycidae family (Inoue et al., 2007). Basic structure of SF consists of alanine (Ala) (35%), glycine (Gly) (38%), and serine (Ser) (12%) (Herrera et al., 2017) (Figure 2.4). SF is a heterodimeric protein with a heavy (H) chain (~325 kDa) and a light (L) chain (~25 kDa) connected at Cys-172 of the L-chain and Cys c-20 of the H-chain by forming (Mondal et al., 2007). Polar amino acids, particularly tyrosine, valine, and acidic amino acids, are also present in the SF chain (Vepari and Kaplan, 2007). Fibrous protein of SF has been used for the formation of films, 3D scaffolds, and microspheres because of its excellent biostability, biocompatibility, slow biodegradability, oxygen permeability, good mechanical properties, and minimal inflammatory and immunogenic response (Zuo et al., 2006; Numata and Kaplan, 2010; Nazarov et al., 2004).

Spider silk-based nanopolymers conjugate with DNA-binding poly-L-lysine. Plasmid DNA (pDNA) encoded with green fluorescent protein assembles into pDNA complexes with nanopolymer of silk via ionic interactions and has the highest transfection efficiency (Zhao et al., 2013).

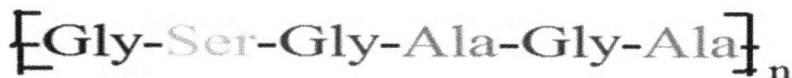

$$\left[\text{Gly-Ser-Gly-Ala-Gly-Ala}\right]_n$$

FIGURE 2.4 Sequence of amino acids present in silk fibroin.

2.3.5 GELATIN

Gelatin (or gelatine, from Latin: gelatus = stiff, frozen) is a naturally versatile biopolymer, colorless, flavorless, solid substance, brittle (when dry), and derived from irreversible denaturation of collagen (Figure 2.5). Acidic or alkaline treatment of cellulose not only gives gelatin but also thermal or enzymatic degradation of the collagen. It is commonly used in pharmaceuticals, gelling agent in food, and cosmetic manufacturing.

The approximate amino acid compositions of gelatin is by weight are glycine (25%), proline (27.5%), hydroxyproline (16%), glutamic acid (12.1%), alanine (11.8%), arginine (9.1%), aspartic acid (5.6%), lysine (4.1%), leucine (3.2%), valine (2.5%), phenylalanine (2.0%), threonine (1.9%), isoleucine (1.4%), methionine (1.2%), histidine (0.8%), tyrosine (0.5%), serine (0.4%), and cysteine (0.1%) (Digenis et al., 1994). These percentage values may vary, depending on the source of the raw material obtained and processing technique (Singh and Mishra, 2014). A and B are two types of gelatins, with different isoelectric points (IEPs). Type A is formed by acid and type B is formed by base hydrolysis of collagen, resulting in a difference in IEPs, being 7–9 for gelatin type A and 4–5 for gelatin type B (Jahanshahi et al., 2008).

In terms of nanopharmaceutics, gelatin is considered as important biodegradable base biomaterial in the last two decades of nanocarrier development because gelatin has low immunogenicity for many years and can be administered intravenously since it is an ingredient of various registered blood substitutes (Marty et al., 1978).

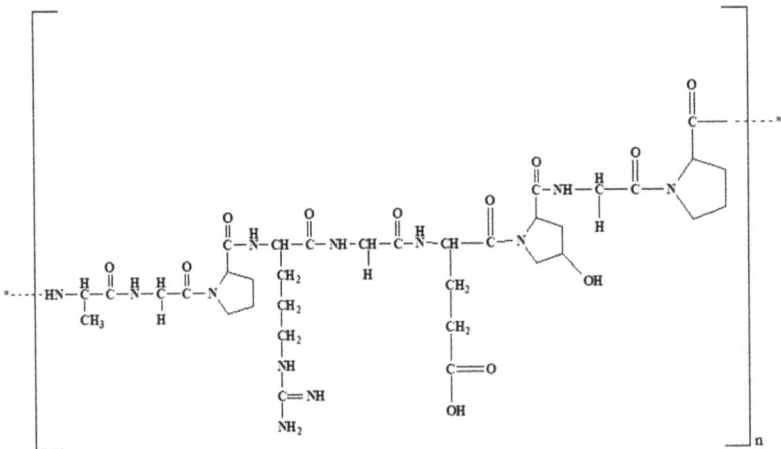

FIGURE 2.5   General component of gelatin (Ala-Gly-Pro-Arg-Gly-Glu-4Hyp-Gly-Pro).

2.3.6 *CHONDROITIN SULFATE*

Chondroitin sulfate is one of the ECM components and well-known GAGs (Figure 2.6). It is biologically active biomaterial and has properties such as antithrombogenic, anti-inflammatory (Gustafson, 1997), and anti-coagulant activity (Mourão et al., 1996). Chondroitin sulfate stabilizes gold nanoparticles and provides greater stability and biocompatibility to synthesized nanoparticles (Ghosh et al., 2014). Combination of chondroitin sulfate and poly(L-lactide) (PLLA) forms amphiphilic copolymeric micelle used for drug delivery applications (Li et al., 2011). Recently, polyvinyl alcohol (PVA)-chondroitin sulfate hybrid nanofibers loaded with combretastatin A4 phosphate were developed as a drug delivery formulation (Guo et al., 2016).

Chondroitin sulfate A (CSA) of glycosaminoglycan placental CSA (plCSA) is expressed on cancer cells and VAR2CSA is a malarial protein bind to plCSA. Placental chondroitin sulfate A binding peptide (plCSA-BP) specifically binds to plCSA on cancer cells. Hence, the nanoparticles are based on plCSA-BP-conjugate loaded with doxorubicin and studied on placental choriocarcinoma (JEG3) cells (Finkenstadt, 2005).

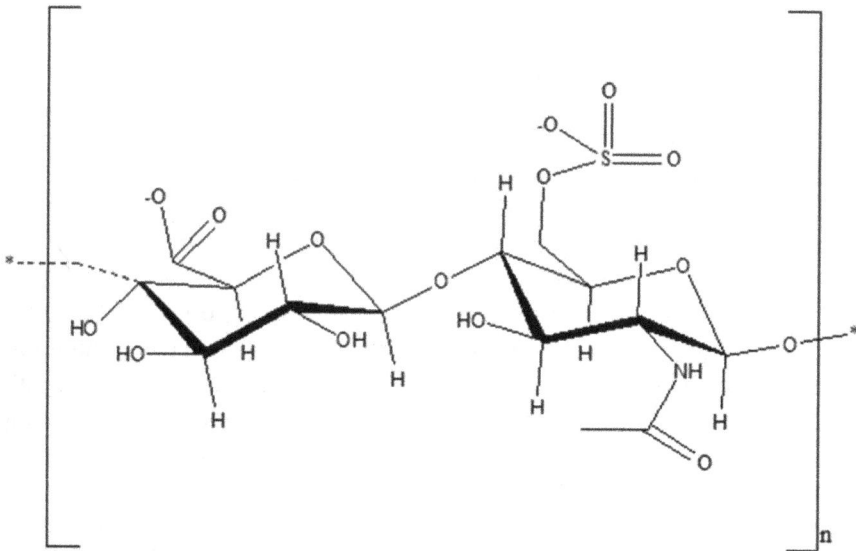

FIGURE 2.6   Chondroitin sulfate—monomeric unit.

2.4   SYNTHETIC BIOPOLYMERIC MATERIALS

Synthetic (chemically synthesized) or artificial polymers are man-made polymers. Various types of man-made biopolymers are present with different functional group's side chains and main chains. Synthetic polybiomaterials have potential to improve the quality of life; therefore, it has great importance in the medical field (Wnek, 2004). Biochemists are now capable of synthesizing number of synthetic biopolymers. Synthetic polymers offer several advantages over their natural counterparts, including improved chemical resistance, mechanical durability, and tunability of their properties. Biodegradable materials which have hydrophilic and nonhydrolytic properties such as polyethylene glycol (PEG), PVA, and polyacrylamide (PAM), amphiphilic block polymers such as PEG-*b*-PPG-*b*-PEG, hydrophobic polymers such as poly(*n*-butyl acrylate) as well as biomaterials which are hydrophobically and hydrolytically susceptible such as poly(α-esters), and thermally sensitive polymers such as PNIPAM have also been widely used as biomaterials (Fields et al., 2012).

2.4.1 POLY(ETHYLENE-CO-VINYL ACETATE)

Poly(ethylene-*co*-vinyl acetate) (PEVA) can be prepared using semicrystalline polyethylene (PE) and polyvinyl acetate (PVA) (Figure 2.7). PEVA is a good biodegradable, biostable, and biocompatible synthetically derived polymer and has been used in biomedical applications such as tissue engineering, drug delivery, sustained-release, etc. PEVA has organized arrangements of linear PE chains and is crystalline in nature. PEVAs can be cross-linked by cross-linker such as peroxide or by the exposure of high-energy ray such as electron beam or γ-ray (Wang and Deng, 2019). Composite materials of PEVA can be prepared using different compositions such as composite material of PEVA-chitosan, PEVA-aluminum hydroxide, PEVA-cellulose, PEVA-HA, PEVA-clay, etc. (Marty et al., 1978). PEVA–chitosan nanocomposite materials can be fabricated by using chitosan aqueous solution with 2% v/v of acetic acid and PEVA composite (Varshosaz and Moazen, 2014).

Ethylene vinyl acetate polymer (PEVA) has been used to prepare various medical appliances such as catheters, intravitreal devices, artificial organs, mouthguards etc. Chlorhexidine hexametaphosphate-PEVA nanocomposites has been inhibit the growth of methicillin-resistant *Staphylococcus aureus* (Varshosaz et al., 2014). PEVA blended with polyvinyl acetate polymer loaded with drugs such as paracetamol has an excellent stability and controlled release of oral administrated drugs (Wood et al., 2014). Mucoadhesion property of lectin-modified PEVA nanocomposites with mucin has been studied by *in vitro* analysis. The results illustrate the potential utility of lectin-modified PEVA nanocomposites for oral delivery of poorly water-soluble drugs with high first-pass metabolism. However, further *in vivo* pharmacokinetic and toxicity studies of these biomaterials were performed (Domb et al., 1994).

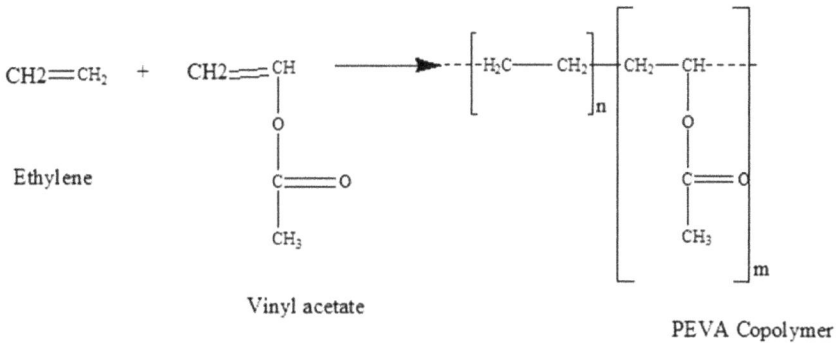

FIGURE 2.7   Formation of poly(ethylene-*co*-vinyl acetate) (PEVA).

2.4.2 POLYANHYDRIDES

Polyanhydrides, rediscovered in detail by Hill and Carothers in 1932, is a copolymer of methyl-vinyl and maleic anhydride and links by anhydride linkage (Figure 2.8). High-molecular weight polyanhydrides have been synthesized (Laurencin et al., 1990) and it possessed an excellent *in vivo* biocompatibility that was found to noncytotoxic and nonmutagenic (Tan et al., 2012). Polyanhydrides are one of the most considered biodegradable polymers and polyanhydride shows physicochemical properties such as hydrophilicity and crystallinity that affect the immune responses (Katti and Laurencin, 2003).

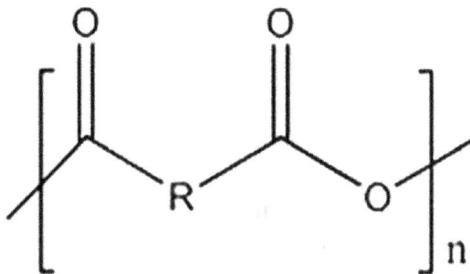

FIGURE 2.8   General structure of polyanhydride.

The most recent applications for polyanhydrides are the drug delivery and tissue engineering (Mathiowitz et al., 1988). Drug-loaded devices can be prepared by compression molding and microencapsulation (Tang et al., 2014). Nanocarrier of polyanhydride and sebacic acid, that is, polysebasic anhydride has been loaded with salbutamol and releases more constantly with 95% of total amount within 6–10 h (Santoro and Perale, 2012). Poly(anhydride-*co*-imides) matrices have strengths similar to human bone that showed excellent osteocompatibility. The poly(anhydride-*co*-imides) polymer matrices support endosteal and cortical bone regeneration and show minimal inflammation with dense fibrosis (Jae, 2012).

2.4.3 POLY(LACTIC-CO-GLYCOLIC ACID) (PLGA)

Copolymers of PLA and PGA, that is, PLGA, are biodegradable and widely used synthetic polymeric biomaterial in medical field (Figure 2.9A and B) (Astete and Sabliov, 2006). PLGA is crystalline in nature and is biocompatible and able to degrade into nontoxic byproducts. Biopolymer of PLGA is effectively used as nanocarrier of medicine and in tissue engineering because it hydrolyzes in the body and produces lactic acid and glycolic acid monomers and easily metabolized in the body via the citric acid cycle (Rezwan et al., 2006). Combination of PLGA copolymer and ceramics such as HA bioglass stimulates bone tissue regeneration and provides great mechanical strength. Composite of PLGA and bioglass shows angiogenic activity used in vascular supply implant (Day et al., 2005).

Polymeric composite of PLGA has been used in the encapsulation of plasmid DNA encoded with siRNA sequence and delivered to methyl-CpG-binding domain protein 1 (MBD1) that showed growth inhibition of cells and apoptotic activity (Hans and Lowman, 2002). Nanomaterials of PLGA are used as immunological adjuvants via nasal route as a safe mode of vaccination (Andersen et al., 2010).

2.4.4 POLYURETHANE

Polyurethanes have repeating unit of urethane moiety (Figure 2.10). Polyurethanes are most medically used synthetic biomaterials comprising medical appliance such as artificial organs, heart valves, wound dressing, catheters, etc. (Infection Control Symposium: Influence of Medical Device Design, US Department of Health and Human Services, Bethesda MD,

January 1995). Polyurethanes have properties such as abrasion resistance, high strength at lower temperature, and fungal resistance (Rajan et al., 2017). Polyurethanes are an important family of synthetic biomaterials in medical field and have excellent biocompatibility. Nonbiodegradable polyurethanes are used in the implantation of artificial pacemaker and breast (Santerre et al., 2005). Biodegradable polyurethanes can be synthesized using diisocyanate compounds such as hexamethylene diisocyanate, which releases nontoxic products such as lysine. Fluoroquinolone, an antimicrobial drug, was incorporated into the polyurethane that releases the drug when degraded by enzymes generated by an inflammatory response known as smart polymer system (Woo et al., 2000).

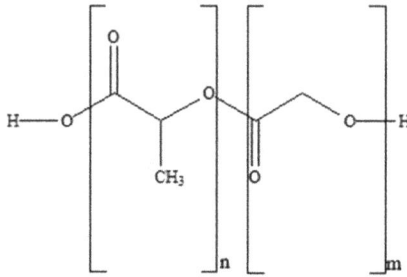

(A)

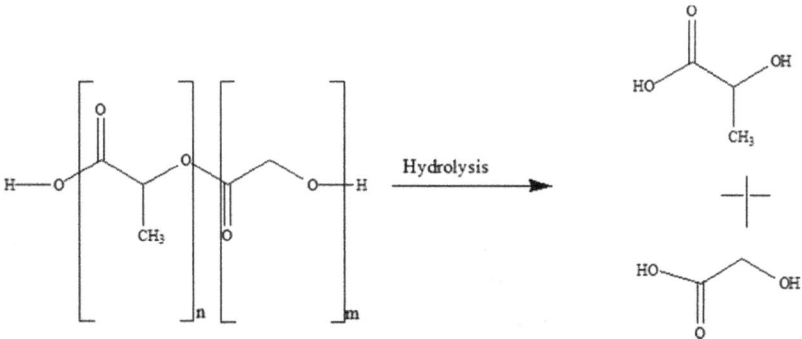

(B)

FIGURES 2.9 (A) Poly(lactic-*co*-glycolic acid) (PLGA) and (B) Hydrolysis of PLGA into lactic acid and glycolic acid.

Segmented polyurethanes are developed with defined degradation and mechanical and chemical properties combined with excellent biocompatibility that can be used in drug delivery, tissue engineering, and medical appliances (Shelke et al., 2014). Encapsulation of antibiotics without molecular modification has been done on biomaterials of polyurethanes and they showed full antimicrobial activity and polyurethanes act as controlled and sustained drug delivery materials (Khambete et al., 2016). Modified polyurethane film can be used as targeted and efficient gene delivery systems (Phaneuf et al., 2001). Polyurethanes are the top biomaterials in the fabrication of all kinds of biomedical devices for cardiovascular applications such as heart valves, catheters, cardiac assist devices, pacemaker leads insulation, vascular prostheses, etc. (Vermette et al., 2001). Due to good oxygen permeability and barrier properties, polyurethanes are used in wound dressing (Wang and Wang, 2012).

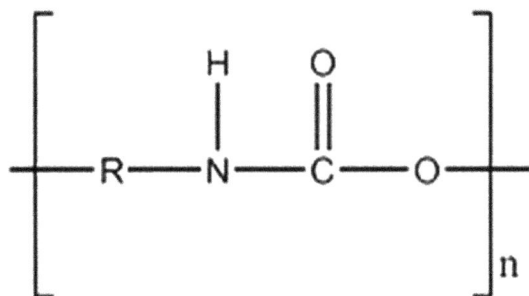

FIGURE 2.10   General structure of polyurethane.

2.5   SMART POLYMERIC BIOMATERIALS

Soft polymeric biomaterials with good mechanical strength and unique properties like human body tissues are called "smart polymeric biomaterials." Self-assembly of protein and natural and synthetic polymers and micro- and nanofabrication technologies have led to the development of advanced or next-generation biomaterials, that is, smart biomaterials (Kaushik et al., 2019). Smart polymers, also known as stimulus-responsive materials, act in controlled manner and can respond to chemical, biological, and physical cues such as enzyme sensitive, temperature, pH, stress, humidity, light, etc. (Aguilar and San Román, 2019; Fenton et al., 2018). Smart polymeric biomaterials may be developed as multifunctional materials to achieve desired biological function with minimum negative response. Some smart biomaterials show unique properties such as shape-memory or self-healing behavior.

Smart polymeric biomaterials are most frequently used in the biomedical field. Smart polymeric biomaterials such as hydrogels are, or may be, pH sensitive with swelling–deswelling and can act as artificial muscles (Figure 2.11). Temperature-responsive polymers such as PNIPAM hydrogels are the recent smart polymeric biomaterial (Holzapfel et al., 2013; Dong and Hoffman, 1987). pNIPAM can be stimulated by temperature, enzymatic sensitivity, pH, humidity, light, magnetic fields, mechanical forces, and ionic strength. PNIPAM has been used in thermoregulated biotin binding and release (Wei et al., 2017), antibiotic, and/or insulin delivery via ultrasound (Ding et al., 1999). For medical application and tissue engineering, biomaterial should possess cell and tissue compatibility, nontoxic, biologically degradable, and biologically stable (James et al., 2014). Smart polymeric scaffolds have been developed with the incorporation of biologically active molecules and nanoparticles. Smart scaffolds can be developed by natural or synthetic biomaterials or by combination of both and can be incorporated in bone progenitor cells (Kowalski et al., 2018; Motamedian et al., 2015).

Designing of smart biopolymeric materials with desired properties and physical and chemical structure depends on ratio of components and nature of functional groups in monomeric forms. Smart 3D structure/scaffold for tissue engineering can be developed by incorporation of proteins and/or peptides. For example, genetically engineered type II collagen has been used for 3D fabrication to reduce migration and proliferation of chondrocytes and artificial cartilage formation (Kaigler et al., 2006; Anderson et al., 2004). Thermosensitive nanoparticles of polyurethanes with different compositions have been reported. Degree of crystallization and strength of hydrogen bond in segment composition of polyurethane nanoparticle provide smartness in morphological and rheological behavior and can be used as cell delivery vehicles (Ito et al., 2006; Ou et al., 2014).

Smart biomaterials with stimuli responsive have been fabricated that can enable minimally invasive drug delivery and monitoring (Hsieh et al., 2015). Smart hydrogel drug delivery systems have been developed with predictable and tunable degradation and rate of drug release (Gu, 2016). Highly porous hydrogels of bacterial cellulose-g-poly(acrylic acid-*co*-acrylamide) with pH sensitivity have been developed for parental route drug delivery carrier (Ashley et al., 2013).

Nanocomposite of butyl methacrylate, 2-propylacrylic acid (PAA), and 2-(dimethylamino)ethyl methacrylate have been synthesized with pH-responsive behavior (Mohd Amin et al., 2014). Lower critical solution temperatures (LCSTs) are a biologically relevant range and depend on type of polymers used. Smart biomaterials fall within this range and for different composition of biomaterial it may be different. Hydrogels/biomaterials such as poly[oligo(ethylene glycol)methyl ether methacrylate] (POEGMA) (Horev et al., 2015), PNIPAM, pluronics [PEG-poly(propylene oxide) copolymers], etc., fall in the LCSTs (Bakaic et al., 2015; Ko et al., 2018). Naturally derived biopolymers show LCSTs behavior after modification such as methylcellulose, galactose-modified xyloglucan, hydroxybutyl CS, and CS-β-glycerophosphate blends (Spicer, 2020).

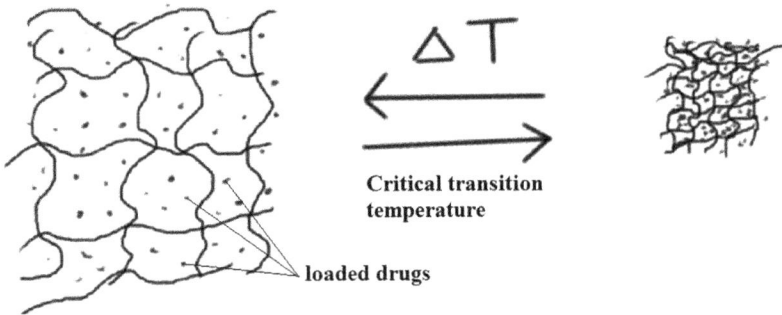

FIGURE 2.11 Hydrogels/smart polymer showing swelling and deswelling behavior at critical transition temperature.

2.5.1 ENZYME-RESPONSIVE SMART BIOPOLYMER

Enzyme responsiveness in the smart biomaterials is associated with the increasing interest to use naturally evolved process as inspiration for synthetic biomaterials. Enzymes induce macro- and/or microscopic change in the chemical and physical properties of biomaterials. Enzymes have advantage of selectivity and specificity for their smart biomaterials. These inherent biocompatibilities of enzymes make enzyme-responsive biomaterials suitable for development of smart biomaterials for medical applications (Zelzer et al.; Ulijn, 2013). Interactions between enzyme-responsive biomaterials and enzymes are very different from enzymatic reactions of the enzymes and substrates. Enzyme-responsive biomaterials are able to operate under conditions that maintain particular enzymatic activity.

Various synthetic biomaterials such as polymer or metal particles have been developed as enzyme-responsive biomaterials; for example, dextran (Itoh et al., 2006), amylase (Chambin et al., 2006) PEG (Lutolf et al., 2003), and silica and gold (Laromaine et al., 2007; Patel et al., 2008) nanoparticles.

2.5.2 pH-RESPONSIVE SMART BIOMATERIALS

pH-sensitive smart biopolymers are polymer of electrolyte that bear weak acidic or basic groups that either gives or takes protons in response to change in surrounding pH. Weakly acidic (anionic) groups in pH-sensitive polymers increase the swelling of biomaterials as the external pH increases but swelling decreases if polymer contains weakly basic groups. pH-sensitive biomaterials may be in variety of forms such as nanoparticles, hydrogels, 3D porous structures, and beads (Li et al., 2014; Tekade et al., 2015; Aycan and Alemdar, 2018; Li et al., 2017; Majumdar et al., 2016). Examples of pH-sensitive smart polymers are polymethacrylic acid, polyethyleneimine, poly(N,N-dimethyl-aminoethyl methacrylamide), poly(N,N-dialkyl aminoethyl methacrylates), and CS (Ouyang et al., 2018; Hester et al., 2002).

2.5.3 THERMORESPONSIVE SMART BIOPOLYMERS

The polymeric biomaterials are responsive or sensitive to change in temperature. These are most used and safest biomaterials in drug administration systems. Thermosensitive biomaterials have very sensitive balance between the hydrophilic and hydrophobic groups and can create new adjustment of structure with small change in temperature (Park and Bae, 1999) and have unique property of sol–gel transition above certain temperature. Some polymeric biomaterials show phase transition near the physiological temperature of human body. On the basis of response of polymer to change in temperature, polymers are categorized in two classes; first, upper critical solution temperature (UCST)—polymers which precipitate and undergo phase change below a critical temperature and second, LCST—polymers which become insoluble above a critical temperature (Bajpai et al., 2008). UCST-type polymer solutions are heterogeneously cloudy and opaque below the UCST, "positive temperature-sensitive polymers," i.e., polyacrylic acid (PAA), PAM, and poly(acrylamide-*co*-butyl methacrylate), while LCST-type polymer solutions are homogeneously clear and transparent below the LCST, "negative temperature-sensitive polymers," that is, PNIPAM (Teotia et al., 2015; Aoki et al., 1999). UCSTs of interpenetrating networks (IPNs) of PAM and PAA are at 25 °C. Poly(allylurea-*co*-allylamine) (PU-Am)-based polymers have 8–65 °C UCST (Glatzel et al., 2011; Owens et al., 2007). LCST of PNIPAM is at 32 °C in aqueous media; below the LSCT, it shows extended, swelling chain conformation and above the LCST, it shows shrinking behavior (Chu et al., 2005). Many other polymers have been synthesized, which show thermoresponsive behavior and used in the drug delivery application.

2.6 CONCLUSION AND FUTURE IN BIOMATERIALS

More functional medical materials will develop with advancement in biomaterials; thus, the use in new fields of application of biomaterials can expand. Understanding of biomaterials and complex dynamic behaviors may be accomplished in nature, which shall lead to the fabrication and design of novel biomaterials that can mimic nature not through presenting active motifs replicated exactly from biological molecule but rather by propagating the functional behaviors of these biomaterials to obtain the new properties with more medical application that are currently unavailable (Ratner, 2004). For example, molecular tempering application of viruses to optoelectronic device fabrication (Nam et al., 2006). Smart multifunctional nanoparticles will develop on the focus of next-generation biomaterials research. Such materials would target the desired anatomical regions for delivery, monitor health, etc. Fertile environment can flourish the future of biomaterial. History of medical sciences has shown that development of new materials was connected to visionary humans who were willing to take risks for advancement.

Biomaterials have a bright history and it shows continuous development and advancement in the biomaterials from natural to synthetic and natural–synthetic composite biomaterials. In next-generation biomaterials, various polymers with different functional groups and various medical applications shall be developed. In the present, stimuli-responsive biomaterials, known as "smart biomaterial," have been developed with new advancements. Smart polymers are used as controlled and targeted drug delivery and other field of medical applications. Smart bipolymers response with specific stimuli at special conditions such as pH, temperature, light, magnetic effect, enzymes, etc. However, tremendous research work and opportunities remain to be explored to find new biomaterials with more advancement and biocompatible.

ACKNOWLEDGEMENT

Authors thanks to Ministry of Education Government of India and Indian Institute of Information Technology for providing fund and lab space to carrying out the research work.

KEYWORDS

- **smart polymer**
- **biomaterial**
- **tissue engineering**
- **synthetic biomaterial**
- **natural biomaterial**

REFERENCES

Aguilar, M. R. and San Román, J. Introduction to smart polymers and their applications. *Smart Polymers and Their Applications*. Woodhead Publishing, **2019**, pp. 1–11.

Andersen, M. Ø., Lichawska, A., Arpanaei, A., Jensen, S. M. R., Kaur, H., Oupicky, D. et al. A. surface functionalisation of PLGA nanoparticles for gene silencing. *Biomaterials*. **2010,** 31(21): 5671–5677.

Anderson, D. G., Burdick, J. A. and Langer, R. Smart biomaterials. *Science*. **2004,** 305(5692): 1923–1924.

Anderson, J. M., Rodriguez, A. and Chang, D. T. Foreign body reaction to biomaterials. *Semin Immunol*. **2008,** 20: 86–100.

Aoki, T., Nakamura, K., Sanui, K., Kikuchi, A., Okano, T., Sakurai, Y. et al. Adenosine-induced changes of the phase transition of poly(6-(acryloyloxymethyl) uracil) aqueous solution. *Polym J*. **1999,** 31(11): 1185–1188.

Ashley, G. W., Henise, J., Reid, R. and Santi, D. V. Hydrogel drug delivery system with predictable and tunable drug release and degradation rates. *Proc Natl Acad Sci U S A*. **2013,** 110(6): 2318–2323.

Astete, C. E. and Sabliov, C. M. Synthesis and characterization of PLGA nanoparticles. *J Biomater Sci Polym Ed*. **2006,** 17(3): 247–289.

Aycan, D. and Alemdar, N. Development of pH-responsive chitosan-based hydrogel modified with bone ash for controlled release of amoxicillin. *Carb Polym*. **2018,** 184: 401–407.

Azuma, K., Izumi, R., Osaki, T., Ifuku, S., Morimoto, M., Saimoto, H. et al. Chitin, chitosan, and its derivatives for wound healing: old and new materials. *J Funct Biomater*. **2015,** 6(1): 104–142.

Badeau, B. A., Comerford, M. P., Arakawa, C. K., Shadish, J. A. and DeForest, C. A. Engineered modular biomaterial logic gates for environmentally triggered therapeutic delivery. *Nat Chem*. **2018,** 10(3): 251.

Bajpai, A. K., Shukla, S. K., Bhanu, S. and Kankane, S. Responsive polymers in controlled drug delivery. *Prog Polym Sci*. **2008,** 33(11): 1088–1118.

Bakaic, E., Smeets, N. M., Dorrington, H. and Hoare, T. "Off-the-shelf" thermoresponsive hydrogel design: tuning hydrogel properties by mixing precursor polymers with different lower-critical solution temperatures. *RSC Adv*. **2015,** 5(42): 33364–33376.

Belabassi, Y., Moreau, J., Gheran, V., Henoumont, C., Robert, A., Callewaert, M. et al. Synthesis and characterization of PEGylated and fluorinated chitosans: application to the synthesis of targeted nanoparticles for drug delivery. *Biomacromolecules*. **2017,** 18(9): 2756–2766.

Bobbio, A. M. A. D. E. O. The first endosseous alloplastic implant in the history of man. *Bull Hist Dent*. **1972**, 20(1): 1.

Chambin, O., Dupuis, G., Champion, D., Voilley, A. and Pourcelot, Y. Colon-specific drug delivery: influence of solution reticulation properties upon pectin beads performance. *Int J Pharm*. **2006**, 321(1–2): 86–93.

Chu, L. Y., Li, Y., Zhu, J. H. and Chen, W. M. Negatively thermoresponsive membranes with functional gates driven by zipper-type hydrogen-bonding interactions. *Angew Chem Int Ed Engl*. **2005**, 44(14): 2124–2127.

Clark, R. A. (Ed.). *The Molecular and Cellular Biology of Wound Repair*. Springer Science and Business Media, **2013**.

Critchley, L. A., Yang, X. X. and Lee, A. Assessment of trending ability of cardiac output monitors by polar plot methodology. *J Cardiothorac Vasc Anesth*. **2011**, 25(3): 536–546.

Crubzy, E., Murail, P., Girard, L. and Bernadou, J. P. False teeth of the Roman world. *Nature*. **1998**, 391(6662): 29–29.

Day, R. M., Maquet, V., Boccaccini, A. R., Jérôme, R. and Forbes, A. *In vitro* and *in vivo* analysis of macroporous biodegradable poly(D,L-lactide-co-glycolide) scaffolds containing bioactive glass. *J Biomed Mater Res A*. **2005**, 75(4): 778–787.

Dhert, W. J. Retrieval studies on calcium phosphate-coated implants. *Med Prog Technol*. **1994**, 20(3–4): 143–154.

Digenis, G. A., Gold, T. B. and Shah, V. P. Cross-linking of gelatin capsules and its relevance to their *in vitro-in vivo* performance. *J Pharm Sci*. **1994**, 83(7): 915–921.

Ding, Z., Long, C. J., Hayashi, Y., Bulmus, E. V., Hoffman, A. S. and Stayton, P. S. Temperature control of biotin binding and release with a streptavidin-poly(N-isopropylacrylamide) site-specific conjugate. *Bioconjug Chem*. **1999**, 10(3): 395–400.

Domb, A.J., Amselem, S., Langer, R. and Maniar, M. Polyanhydrides as carriers of drugs. *Biomedical Polymers Designed to Degrade Systems*. New York: Hanser, **1994**, p. 69.

Dong, L. C. and Hoffman, A. S. Thermally reversible hydrogels: Swelling characteristics and activities of co-poly(*N*-isopropylacrylamide-acrylamide) gels containing immobilized. *ACS Symp Series*. **1987**, Vol. 350.

Fenton, O. S., Olafson, K. N., Pillai, P. S., Mitchell, M. J. and Langer, R. Advances in biomaterials for drug delivery. *Adv Mater*. **2018**, 30(29): 1705328.

Ferrari, F. A. and Cappello, J. *Protein-based Naterials*. Springer, 1997.

Fields, R. J., Cheng, C. J., Quijano, E., Weller, C., Kristofik, N., Duong, N. et al. Surface modified poly(β-aminoester)-containing nanoparticles for plasmid DNA delivery. *J Control Release*. **2012**, 164(1): 41–48.

Finkenstadt, V.L. Natural polysaccharides as electroactive polymers. *Appl Microbiol Biotechnol*. **2005**, 67(6): 735–745.

Fratzl, P. Biomimetic materials research: what can we really learn from nature's structural materials? *J R Soc Interface*. **2007**, 4(15): 637–642.

Freed, L. E., Guilak, F., Guo, X. E., Gray, M. L., Tranquillo, R., Holmes, J. W. et al. Advanced tools for tissue engineering: scaffolds, bioreactors, and signaling. *Tissue Eng*. **2006**, 12(12): 3285–3305.

Ghosh, S., Ucer, K. B., D'Agostino, R., Grant, K., Sirintrapun, J., Thomas, M. J. et al. Non-covalent assembly of meso-tetra-4-pyridyl porphine with single-stranded DNA to form nano-sized complexes with hydrophobicity-dependent DNA release and anti-tumor activity. *Biol Med*. **2014**, 10(2): 451–461.

Glatzel, S., Laschewsky, A. and Lutz, J. F. Well-defined uncharged polymers with a sharp UCST in water and in physiological milieu. *Macromolecules*. **2011,** 44(2): 413–415.

Gu, Z. Introduction to special issue on "Responsive Materials and Systems: Toward Smart and Precision Medications." *Bioeng Transl Med*. **2016,** 1(3): 235.

Guo, J., Zhou, H., Akram, M. Y., Mu, X., Nie, J. and Ma, G. Characterization and application of chondroitin sulfate/polyvinyl alcohol nanofibres prepared by electrospinning. *Carb Polym*. **2016,** 143: 239–245.

Gupta, S., Yadav, B.S., Kesharwani, R., Mishra, K.P. and Singh, N.K. The role of nanodrugs for targeted drug delivery in cancer treatment. *Arch Appl Sci Res*. **2010,** 2(1): 37–51.

Gustafson, S. The influence of sulfated polysaccharides on the circulating levels of hyaluronan. *Glycobiology*. **1997,** 7(8): 1209–1214.

Hans, M. L. and Lowman, A. M. Biodegradable nanoparticles for drug delivery and targeting. *Curr Opin Solid State Mater Sci*. **2002,** 6(4): 319–327.

Hastings, G., Ducheyne P. Eds. *Macromolecular Biomaterials*. Boca Raton, FL: CRC Press, **1984**.

Hench L. L. Wilson J, editors. *Clinical Performance of Skeletal Prostheses*. London: Chapman and Hall. **1996**.

Hench, L. L. Special report: the interfacial behavior of biomaterials, 1979. *J Biomed Mater Res*. **1980,** 14(6): 803–811.

Hench, L. L. An introduction to bioceramics (Vol. 1). **1993,** *World Scientific*.

Hench, L. L. and Thompson, I. Twenty-first century challenges for biomaterials. *J R Soc Interface*. **2010,** 7: S379–S391.

Hench, L. L., Polak, J. M., Xynos, I. D. and Buttery, L. D. K. Bioactive materials to control cell cycle. *Mater Res Innov*. **2000,** 3(6): 313–323.

Hench, L. L., Polak, J. M. Third-generation biomedical materials. *Science*. **2002,** 295(5557): 1014–1017.

Herrera, M. A., Mathew, A. P. and Oksman, K. Barrier and mechanical properties of plasticized and cross-linked nanocellulose coatings for paper packaging applications. *Cellulose*. **2017,** 24(9): 3969–3980.

Hester, J. F., Olugebefola, S.C. and Mayes, A. M. Preparation of pH-responsive polymer membranes by self-organization. *J Membr Sci*. **2002,** 208(1–2): 375–388.

Hildebrand HF. Biomaterials—a history of 7000 years. *Bionanomaterials*. **2013,** 14(3–4): 119–33.

Holzapfel, B. M., Reichert, J. C., Schantz, J. T., Gbureck, U., Rackwitz, L., Nöth, U. et al. How smart do biomaterials need to be? A translational science and clinical point of view. *Adv Drug Deliv Rev*. **2013,** 65(4): 581–603.

Horev, B., Klein, M. I., Hwang, G., Li, Y., Kim, D., Koo, H. et al. pH-activated nanoparticles for controlled topical delivery of farnesol to disrupt oral biofilm virulence. *ACS Nano*. **2015,** 9(3): 2390–2404.

Hsieh, F. Y., Lin, H. H. and Hsu, S. H. 3D bioprinting of neural stem cell-laden thermo-responsive biodegradable polyurethane hydrogel and potential in central nervous system repair. *Biomaterials*. **2015,** 71: 48–57.

https://www.piedmonteye.com/history-contact-lenses/ (3/01/2020)

Huebsch, N. and Mooney, D. J. Inspiration and application in the evolution of biomaterials. *Nature*. **2009,** 462(7272): 426–432.

Ingber, D. E. From cellular mechanotransduction to biologically inspired engineering. *Ann Biomed Eng*. **2010,** 38(3): 1148–1161.

Inoue, S., Tanaka, K., Arisaka, F., Kimura, S., Ohtomo, K. and Mizuno, S. Silk fibroin of Bombyx mori is secreted, assembling a high molecular mass elementary unit consisting of H-chain, L-chain, and P25, with a 6: 6: 1 molar ratio. *J Biol Chem.* **2000,** 275(51): 40517–40528.

Ito, H., Steplewski, A., Alabyeva, T. and Fertala, A. Testing the utility of rationally engineered recombinant collagen-like proteins for applications in tissue engineering. *J Biomed Mater Res Part A.* **2006,** 76(3): 551–560.

Itoh, Y., Matsusaki, M., Kida, T. and Akashi, M. Enzyme-responsive release of encapsulated proteins from biodegradable hollow capsules. *Biomacromolecules.* **2006,** 7(10): 2715–2718.

Jae, H. P. (2012). Hyaluronic acid-based nanoparticles: implications for drug delivery and molecular imaging. *2nd International Conference on Pharmaceutics and Novel Drug Delivery Systems*, 20–22 February 2012, San Francisco Airport Marriott Waterfront, USA Pharmaceutica Analytica Acta.

Jahanshahi, M., Sanati, M.H. and Babaei, Z. Optimization of parameters for the fabrication of gelatin nanoparticles by the Taguchi robust design method. *J Appl Stat.* **2008,** 35(12): 1345–1353.

James, H. P., John, R., Alex, A. and Anoop, K. R. Smart polymers for the controlled delivery of drugs—a concise overview. *Acta Pharm Sin B.* **2014,** 4(2): 120–127.

Jandt, K. D. Evolutions, revolutions and trends in biomaterials science—a perspective. *Adv Eng Mat.* **2007,** 9(12): 1035–1050.

Kaigler, D., Wang, Z., Horger, K., Mooney, D. J. and Krebsbach, P. H. VEGF scaffolds enhance angiogenesis and bone regeneration in irradiated osseous defects. *J Bone Miner Res.* **2006,** 21(5): 735–744.

Katti, D. S. and Laurencin, C. T. Synthetic biomedical polymers for tissue engineering and drug delivery. *Adv Polym Mat.* **2003,** 3(2): 479–525.

Kaushik, A., Mujawar, M. A. and Sharma, K. State-of-art functional biomaterials for tissue engineering. *Front Mat.* **2019,** 6: 172.

Kean, T. and Thanou, M. Biodegradation, biodistribution and toxicity of chitosan. *Adv Drug Del Rev.* **2010,** 62(1): 3–11.

Keservani, R. K. and Sharma, A. K. Nanobiomaterials involved in medical imaging technologies. *Nanobiomaterials in Medical Imaging,* William Andrew Publishing, **2016,** pp. 303–337.

Khambete, H., Keservani, R. K., Kesharwani, R. K., Jain, N. P. and Jain, C. P. Emerging trends of nanobiomaterials in hard tissue engineering. *Nanobiomaterials in Hard Tissue Engineering,* William Andrew Publishing. **2016,** pp. 63–101.

Khan, F. and Tanaka, M. Designing smart biomaterials for tissue engineering. *Int J Mol Sci.* **2018,** 19(1): 17.

Ko, D. Y., Patel, M., Lee, H. J. and Jeong, B. Coordinating thermogel for stem cell spheroids and their cytoeffectiveness. *Adv Funct Mat.* **2018,** 28(7): 1706286.

Konstantinov, I. E. At the cutting edge of the impossible: a tribute to Vladimir P. Demikhov. *Tex Heart J.* **2009,** 36(5): 453.

Kowalski, P. S., Bhattacharya, C., Afewerki, S. and Langer, R. Smart biomaterials: recent advances and future directions. *ACS Biomater Sci Eng.* **2018,** 4(11): 3809–3817.

Kozlowski, R. M. (Ed.). *Handbook of Natural Fibres: Volume 2: Processing and Applications.* Elsevier, **2012.**

Kukreja, N., Onuma, Y., Daemen, J. and Serruys, P. W. The future of drug-eluting stents. *Pharmacol Res Commun.* **2008,** 57(3): 171–180.

Kundu, S., Editor. *Silk Biomaterials for Tissue Engineering and Regenerative Medicine.* Elsevier, **2014**.

Laromaine, A., Koh, L., Murugesan, M., Ulijn, R. V. and Stevens, M. M. Protease-triggered dispersion of nanoparticle assemblies. *J Am Chem Soc.* **2007**, 129(14): 4156–4157.

Laurencin, C., Domb, A., Morris, C., Brown, V., Chasin, M., McConnell, R. et al. Poly(anhydride) administration in high doses *in vivo*: studies of biocompatibility and toxicology. *J Biomed Mater Res.* **1990**, 24(11): 1463–1481.

Lee, K. Y., Aitomäki, Y., Berglund, L. A., Oksman, K. and Bismarck, A. On the use of nanocellulose as reinforcement in polymer matrix composites. *Compos Sci Technol.* **2014**, 105: 15–27.

Li, S., Hu, K., Cao, W., Sun, Y., Sheng, W., Li, F. et al. pH-responsive biocompatible fluorescent polymer nanoparticles based on phenylboronic acid for intracellular imaging and drug delivery. *Nanoscale.* **2014**, 6(22): 13701–13709.

Li, W., Li, X., Su, H., Zhao, S., Li, Y. and Hu, J. Facile synthesis of chondroitin sulfate-stabilized gold nanoparticles. *Mat Chem Phy.* **2011**, 125(3): 518–521.

Li, X., Fu, M., Wu, J., Zhang, C., Deng, X., Dhinakar, A. et al. pH-sensitive peptide hydrogel for glucose-responsive insulin delivery. *Acta Biomater.* **2017**, 51: 294–303.

Lin, N. and Dufresne, A. Nanocellulose in biomedicine: Current status and future prospect. *Eur Poly J.* **2014**, 59: 302–325.

Lutolf, M. P., Lauer-Fields, J. L., Schmoekel, H. G., Metters, A.T., Weber, F. E., Fields, G. B. et al. Synthetic matrix metalloproteinase-sensitive hydrogels for the conduction of tissue regeneration: engineering cell-invasion characteristics. *Proc Natl Acad Sci.* **2003**, 100(9): 5413–5418.

Majumdar, S., Krishnatreya, G., Gogoi, N., Thakur, D. and Chowdhury, D. Carbon-dot-coated alginate beads as a smart stimuli-responsive drug delivery system. *ACS Appl Mater Int.* **2016**, 8(50): 34179–34184.

Marty, J. J., Oppenheim, R.C., Speiser, P. Nanoparticles—a new colloidal drug delivery system. *Pharm Acta Helv* **1978**, 53(1): 17–23.

Mathiowitz, E., Saltzman, W. M., Domb, A., Dor, P., and Langer, R. Polyanhydride microspheres as drug carriers. II. Microencapsulation by solvent removal. *J Appl Polym Sci.* **1988**, 35(3): 755–774.

Mikos, A. G., Herring, S. W., Ochareon, P., Elisseeff, J., Lu, H. H., Kandel, R. et al. *Tissue Eng.* **2006**, 12: 3307–3339.

Mohd Amin, M. C. I., Ahmad, N., Pandey, M. and Xin, C. J. Stimuli-responsive bacterial cellulose-g-poly(acrylic acid-co-acrylamide) hydrogels for oral controlled release drug delivery. *Drug Dev Ind Pharm.* **2014**, 40(10): 1340–1349.

Mondal, M., Trivedy, K. and Nirmal, K. S. The silk proteins, sericin and fibroin in silkworm, *Bombyx mori Linn*—a review. Caspian J. Env. Sci. **2007**, 5, 63–76.

Motamedian, S. R., Hosseinpour, S., Ahsaie, M. G. and Khojasteh, A. Smart scaffolds in bone tissue engineering: a systematic review of literature. *World J Stem Cells.* **2015**, 7(3): 657.

Motiei, M., Kashanian, S., Lucia, L. A., and Khazaei, M. Intrinsic parameters for the synthesis and tuned properties of amphiphilic chitosan drug delivery nanocarriers. *J Control Release.* **2017**, 260: 213–225.

Mourão, P. A., Pereira, M. S., Pavão, M. S., Mulloy, B., Tollefsen, D. M., Mowinckel, M. C. et al. Structure and anticoagulant activity of a fucosylated chondroitin sulfate from echinoderm sulfated fucose branches on the polysaccharide account for its high anticoagulant action. *J Biol Chem.* **1996**, 271(39): 23973–23984.

Nakanishi, K. A brief history of natural products chemistry. In *Comprehensive Natural Products Chemistry* (D. Barton, O. Meth-Cohn, editors), Newnes **1999**, pp. 21–48.

Nam, K. T., Kim, D. W., Yoo, P. J., Chiang, C. Y., Meethong, N., Hammond, P. T. et al. Virus-enabled synthesis and assembly of nanowires for lithium ion battery electrodes. *Science.* **2006,** 312(5775): 885–888.

Narayan, R. J. The next generation of biomaterial development. *Philos Trans A Math Phys Eng Sci.* **2010,** 368: 1831–1837.

Nazarov, R., Jin, H. J., and Kaplan, D. L. Porous 3-D scaffolds from regenerated silk fibroin. *Biomacromolecules.* **2004,** 5(3): 718–726.

Numata, K. and Kaplan, D. L. Silk-based delivery systems of bioactive molecules. *Adv Drug Del Rev.* **2010,** 62(15): 1497–1508.

Ou, C. W., Su, C. H., Jeng, U. S. and Hsu, S. H. Characterization of biodegradable polyurethane nanoparticles and thermally induced self-assembly in water dispersion. *ACS Appl Mater Interfaces.* **2014,** 6(8): 5685–5694.

Ouyang, L., Sun, Z., Wang, D., Qiao, Y., Zhu, H., Ma, X. et al. Smart release of doxorubicin loaded on polyetheretherketone (PEEK) surface with 3D porous structure. *Colloids Surf B Biointerfaces.* **2018,** 163: 175–183.

Owens, D. E., Jian, Y., Fang, J. E., Slaughter, B. V., Chen, Y. H., and Peppas, N. A. Thermally responsive swelling properties of polyacrylamide/poly(acrylic acid) interpenetrating polymer network nanoparticles. *Macromolecules.* **2007,** 40(20): 7306–7310.

Pääkkö, M., Ankerfors, M., Kosonen, H., Nykänen, A., Ahola, S., Österberg, M. et al. Enzymatic hydrolysis combined with mechanical shearing and high-pressure homogenization for nanoscale cellulose fibrils and strong gels. *Biomacromolecules.* **2007,** 8(6): 1934–1941.

Park, S. Y. and Bae, Y. H. Novel pH-sensitive polymers containing sulfonamide groups. *Macromol Rap Commun.* **1999,** 20(5): 269–273.

Patel, K., Angelos, S., Dichtel, W. R., Coskun, A., Yang, Y. W., Zink, J. I. et al. Enzyme-responsive snap-top covered silica nanocontainers. *J Am Chem Soc.* **2008,** 130(8): 2382–2383.

Phaneuf, M. D., Bide, M. J., Szycher, M., Gale, M. B., Huang, H., Yang, C. et al. Development of infection-resistant polyurethane biomaterials using textile dyeing technology. *ASAIO J.* **2001,** 47(6): 634–640.

Pignatello, R. (Ed.). Biomaterials science and engineering. *BoD—Books on Demand.* **2011.**

Rajan, K. P., Thomas, S. P., Gopanna, A. and Chavali, M. Polyurethane nanostructures for drug delivery applications. *Nano Micros Drug Del Syst.* **2017,** 2: 299–319.

Ratner, B. D. A history of biomaterials. *Biomaterials.* **2004,** 2.

Ratner, B. D. and Bryant, S. J. Biomaterials: where we have been and where we are going. *Ann Rev Biomed Eng.* **2004,** 6: 41–75.

Ratner, B. D., Hoffman, A. S., Schoen, F. J. and Lemons, J. E. *Biomaterials Science: An Evolving, Multidisciplinary Endeavor Biomaterials Science.* Academic Press**. 2013.**

Rea, S. M. and Bonfield, W. Biocomposites for medical applications. *J Australas Ceram Soc.* **2004,** 40(1): 43–57.

Rezwan, K., Chen, Q. Z., Blaker, J. J. and Boccaccini, A. R. Biodegradable and bioactive porous polymer/inorganic composite scaffolds for bone tissue engineering. *Biomaterials.* **2006,** 27(18): 3413–3431.

Rose, E. A., Gelijns, A. C., Moskowitz, A. J., Heitjan, D. F., Stevenson, L. W., Dembitsky, W. et al. Long-term use of a left ventricular assist device for end-stage heart failure. *N Engl J Med.* **2001,** 345(20): 1435–1443.

Sahni, A. and Francis, C. W. Vascular endothelial growth factor binds to fibrinogen and fibrin and stimulates endothelial cell proliferation. *J Am Soc Hematol.* **2000,** 96(12): 3772–3778.

Sahu, P., Kashaw, S. K., Jain, S., Sau, S. and Iyer, A. K. Assessment of penetration potential of pH-responsive double-walled biodegradable nanogels coated with eucalyptus oil for the controlled delivery of 5-fluorouracil: *In vitro* and ex vivo studies. *J Control Release.* **2017,** 253: 122–136.

Santerre, J. P., Woodhouse, K., Laroche, G. and Labow, R. S. Understanding the biodegradation of polyurethanes: from classical implants to tissue engineering materials. *Biomaterials.* **2005,** 26(35): 7457–7470.

Santoro, M. and Perale, G. Using synthetic bioresorbable polymers for orthopedic tissue regeneration.*Durability and Reliability of Medical Polymers.* Woodhead Publishing. **2012,** pp. 119–139.

Sharma, A. K., Keservani, R. K. and Kesharwani, R. K. eds., *Nanobiomaterials: Applications in Drug Delivery.* Apple Academic Press*,* CRC Press, **2018,** 550 pages.

Sheikhi, A. Emerging cellulose-based nanomaterials and nanocomposites.*Nanomaterials and Polymer Nanocomposites,* Elsevier. **2019.** 307–351.

Shelke, N. B., Nagarale, R. K. and Kumbar, S. G. Polyurethanes.*Natural and Synthetic Biomedical Polymers,* Elsevier. **2014,** 123–144.

Silva, R., Singh, R., Sarker, B., Papageorgiou, D. G., Juhasz, J. A., Roether J. A. et al. Hybrid hydrogels based on keratin and alginate for tissue engineering. *J Mater Chem.* **2014,** 2: 5441–5451.

Silva, S. S., Fernandes, E. M., Pina, S., Silva-Correia, J., Vieira, S., Oliveira, J. M. et al. Natural-origin materials for tissue engineering and regenerative medicine. *Comp Biomater II.* **2018,** 5(2): 228–252.

Simionescu, B. C. and Ivanov, D. Natural and synthetic polymers for designing composite materials. *Handbook of Bioceramics and Biocomposites,* Berlin: Springer. **2016,** pp. 233–286.

Singh, K. and Mishra, A. Gelatin nanoparticle: preparation, characterization and application in drug delivery. *Int J Pharm Sci Res.* **2014,** 5(6): 2149.

Sitterley, G. Attachment and matrix factors. *Biofiles* (*Sigma-Aldrich*). **2008,** 3: 1–28.

Spicer, C. D. Hydrogel scaffolds for tissue engineering: the importance of polymer choice. *Polym Chem.* **2020,** 11(2), 184–219.

Sun, M., Li, J., Zhang, C., Xie, Y., Qiao, H., Su, Z. et al. Arginine-modified nanostructured lipid carriers with charge-reversal and pH-sensitive membranolytic properties for anticancer drug delivery. *Adv Healthc Mater.* **2017,** 6(8).

Tan, Q. Y., Xu, M. L., Wu, J. Y., Yin, H. F. and Zhang, J. Q. Preparation and characterization of poly(lactic acid) nanoparticles for sustained release of pyridostigmine bromide. *Pharmazie.* **2012,** 67(4): 311–318.

Tang, W. J., Fernandez, J. G., Sohn, J. J. and Amemiya, C. T. Chitin is endogenously produced in vertebrates. *Curr Biol.* **2015,** 25(7): 897–900.

Tang, X., Thankappan, S. K., Lee, P., Fard, S. E., Harmon, M. D., Tran, K. et al. Polymeric biomaterials in tissue engineering and regenerative medicine. *Natural and Synthetic Biomedical Polymers,* Elsevier. **2014,** 351–371.

Tekade, R. K., Tekade, M., Kumar, M. and Chauhan, A. S. Dendrimer-stabilized smart-nanoparticle (DSSN) platform for targeted delivery of hydrophobic antitumor therapeutics. *Pharm Res.* **2015,** 32(3): 910–928.

Teotia, A. K., Sami, H. and Kumar, A. Thermo-responsive polymers. Switchable and responsive surfaces and materials for biomedical applications. *J Mater Chem B.* **2015,** 2: 3–43.

Tomić, S., Kokol, V., Mihajlović, D., Mirčić, A. and Čolić, M. Native cellulose nanofibrils induce immune tolerance *in vitro* by acting on dendritic cells. *Sci Rep.* **2016,** 6(1): 1–14.

Varshosaz, J. and Moazen, E. Novel lectin-modified poly(ethylene-co-vinyl acetate) mucoadhesive nanoparticles of carvedilol: preparation and *in vitro* optimization using a two-level factorial design. *Pharm Dev Technol.* **2014,** 19(5): 605–617.

Varshosaz, J., Taymouri, S. and Hamishehkar, H. Fabrication of polymeric nanoparticles of poly(ethylene-co-vinyl acetate) coated with chitosan for pulmonary delivery of carvedilol. *J Appl Polym Sci.* **2014,** 131(1).

Vepari, C. and Kaplan, D. L. Silk as a biomaterial. *Prog Polym Sci.* **2007,** 32(8–9): 991–1007.

Vermette, P., Griesser, H. J., Laroche, G. and Guidoin, R. *Biomedical Applications of Polyurethanes.* Georgetown, TX: Landes Bioscience. **2001,** 6.

Wang, K. and Deng, Q. The thermal and mechanical properties of poly(ethylene-co-vinyl acetate) random copolymers (PEVA) and its covalently cross-linked analogues (cPEVA). *Polymers.* **2019,** 11(6): 1055.

Wang, W. and Wang, C. Polyurethane for biomedical applications: A review of recent developments.*The Design and Manufacture of Medical Devices.* Woodhead Publishing. **2012,** pp. 115–151.

Wang, Z., Sun, J., Qiu, Y., Li, W., Guo, X., Li, Q. et al. Specific photothermal therapy to the tumors with high EphB4 receptor expression. *Biomaterials.* **2015,** 68: 32–41.

Wei, M., Gao, Y., Li, X. and Serpe, M. J. Stimuli-responsive polymers and their applications. *Polym Chem.* **2017,** 8(1): 127–143.

Wnek, G. E. *Encyclopedia of Biomaterials and Biomedical Engineering.* **2004.**

Woo, G. L. Y., Mittelman, M. W. and Santerre, J. P. Synthesis and characterization of a novel biodegradable antimicrobial polymer. *Biomaterials.* **2000,** 21(12): 1235–1246.

Wood, N. J., Maddocks, S. E., Grady, H. J., Collins, A. M. and Barbour, M. E. Functionalization of ethylene vinyl acetate with antimicrobial chlorhexidine hexametaphosphate nanoparticles. *Int J Nanomed.* **2014,** 9: 41–45.

Woraphatphadung, T., Sajomsang, W., Rojanarata, T., Ngawhirunpat, T., Tonglairoum, P. and Opanasopit, P. Development of chitosan-based pH-sensitive polymeric micelles containing curcumin for colon-targeted drug delivery. *AAPS Pharm Sci Tech.* **2018,** 19(3): 991–1000.

Yamamuro, T. A/W glass-ceramic: clinical applications. *An Introduction to Bioceramics.* World Scientific: Singapore, **1993,** pp. 89–103.

Yamamuro, T., Hench, L. L. and Wilson, J. (Eds.). *CRC Handbook of Bioactive Ceramics.* Boca Raton, FL, USA: CRC Press. **1990.**

Zelzer, M., Todd, S. J., Hirst, A. R., McDonald, T. O. and Ulijn, R. V. Enzyme-responsive materials: design strategies and future developments. *Biomater Sci.* **2013,** 1(1): 11–39.

Zhao, Z., Li, Y., Chen, A. Z., Zheng, Z. J., Hu, J. Y., Li, J. S. et al. Generation of silk fibroin nanoparticles via solution-enhanced dispersion by supercritical CO_2. *Ind Eng Chem Res.* **2013,** 52(10): 3752–3761.

Zuo, B., Dai, L. and Wu, Z. Analysis of structure and properties of biodegradable regenerated silk fibroin fibers. *J Mater Sci.* **2006,** 41(11): 3357–3361.

CHAPTER 3

Gene Therapy in Tissue Engineering: Prospects and Challenges

SOMA MONDAL GHORAI[1*] and HARDEEP KAUR[2]

[1]Department of Zoology, Hindu College, University of Delhi, Delhi 110007, India

[2]Department of Zoology, Ramjas College, University of Delhi, Delhi 110007, India

*Corresponding author. E-mail: somamghorai@hindu.du.ac.in

ABSTRACT

Humanity hopes for a better future in clinical therapeutics where one wishes to overcome challenges such as long and painful wait for right donor for organ transplant, problems in plastic surgery, impaired wound healing and dysfunctional operations, and debilitating genetic disorders. Tissue engineering is still at baby steps as it deliberates to combine principles of engineering and life sciences to give people hope. This technique aims to repair, restore, and regenerate damaged and diseased cells and organs of the human body. Among many approaches that are employed alongside, "gene therapy" holds great prospects for future clinical therapeutics as it can be effortlessly united with tissue engineering and can repair the damaged tissue at the cellular and molecular level. This hybrid approach of conjunction between tissue engineering and gene therapy provides the optimum environment for therapeutic protein expression for regeneration of cells and tissues, thereby holds immense potential in areas of skin, bone, and cartilage repair. The aim of this chapter is to provide the readers with the varied aspects of tissue engineering and gene therapy, their advantages and future prospects as well as the challenges pertaining to the combination of the two.

3.1 INTRODUCTION TO TISSUE ENGINEERING

Having reduced mortality from starvation, disease, and wars, humankind has set itself even more daring goals. With secured unprecedented levels of prosperity, health, and given our past records and our current values, humanity's next targets are likely to be immortality. So, some very able researchers in the world are nicknamed as Dr Frankenstein as they regularly harvest heart and lungs from the freshly dead, re-engineers them, and attempts to bring them back to life in the hope that they might be able to beat or breathe in the living once again. So, this is what in biotechnological term is called "tissue engineering," first introduced by Professor Robert Nerem in 1988 at UCLA Symposia on Molecular and Cellular Biology (Lanza et al., 2011).

Tissue engineering should not be confused with organ transplantation. Indeed, it is an attractive compromise between the conventional medical practices and organ transplantation. As the name suggests, tissue engineering combines principles of engineering and polymer chemistry with biology. This technique aims to enable tissue or organ transplantation without the risk of rejection by the recipient's immune system. In the current scenario, there is a long waiting list of patients for organ transplantation. Besides social stigma associated with organ donation, another challenge in this case is nonavailability of perfect donor, whose tissue's histocompatibility complex matches with the recipient's histocompatibility complex. Thus, to overcome this hurdle and solve the crippling problem of shortage of transplantable organs, "tissue engineering" is the hope where cells are harvested from dead organ (which may not be even human) and then the protein scaffold is extracted after cleaning off all the cells. The scaffolds are then incubated with mediums containing growth factors and repopulated with stem cells that immunologically match with the patient in need. As the cells grow and divide across the scaffold, a substitute tissue is generated which is finally implanted in the host.

Tissue engineering is a subtype of regenerative medicine, which focuses on restoring, repairing, and maintaining damaged cells albeit outside the body by using synthetic- and naturally-derived materials as scaffolds to provide right environment to help grow tissue in test tubes and later apply them on affected areas. Tissue engineering is, thereby, aimed to promote and advance regenerative engineering, a new field defined as the Convergence of Advanced Materials Sciences, Stem Cell Science, Physics, Developmental Biology, and Clinical Translation for the regeneration of complex tissues and organ systems. Thus, three components are most important for tissue engineering; first is the scaffold (biodegradable structures that hold implanted cells in place until they develop into integrated tissue), second are the cells, and third are the growth factors (Figure 3.1).

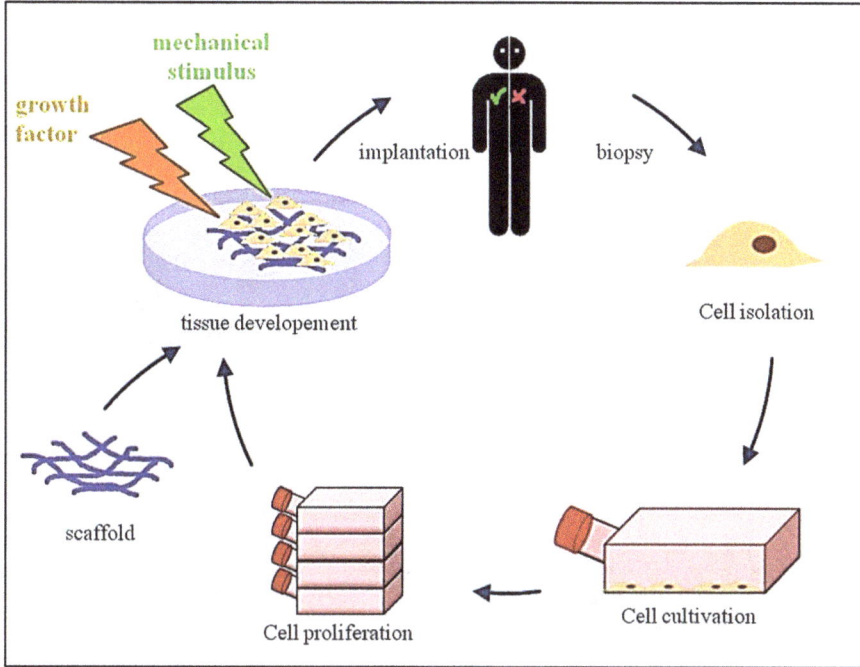

FIGURE 3.1 Schematic representation of basic principles of tissue engineering.
Source: https://commons.wikimedia.org/wiki/File:Tissue_engineering_english.jpg/https://creativecommons.org/licenses/by/3.0/deed.en

In certain genetic disorders such as adenosine deaminase-severe combined immunodeficiency (ADA-SCID), the targeted cells derived for tissue engineering from organs or tissue may be tinkered to express specific genes or proteins to generate long-lived tissue cells. In such a scenario, gene therapy can be combined with tissue engineering which encompasses the growth of genetically modified cells, expanded in sufficient numbers onto the scaffolds *in vitro*, and finally the enriched cells can be administered into the patient's body.

3.2 SCAFFOLDS IN TISSUE ENGINEERING

Consider some obfuscate blob of tissues in a petri plate, finally culminating into a full-fledged heart with its intricate capillaries that supply the heart with oxygen and nutrients as well as remove the waste materials from deep within its tissues. Seems unimaginable, but that is what the scaffold offers in tissue engineering, where a complex structure such as heart can be constructed by organizing the cells in three dimensions, a feat which is beyond the reach of most sophisticated machines. Success stories such as that of artificial trachea have already been achieved (Chaneton et al., 2012). Anthony Atala of Wake Forest University in Winston-Salem, North Carolina had implanted bioengineered bladders into patients and now researching toward building working kidneys (Maher, 2013).

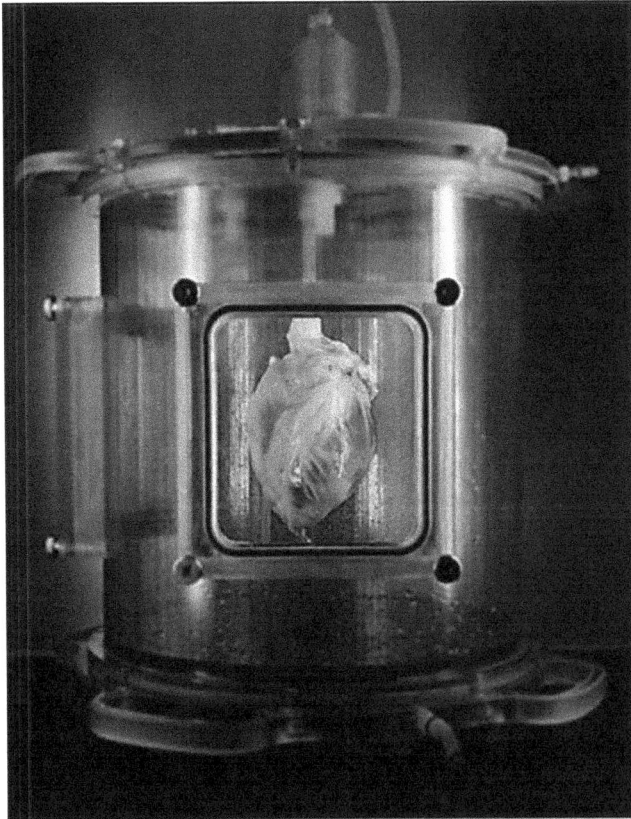

FIGURE 3.2   Heart bioreactor.
Credit: Bernhard Jank, MD/Ott Lab, Center for Regenerative Medicine, Massachusetts General Hospital. https://openwetware.org/wiki/File:Heart_bioreactor.JPG#filelinks

A freshly retrieved heart from once living being that need not be a human (pig heart is a much promising candidate) is suspended by plastic tubes in a drum-shaped glass chamber (Figure 3.2). It is then flushed with detergents and sends through the aortic valve, so that it reaches the entire network of blood vessels, slowly stripping the DNA), sugars, lipids, soluble proteins, and other cellular material till a pale mesh of extracellular matrix (ECM) is left that forms the scaffold. Scaffolds derived from pig heart have many advantages (Ott et al., 2008). The supply is abundant from the local abattoirs; they have all the crucial components of ECM of a human heart, they are tougher and rarely weakened by illness and resuscitation efforts, and most importantly unlikely to carry any human diseases. Dr Stephen Badylak at McGowan Institute for Regenerative Medicine, University of Pittsburgh has done tremendous work in this field.

Decellularization of the organ is the trickiest part as too little of detergent flush may leave certain cell surface molecules, triggering rejection by the recipient's immune system and too much may lead to loss of crucial proteins and growth factors for the scaffolds. It is a complete trial and error process and requires tremendous skill and expertise to achieve the right blend of concentration, timings, and pressure of the detergents used. Once the scaffold is retrieved, it is repopulated with the desired human cells (Figure 3.3) (Zheng et al., 2018).

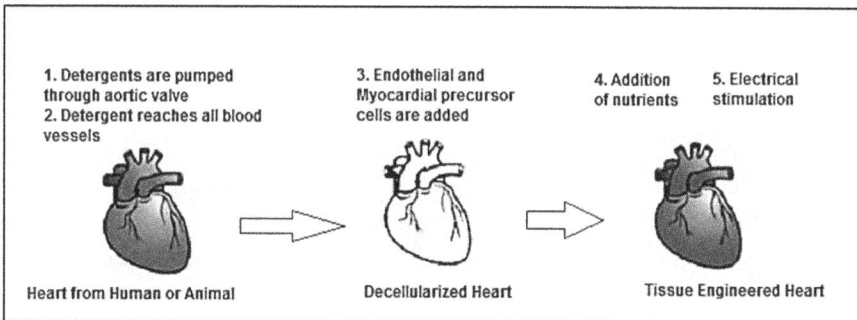

FIGURE 3.3   Chronological steps involved in heart tissue engineering.

Scaffolds are the supporting structures that provide the optimum environment to colonize the host cells and get selectively expanded ex vivo with the help of growth factors for specific lineage before being implanted at the target site (Roseti et al., 2017). Once implanted, it biodegrades during the healing process of the tissue and gradually makes way for freshly generated tissues of desired shape and properties. Its dissolvable properties ensure that no immunological hyperactivity occurs due to the presence of foreign tissue (Aldana and Abraham, 2017). To avoid elicitation of host immune defenses against the implanted scaffold, the immune-inert biomaterial is conceptualized which is based on downregulating the natural killer (NK) cell activity along with T- and B-cell-mediated immunity (Roseti et al., 2017). Apart from immune inertness, a good scaffold should meet the precise physical (adhesion), chemical (nontoxic), and mechanical (cross-linking) requirements to gain 3D tissue formation. Idyllically, scaffold should possess four significant characteristics: (1) interconnected pore network to support 3D building of cell and enable flow of nutrients and wastes; (2) rate of degradation and bioresorption should match with the growth of cell/tissue *in vitro* and/or *in vivo*; (3) optimum surface chemistry for cell adhesion, proliferation, and differentiation; and (4) mechanical support to the cells/tissues to match with the position of implantation (Hutmacher, 2000).

Nevertheless, the choice of scaffold finally depends on its vascularization ability and has remained the major challenge in tissue engineering. The scaffold should be able to abridge the structural complexity and provide for cells, proteins, and genes for tissue reconstruction. We are still far behind in designating a scaffold from any biomaterial that can mimic the complex interaction among the various cell types and the cytokines present within the tissue microenvironment (Meyer et al., 2009). There are pertinent concerns of biocompatibility and decomposition properties. Moreover, biological material has low capacity to interact with the scaffold, thus efforts are made to promote bioactive scaffolds for effective cross-talk with the environment, cells colonization, migration, and tissue differentiation. Nowadays, most scaffolds are bioceramics, polymers, or hybrid materials (Yang et al., 2017). Scaffolds made from natural or synthetic polymers are the probable choice and the matrices closest to the natural ECM are the most promising in tissue engineering. Hyaluronic acid, fibrin, collagen, and chitosan are the commonly used natural polymers that are low in immunogenicity and osteoconductivity and possess good biocompatibility, but they have erratic degradation rates and low mechanical stability, whereas synthetic polymers such as polyglycolic acid (PGA), polypropylene fumarate, polylactic acid (PLA), polyetheretherketone, polycaprolactone, polyanhydride, and polyphosphazene overcome the inability of cell attachment and degradation, have a longer shelf-life, abundantly produced, and cost-effective, but they are shown to destroy ex vivo cells, elicit strong immune reactions, and unexpected degradation compared to natural tissue matrices (Roseti et al., 2017). Thus, ECM has gained propensity in 3D printing due to its high remodeling ability, biological compatibility, and degradability (Celikkkin et al., 2017). In fact, decellularized ECM (dECM) has been extensively reconnoitered in Regenerative Medicine (Taylor et al., 2018). These dECM preserves not only the native tissue composition, but also the structural proteins, growth factors, and cytokines. The procurement of dECM is also direct from a variety of tissues namely such as bone, cartilage, meniscus, tendons, skin and adipose tissue, urinary bladder, small intestinal submucosa, liver, and brain (Abedin et al., 2018; Cho et al., 2019; Grant et al., 2019; Parmaksiz et al., 2019; Ghazanfari et al., 2019; Zhang et al., 2019). Thus, functionalized scaffolds from ECM can mimic the *in vivo*-like microenvironment required for cell-specific tissue regeneration and repair (Sultana, 2003; Aldana and Abraham, 2017). For example, with the help of robocasting techniques, 3D-printed scaffolds coated with dECM have been shown much promise as they resulted in enhanced osteogenic differentiation and new bone formation (Goodman et al., 2013).

Tissue engineering is a complex technique and the construction of the right kind of scaffold is a challenging task. Biomedical 3D scaffold fabrication techniques involve some conventional and current technologies. The conventional methods are thermally induced phase separation, gas foaming, freeze drying, electrospinning, solvent casting, and particle leaching while modern methods comprise rapid prototyping, fused deposition modeling, stereolithography, selective laser sintering, and 3D printing (Eltom et al., 2019). Nowadays, tissue engineering employs more sophisticated strategies such as 3D scaffolds and hydrogels which are porous so as to pass the gases, nutrients, and regulatory factors, have good tensile strength, help in cell-biomaterial attachment, growth, and migration and controlled degradation rates (Thorrez et al., 2008). Using salt-leaching and a freeze-drying technique, natural 3D scaffolds are made from natural biopolymer obtained from marine sources (shark skin) or silk fibroin (SF) blended with β-tricalcium phosphate, strontium, zinc, and manganese (Pina et al., 2017). SF has been gradually known as a likely material for tissue engineering due to the effortlessness of processing, its exceptional biocompatibility, and efficient mechanical properties (Figure 3.4). 3D-bioprinting techniques have enabled 3D scaffolds with diverse cell and biomolecules positioning with favored design and geometrics (Jang et al., 2018; Park et al., 2018). Among the biomolecules used for 3D bioprinting, the preferred ones are the alginate enriched with surface peptides such as arginine-glycine-aspartate (RGD) (Lee and Mooney, 2012) and collagen type I or agarose (AG) with sodium alginate (SA). Collagen facilitated cell adhesion, accelerated cell proliferation, and can enhance the expression of the cartilage-specific genes, namely *Acan*, *Sox9*, and *Col2al* (Yang et al., 2018).

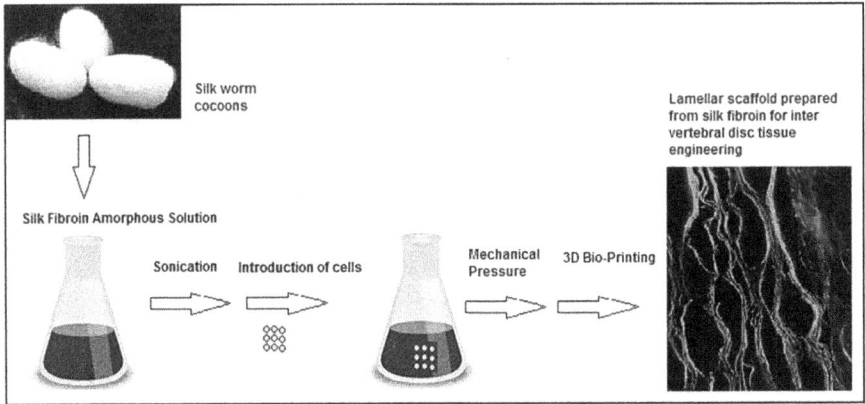

FIGURE 3.4   3D cell-laden scaffolds prepared from natural biopolymer such as silk fibroin (SF) through the 3D bioprinting method to promote intervertebral disk tissue regeneration.

As compared to the nonbiological 3D printing which has some technical challenges related to sheer stress and biocompatibility, fabrication of 3D hydrogel-based scaffolds has emerged as highly precise biomimetic matrices (Garcia et al., 2018). With the help of high-throughput *in vitro* platforms, tissue engineering has been able to address high levels of precision medicine by introducing hydrogel scaffolds from healthy and diseased tissues of human body (Devarasetty et al., 2018). Scaffolds from hydrogel have been proposed for transplantation of a number of tissues including meniscus and cartilage (Garcia et al., 2018), bone (Ashammakhi et al., 2019), vascular grafts (Miri et al., 2019), skin (Velasco et al., 2018), and intervertebral disk (Costa et al., 2018). A hydrogel scaffold enables better interaction between cells and the ECM and establishes a dynamic regulatory system for regeneration (Figure 3.5). Nowadays, different processing methodologies are being employed to structure hydrogels for more porosity and superior mechanical characteristics that led to their use as aqueous-based system for cell encapsulation (Bryant and Vernerey, 2018), as injectable filters (Varma et al., 2014), and as bioprinting system (Wang et al., 2015).

Additionally, the fabricated scaffold properties depend on its specific application and the type of tissues that needs repair, whether soft tissues such as neural or hard tissues such as bones. It also depends upon factors such as anatomical location, trauma severity, pathological conditions, and the patient age. Scaffolds required for hard tissue, such as in bone regeneration, must be resistant to physiological stress and reduce stress shielding. It should also possess the exact size, shape, wall thickness and surface pores, resorption kinetics, cell adhesion properties, and mechanical strength (Sanzherrera et al., 2009). In case of soft tissues such as spinal cord, scaffolds are usually made of hydrogels as they can adapt to the mechanical milieu and viscoelasticity of the neural tissues (Gregor et al., 2017; Foong and Sultana, 2017). For scaffolds in cell regeneration, extended or nonextended cell types are derived from donor or patient. Sources of extended cells are adult stem cells (such as bone marrow, fatty tissue, teeth, and blood cells) or embryonic stem cells (ESCs), induced pluripotent stem cells (iPSCs), and the genetically engineered cells while the sources of nonextended cells are bone marrow aspirate-derived platelet-rich plasma cells (Roseti et al., 2017).

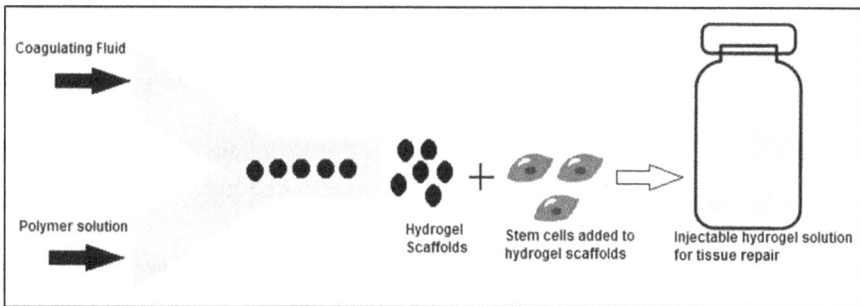

FIGURE 3.5   Use of hydrogel scaffold for tissue repair.

3.3   CELLS IN TISSUE ENGINEERING

At the dawn of the third millennium, humanity wakes up to an amazing realization that he can have "spare parts" not only for his machines, but also for replacement of damaged or lost organs; thanks to modern technological practices such as tissue engineering. This amazing realization was made possible by certain cells called "stem cells", which have the potential to significantly alter the perspective of tissue engineering. These extensively self-renewing cells can repair and restore injured tissues, if provided with the appropriate growth factors and environment. They also can be targeted for prospective gene therapies. Cells involved in tissue engineering must be able to deliver effective and long-lasting tissue repair, thus they should possess certain characteristics: (1) must be in sufficient amount to be able to colonize; (2) should possess good differentiation capability into desired phenotypes; (3) should be able to adopt to the 3D structural scaffold and generate extracellular matrices; (4) should be compliant to the native cells both in terms of adhesion and mechanical support; and (5) should be able to overcome immunological rejection and be biologically safe (Vats et al., 2002). There are three approaches toward tissue engineering by stem cell therapy: (1) substitutive, where whole organ replacement is done ex vivo; (2) histioconductive, where damaged or injured tissue is replaced by ex-vivo constructs; and (3) histioinductive, where self-repair is facilitated via gene therapy.

Stem cells can be either multipotent or pluripotent where the former is able to differentiate into limited number of tissue types and the latter can generate every cells and organs of the body. Surprisingly, stem cells are found throughout the body in one's lifetime. Every tissue hosts some amount of stem cells for its general purpose of maintenance and repair of dead and injured cells and tissues such as those found in heart, kidney, gut, brain, muscle, etc. The source of cells for tissue engineering can be derived from the patient's own body (autologous) or from another immunological incompatible person (allogenic) or from different species (xenogenic) (Knight and Evans, 2004).

Stem cells are further categorized into: (1) ESCs, obtained from human blastocyst (150-celled). These are pluripotent and can give rise to any cells and tissue; (2) *adult stem cells*, are fewer in number, present in most adult tissues, and are multipotent in nature; and (3) iPSCs, where adult cells are genetically modified and reprogrammed for specific functions. These are mostly pluripotent cells and hold much promise as they can be altered to evade host's immune responses (Figure 3.6A and B). Stem cell sources have their own merits and demerits (Table 1).

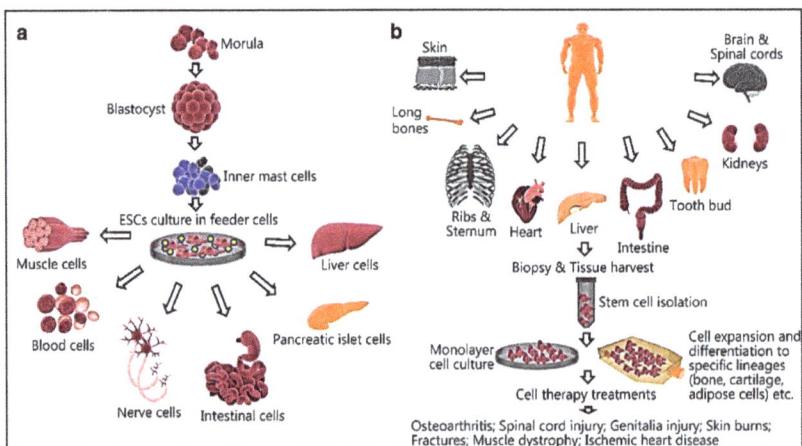

FIGURES 3.6   Types of stem cells used in tissue engineering. (A) Embryonic stem cells (ESCs) and (B) Adult stem cells [mesenchymal stem cells (MSCs), etc.].
Source: Ude et al. (2018); https://europepmc.org/articles/PMC6389246/figure/Fig2/(http://creativecommons.org/licenses/by/4.0/)

TABLE 3.1 List of Advantages and Disadvantages of Different Cell Source(S) in Tissue Engineering

Cell sources	Advantages	Disadvantages
A. Embryonic stem cells (ESCs)	1. Pluripotency 2. Self-renewal 3. Can differentiate into any cell type	1. Have high propensity to transform into teratomas when transplanted *in vivo* 2. Have ethical and regulatory restraints
B. Adult stem cells		
1. Bone-marrow derived mesenchymal stem cells (BM-MSCs)	1. High osteogenic potential	1. Low retrieval capacity 2. Requires extensive *in vitro* expansion
2. Neural stem cells (NSCs)	1. Good proliferative potential 2. Low immunogenicity	1. Difficult to harvest 2. Low differentiation capacity
3. Adipose-derived stem cells (ASCs)	1. Good growth potential 2. Easy to harvest 3. Abundantly present	1. Fewer studied
4. Adipose-derived stromal vascular fraction (SVF)	1. Abundant 2. Can easily be derived through liposuction	1. Cell population varies in donors 2. ii. Multiple procedural steps
5. Umbilical cord-derived mesenchymal stem cells (UC-MSCs)	1. Abundantly obtained 2. Broad differentiation capacity and proliferation potential 3. High *in vivo* safety than ESCs	1. Difficult to isolate 2. Fewer studied
C. Induced pluripotent stem cells (iPSCs)	1. Pluripotency 2. Capable of differentiating into all cell types	1. Low reprogramming efficacy 2. Extensive expansion required 3. Have safety concerns, thereby less clinical application

Though USA leads in tissue engineering and stem cell therapy, India too has her own success stories. It is among the top 10 leading countries engaged in stem cell industry with an estimated worth of approximately $500 million in 2010 and a growth rate of 15% in both military and civilian research.

Among the leading institutes are National Centre for Biological Sciences (NCBS), Bangalore; Centre for Cellular and Molecular Biology, Hyderabad; L V Prasad Eye Institute, Hyderabad; Centre for Stem Cell Research, Vellore; National Brain Research Centre, New Delhi; and National Centre for Cell Science, Pune (Prasad et al., 2014). Successful clinical trials were conducted on ailments such as cerebral artery infarction, strokes, spinal injuries, partial paralysis, etc. (Pollard, 2017). Army Hospital for Research and Referral, New Delhi and Armed Forces Medical College, Pune have collaborated in 2009 and successfully cured subacute ischemic stroke by infusing 30–500 million autologous bone marrow-derived mesenchymal stem cells (BM-MSCs) derived from the patient's own body (Prasad, 2014). Another feat was achieved by a private company, Nutech Mediworld, based in Green Park in South Delhi that successfully treated severe spinal injuries without any immunosuppressants by introducing isolated ESCs (Ian, 2015).

3.3.1 *EMBRYONIC STEM CELLS IN TISSUE ENGINEERING*

Embryonic stem cells hold immense possibilities in healthcare from treating patients with neurological disorders to Parkinson's disease and even provide insight into the molecular processes that drive a normal cell to develop into a tumorous mass. ESCs are obtained from the blastocysts before implantation, hence mostly human ESCs are derived from discarded embryos from *in vitro* fertilization clinics. The physiognomies that define ESCs are: (1) embryo is 4–5 days old; (2) they are an undifferentiated mass of cells capable of self-renewal; (3) they maintain pluripotency even after prolonged culture; (4) capable of differentiating into three germ layers—ectoderm, endoderm, and mesoderm; and (5) capable to differentiate into any cell types and can colonize tissues of interest. ESCs can be maintained for unlimited time period in their pluripotent state by providing with leukemia inhibitory factor (LIF) or embryonic fibroblast feeder layers and withdrawal of LIF leads to the formation of embryoid mass comprising of ectodermal, mesodermal, and endodermal cells (Wiles and Johansson, 1999; Thompson et al., 1998). Human ESCs showed considerable promise in generating myocardial infarcts as they are able to differentiate into cardiomyocytes (Kehat et al., 2001). Similarly, smooth muscle cells can be procured from human ESCs by isolating the progenitor cells (CD34+) from embryoid bodies (EBs) and then treating with transforming growth factor-β1 (TGF-β1), PDGF-BB (the two B subunits of platelet-derived growth factor), and retinoic acid (Hill et al., 2010) or seeding the human ESCs with extracellular matrices such as collagen IV or Matrigel (Xie et al., 2007). Using 2D and 3D cultures in tissue engineering, ESCs have also shown success in differentiating into functional vascularized skeletal tissue and implantable blood vessels (Levenberg et al., 2005), thus paving way to be able to form tube-like structures and form microvessels (Wang et al., 2007).

3.3.2 ADULT STEM CELLS

Unlike ESCs, research in adult stem cells does not call for ethical issues as no killing of embryo is involved; rather the cells are obtained from human body. Also known as somatic stem cells, these are undifferentiated cells present in every tissue and organ of the body that helps to maintain homeostasis and replenish damaged and injured tissues. Adult stem cells are multipotent cells that give rise to cell types of one particular tissue and are believed to reside in specific niches. They exhibit tissue-specific characteristics and are defined by expression of specific cell-surface markers and transcription factors (Figure 3.7). These cells mostly remain dormant throughout the lifespan of an individual in certain organs such as brain and heart, till they are triggered by a tissue injury, disease, or other factors to replenish the tissue. While in other tissues such as blood marrow and gut lining, it is continuously being replenished. Though they hold a lot of promise for future therapeutics, many limitations need to be overcome to consider them for clinical application.

Bone marrow-derived mesenchymal cells are the adult stem cells for bone and cartilage repair and are derived from the generic marrow of the osteogenic lineage (Bruder et al., 1998; Yang et al., 2001; Howard et al., 2002). These can be isolated via antibody selection procedure by targeting cell surface receptor on the marrow tissues such as endoglin (Haynesworth et al., 1992; Majumdar et al., 2000) and Stro-1 (Simmons and Torok-Storb, 1991; Howard et al., 2002; Stewart et al., 2003). Stromal vascular fraction (SVF) is the source for *adipose-derived stem cells* (ADSCs) harvested during liposuction. A processed lipoaspirate filtrate generates ADSCs after subsequent digestion, washing, and filtration in the presence of fetal bovine serum (Zuk et al., 2001). Analogous to mesenchymal stem cells, ADSCs exhibit tremendous potential to differentiate into all mesenchymal lineages and possess MSC-like immunophenotypes (Boquest et al., 2005). They are also known to support allogenic transplantations by immunosuppression of mixed lymphocyte reaction and lymphocyte proliferation (Puissant et al., 2005). These can also differentiate into smooth muscle cells as well as endothelial cells by treating with TGF-β1 and bone morphogenetic protein

4 (BMP4), leading to synthesis of collagen and vessel walls, thus is an important source for vascular regeneration (Chang et al., 2010; Zang et al., 2011). Recently, research is more focused toward the applicability quotient since the discovery that *umbilical cord-derived mesenchymal stem cells* (UC-MSCs) can undergo multilineage differentiation. Umbilical cord cells (UB-MSCs) are very similar to mesenchymal stem cells, as they can differentiate into many cell types such as adipocytes, osteoblasts (Lee et al., 2004), hepatocytes (Kang et al., 2006), and neuronal-like cells (Hou et al., 2003).

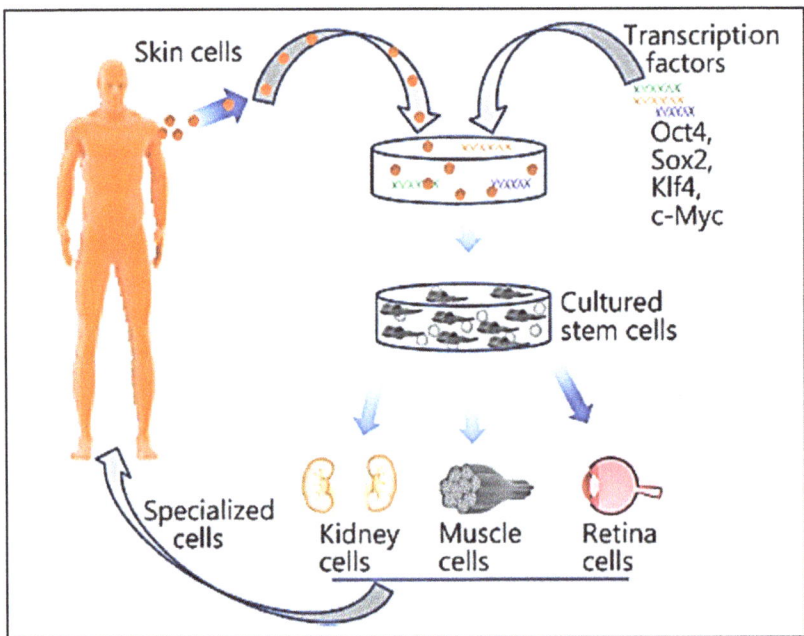

FIGURE 3.7   Schematic representation of the procedure involved in adult stem cell therapy. *Source:* https://europepmc.org/articles/PMC6389246/figure/Fig12/(http://creativecommons. org/licenses/by/4.0/)

3.3.3   INDUCED PLURIPOTENT STEM CELLS

Shinya Takahashi, an Alchemist at work, received Nobel Prize in the year 2012 for his path-breaking work on reprogramming adult stem cells to behave like ESCs. He took adult skin cells and infected them with virus carrying 24 carefully chosen genes and transforming them into pluripotent embryonic cells capable to give rise to any cell types (Figure 3.8) (Takahashi and Yamanaka, 2006). This paved way for a new research field called "personalized therapy", which has the advantage of no risk of immune rejection and also sidestep the ethical concerns of using embryos. With the aid of gene-editing technologies, iPSCs have become a source of unlimited supply of human tissues for research. Though iPSCs behaved like ESCs, they carried an "epigenetic memory"—a pattern of chemical marks on their DNA that reflects their original cell type, but that did not came in way of regenerative medicine especially for neurodegenerative disorders. Till date, iPSCs have been able to differentiate into endothelial cells (ECs), endothelial progenitor cells (EPCs) as well as mesenchymal cells (Lian et al., 2010). As compared to BM-MSCs, iPSCs sorted with CD24−/CD105+ receptors have incredible proliferative and differentiation capacity into adipocyte, chondrocyte, and osteocyte lineages (Lee et al., 2010).

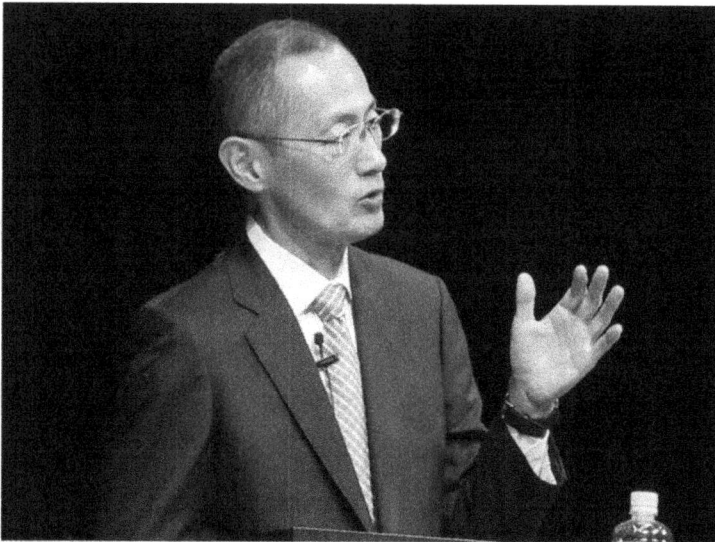

FIGURE 3.8   Nobel winning file photo of Prof Shinya Yamanaka.
Source: https://upload.wikimedia.org/wikipedia/commons/4/49/Lecture_by_Nobel_Laureate_Dr._Shinya_Yamanaka_%E2%80%9CNew_Era_of_Medicine_with_iPS_Cells-_Message_to_Future_Scientists%E2%80%9C_%2846596989145%29.jpg (https://creativecommons.org/licenses/by/2.0/)

3.4   RECONSTRUCTION VERSUS CORRECTION

It has been a long battle to ensure that stimulation of stem cells in situ should lead to specific regeneration and not to scar formation or teratogenesis. There are persistent challenges namely inability to sustain growth factors' presence in the culture media for indefinite period of time, correct dosage, and lack of activity of recombinant factors. Thus, research nowadays is focused on overcoming the hurdles and transduce cell *in vivo* to bring about suitable regeneration processes by investigating "gene-activated matrices" using plasmids coding as delivery vehicles (Bonadio, 2000). Stems cells herald the backbone of tissue engineering, but they are also the critical targets for correcting any genetic defects. Many of the hazards caused by direct gene transfer in human are now been avoided by genetically modifying these cells ex vivo using viral and nonviral transducing agents (Asahara et al., 2000). Gene therapy is the answer to the successful cure of junctional epidermolysis bullosa, a debilitating skin disease by transducing epidermal cells (Dellambra et al., 2000). Undoubtedly, care should be taken to avoid mutagenesis by silencing the gene. Strategies such as site-directed mutagenesis and homologous recombination should be the crucial goal, though many intermediate methods can also be employed such as antisense RNA, RNA interference, and hammerhead and hairpin RNase(s) to preclude expression of mutant gene. Thus, in an attempt to revolutionize tissue engineering, frontiers of genetic engineering are being merged, so that reconstruction is now termed as "correction". tissue engineering has a new definition as engineering of tissue function via stem cell-mediated gene therapy and holds tremendous prospects in clinical application. The next section of the chapter provides an understanding to the readers about gene therapy.

3.5   INTRODUCTION TO GENE THERAPY

The concept of gene therapy was introduced almost in the middle of 20th century wherein scientists began to toil around the idea of using good gene to replace the bad defective gene. However, it was Friedmann and Roblin who in 1972 wrote a paper titled "Gene Therapy for Human Genetic Disease?" (Friedmann et al., 1972). In 1980, Martin Cline was the first to transfer rDNA in the bone marrow cells of two patients who had hereditary blood disorders. In 1984, a highly transmissible murine retrovirus shuttle vector was constructed to carry the DNA insert into mammalian chromosomes (Cepko et al., 1984). However, the first approved gene therapy clinical research took place in the US, at the National Institutes of Health (NIH), under the direction of William French Anderson (also called "Father of Gene Therapy") on 14th September, 1990. Ashanti DeSilva, a 4-year-old girl, received treatment for a genetic defect called SCID that had severely impaired her immune system. Ashanti DeSilva actually suffered from ADA deficiency, which is a rarer and slightly less severe form of SCID. In her case, the defective gene was replaced by the functional gene that started expressing the missing enzyme in her cells. Ashanti's immune system was partially restored as not all cells expressed the missing enzyme but she was able to lead normal life subsequently with regular medications (Thompson, 1994).

In the period between the years 1990 and 2000, numerous attempts related to gene therapy were made involving more than thousands of patients (Abbott, 1992; Blaese et al., 1995). Claudio Bordignon, while working at the Vita-Salute San Raffaele University in 1992, successfully performed the first gene therapy procedure in which hematopoietic stem cells were used as vectors to deliver genes with the intention of correcting hereditary diseases. Jesse Gelsinger, one such patient, had ornithine transcarbamylase deficiency, an X-linked genetic disease of the liver, the symptoms of which include an inability to metabolize ammonia, a byproduct of protein breakdown. He was injected with an adenoviral vector carrying a corrected gene on 13th September, 1999. He died 4 days later due to massive immune response triggered by the use of the viral vector. This was a major setback for gene therapy research in the US (Stolberg, 1999). In 2002, gene therapy was used to treat sickle cell anemia in mice (Wilson, 2002). The year 2003 proved very promising with liposome-aided gene insertion in the brain being performed successfully (Ananthaswamy, 2003). In March 2006, two adult patients for X-linked chronic granulomatous disease (a disease which affects myeloid cells and impairs the immune system) were treated by gene therapy (Ott et al., 2006). In November 2006, VRX496, a gene-based immunotherapy, was successfully employed for the treatment of HIV. Lentiviral vector was used in this case to deliver an antisense gene against the HIV envelope (Levine et al., 2006). The first gene therapy trial for inherited retinal disease was done in 2007 (Ghosh, 2007). In 2010, an 18-year-old male patient in France with beta-thalassemia major was successfully treated (Cavazzana-Calvo et al., 2010). In 2011, Neovasculgen was registered in Russia as the first-in-class gene-therapy drug for treatment of peripheral artery disease, including critical limb ischemia; it delivers the gene encoding for vascular endothelial growth factor (VEGF) (Deev et al., 2015). In 2013, scientists reported successful treatment of hemophilia patients using adenovirus-based vectors (Nathwani et al., 2014). The period between 2013 onward has seen immense research being carried out around the world with many successful attempts in certain diseases such as sickle cell disease (Romero et al., 2013), acute lymphoblastic leukemia (ALL) (Qasim et al., 2017), non-Hodgkin lymphoma (Avanzi et al., 2017), Hunter syndrome (Sestito et al., 2018), and many other diseases.

Indeed our genes define who we are, though sometimes a defect in the gene can produce an imperfection that can threaten the existence of an individual. In the last four decades, several genes have been identified that are responsible for different genetic disorders in human. A new field of biology has henceforth emerged called the gene therapy. Gene therapy can, therefore, be defined as a method of treating diseases by either modifying the expressions of an individual's genes or alteration of abnormal genes or introduction of a normal healthy gene. The field holds great promise for treating an extensive range of human diseases. It has been found to be successful especially in single-gene diseases such as sickle cell anemia, hemophilia, etc. However, the therapy is still in its infancy but it brings a new ray of hope for patients who are living with difficult and incurable diseases.

3.6 PROCESS OF GENE THERAPY

Gene therapy can be described as the delivery of nucleic acid into the cells of patient to treat a disease. The nucleic acid here acts as a drug and tries to fix the genetic problem at the source. There are three ways that gene delivery can be performed.

3.6.1 REPLACEMENT OF THE MUTATED GENE THAT IS RESPONSIBLE FOR THE DISEASE WITH ITS HEALTHY COPY

The process is more appropriately called gene augmentation wherein multiple copies of the desired gene are introduced in the cell through transfer vectors and made to express at high levels. However, this is successful only if the disease has not caused irreversible damage in the body, for example, the method has been successfully applied to correct cystic fibrosis (Figure 3.9).

3.6.2 "KNOCKING OUT" OR INACTIVATING THE MUTATED GENE THAT IS FUNCTIONING IMPROPERLY

The process is also called "gene inhibition therapy" and is more suitable for treating infectious diseases, cancer (oncogene is inhibited), and certain inherited diseases (Figure 3.10).

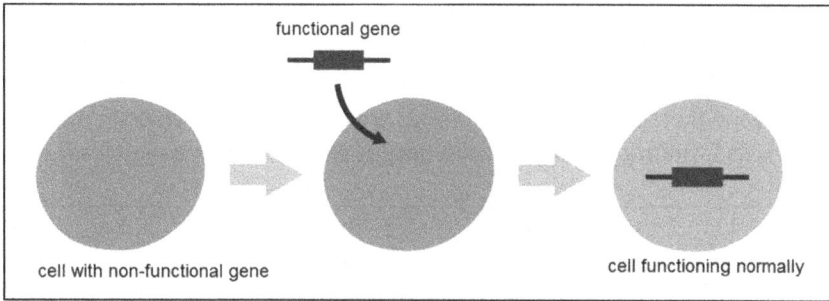

FIGURE 3.9 Gene replacement.
Source: Adapted from https://www.yourgenome.org/facts/what-is-gene-therapy (https://creativecommons.org/licenses/by/4.0/).

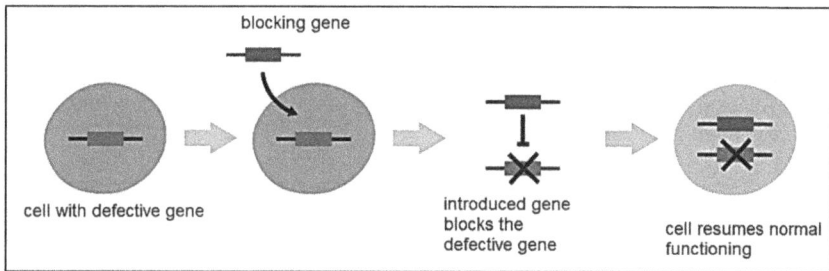

FIGURE 3.10 Gene inhibition.
Source: Adapted from https://www.yourgenome.org/facts/what-is-gene-therapy (https://creativecommons.org/licenses/by/4.0/).

3.6.3 INTRODUCTION OF A NEW GENE INTO THE BODY THAT CAN HELP TO FIGHT THE DISEASE

Gene therapy needs not always aim at replacing a defective gene or suppressing its function, but sometimes a different gene is introduced that can affect the peripheral or epigenetic function of the defective gene. For example, one may not correct or suppress the oncogene rather introduce another gene that has tumor suppressing function such as introducing cytokine gene into tumor cells (Figure 3.11).

3.6.4 INTRODUCTION OF "SUICIDE GENE"

This type of gene therapy involves introduction of a suicide gene into certain target cells that initiate apoptosis in them (Figure 3.12). This technique has been found to be most useful in case of cancer cells and called cancer suicide gene therapy (CSGT). The delivery of the suicide genes involves viral or synthetic vectors, which are guided to the target cancer cells by specific antibodies and ligands. Such vector must have the capability to discriminate between target (cancer) and nontarget (normal) cells. The two major suicide gene therapeutic techniques that are currently followed are: cytosine deaminase/5-fluorocytosine and the herpes simplex virus/ganciclovir.

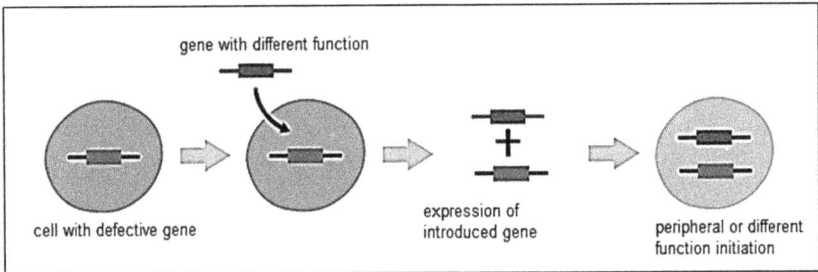

FIGURE 3.11   Gene addition.
Source: Adapted from https://www.yourgenome.org/facts/what-is-gene-therapy (https://creativecommons.org/licenses/by/4.0/).

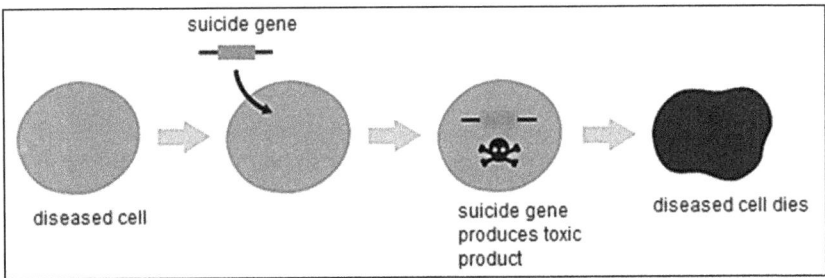

FIGURE 3.12   Suicide gene insertion.
Source: Adapted from https://www.yourgenome.org/facts/what-is-gene-therapy (https://creativecommons.org/licenses/by/4.0/).

3.7   TYPES OF GENE THERAPY

Delivery of the normal foreign gene by gene therapy requires a genetically engineered, efficient carrier or vector and a recipient cell. There are two types of gene therapy depending on the type of cells that are being treated.

3.7.1   *SOMATIC CELL GENE THERAPY (SCGT)*

In this case, the therapeutic genes are transferred into any somatic or body cell other than germ cell or gamete or gametocyte or undifferentiated stem cell. The changes or modifications that might follow will be restricted to the individual patient who has received the gene and not the future generation. Since somatic cells are nonreproductive, there is no inheritance of the character by the offspring of the patient. The technique is, therefore, considered conservative and safer than the germline gene therapy (GGT). In majority of cases, the somatic gene therapy involves integration of therapeutic gene either into the genome of the person or is present as an extrachromosomal plasmid or episome and helps in treating a disease. Certain disorders such as hemophilia, thalassemia, and cystic fibrosis (single gene defects) are excellent candidates for SCGT. It is, however, not possible to target all somatic cells; therefore, complete correction of genetic disorder by this method is not possible (Mavilio et al., 2008). Currently, almost all research directed to correct genetic defects is by SCGT. The technique can be further categorized as follows.

3.7.1.1 EX-VIVO SOMATIC CELL GENE THERAPY

In this case, the sample of patient's cells is removed and exposed to the vector that is carrying the desired gene. The target cells might be bone marrow cells that are easy to isolate and propagate in laboratory. The cells containing the vector are transplanted back or returned to the patient. If the procedure is successful, the therapeutic gene would start expressing and make a functional protein in the transplanted cells (Figure 3.13). Since the cells are treated outside the body of recipient and then transplanted back, the process is called ex-vivo gene therapy. Bone marrow cells generally continue to divide in the body and produce blood cells so are used in correcting those genetic defects involving blood cells. The process can be performed in other somatic cells as well such as lungs, muscle, or liver cells; however, gaining access to these cells can be difficult in many cases. The technique is mostly applied in patients of β-thalassemia and certain cancers.

3.7.1.2 IN-VIVO SOMATIC CELL GENE THERAPY

In this case, the genes are introduced in the cells, when the target cell is within the patient's body, hence called in-vivo therapy. Once inside the body and in contact with the target cells, the injected DNA gets incorporated into the target cell and starts expression of desired protein (Figure 3.14). The vector used in this procedure is mostly viral vector; though liposome or plasmid-mediated transport is also possible. The technique is mostly applied in cases where it is difficult to culture cells *in vitro* from the patient and equally difficult to reimplant the altered cells back into the patient, for example, brain cells. Technique is useful with patients of spinal muscular dystrophy, retinitis pigmentosa, etc.

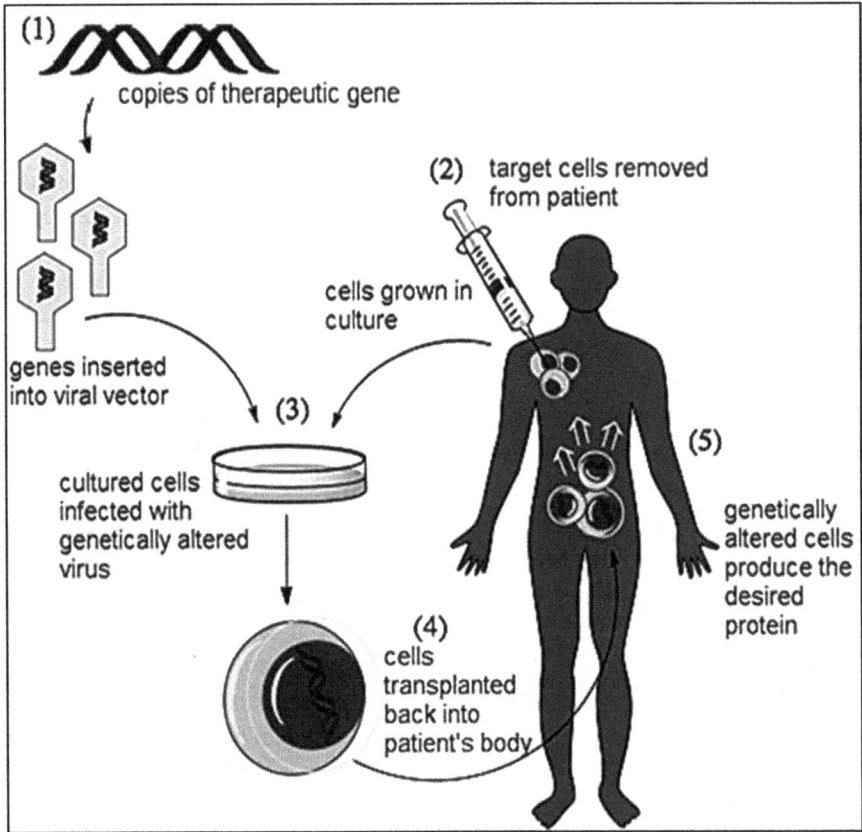

FIGURE 3.13   Ex-vivo somatic cell gene therapy.
Source: Adapted from https://commons.wikimedia.org/wiki/File:ExVivoGeneTherapy.jpg; <a href="https://commons.wikimedia.org/wiki/File:ExVivoGeneTherapy.jpg" title="via Wikimedia Commons">Lizanne Koch</a>/Public domain

3.7.2   GERMLINE GENE THERAPY

In this case, the germ cells, that is, sperm or egg cells are altered by introducing functional genes into their genome. This can result in permanent

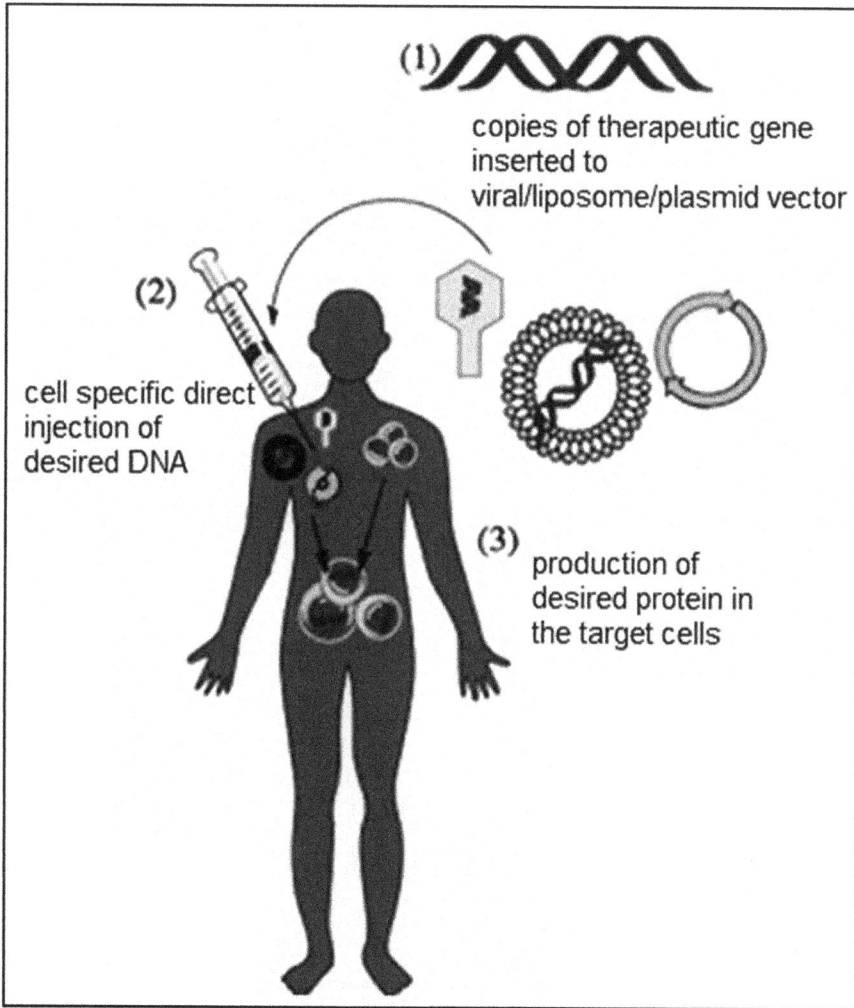

FIGURE 3.14 In-vivo somatic cell gene therapy.
Source: Adapted from https://commons.wikimedia.org/wiki/File:In_vivo_gene_therapy.jpg; <a href="https://commons.wikimedia.org/wiki/File:In_vivo_gene_therapy.jpg" title="via Wikimedia Commons">Lizanne Koch</a>/Public domain

change that is passed down to future generations. It can also be done in early embryological development and can ensure the foreign gene in all cells of the embryo (Figure 3.15). Successful GGT can ensure the possibility of complete removal of certain genetic diseases from some families; however, there are many controversies associated with this technique. Some people view this as unnatural and compare it to "playing God" while some present certain technical problems with concern for certain unforeseen negative effects in later generations as it is sometimes difficult to predict the possible site of insertion of the new gene in the genome and it may lead to harmful consequences. There can also be some ethical issues involved as the therapy can be used for enhancements or in creating "designer babies" or genetically modified babies. The technique is, hence, prohibited in European Union and many other nations around the world.

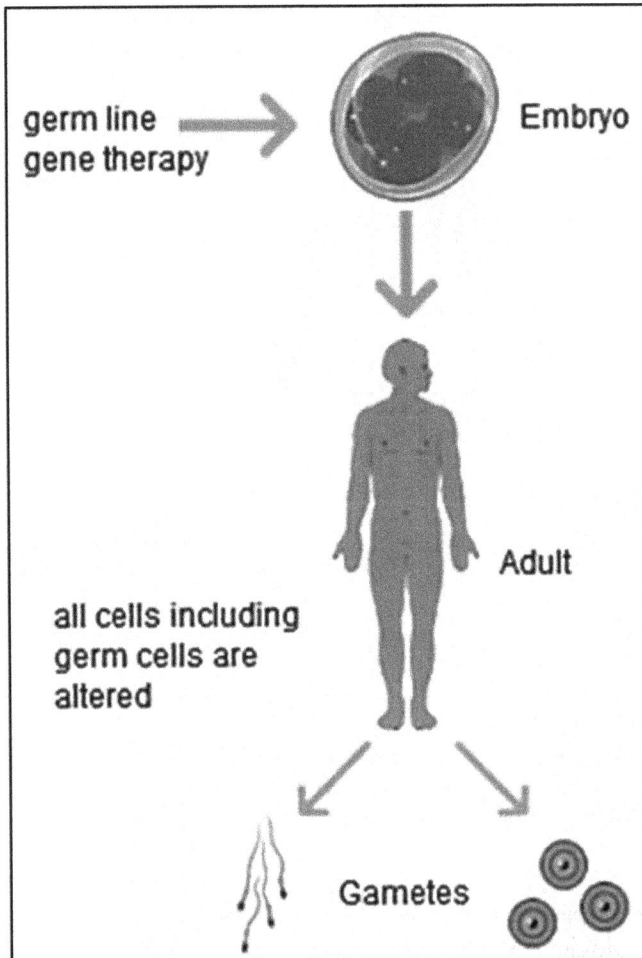

FIGURE 3.15   Germline gene therapy.
Source: Reprinted from https://images.app.goo.gl/grKRTkhXUCFkkeg1A. Image created by Sonya Frazier.

3.8 DISEASES TARGETED FOR GENE THERAPY

Gene therapy was initially considered for disease due to single gene defects, for example, cystic fibrosis and hemophilia. Two types of diseases are now treated by gene therapy which are discussed in the following sections.

3.8.1 MONOGENIC DISEASES

Diseases caused due to defect in single locus (gene), for example, sickle cell anemia, cystic fibrosis, hemophilia, Duchenne muscular dystrophy, Huntington's disease, hypercholesterolemia, emphysema, phenylketonuria, chronic granulomatous disease, Fanconi anemia, and Gaucher disease. These diseases are typically transferred from one generation to next generation. In most cases, the genes for the diseases are carried in heterozygous condition in normal individuals and disease occurs only if recessive allele is present in homozygous condition. However, it gets difficult to perform gene therapy if disease is due to dominant allele as in such cases besides introducing normal allele, removal of dominant allele becomes mandatory.

3.8.2 MULTIFACTORIAL DISEASES

In these diseases, either there are defects present in multiple genes (polygenic) or certain environmental factors (diet, infection, and lack of exercise) are involved, for example, heart disease, cancer, diabetes, Alzheimer's disease, and schizophrenia. Most of these diseases are caused due to combination of both genetic predisposition triggered by environmental factors such as in case of heart diseases, some individuals exhibit some mutation in genes expressing low-density lipoprotein receptors that help in movement of cholesterol inside the cells. This along with environmental factors can trigger development of problems in the normal functioning of heart. All these diseases can be treated with gene therapies. Table 3.2 gives further details about such diseases and the gene therapy employed in each case.

3.9 VECTORS USED IN GENE THERAPY

The gene therapy involves introduction of therapeutic gene into the patient's cell and this can be achieved by two methods: (1) viral vectors and (2) nonviral vectors. The most important characteristic of the vector that is chosen is that it should ensure *regulated* and *sustained* expression of introduced gene in **specific** cells or tissues of the host, without producing any harmful side effects. The vectors that are currently used are as follows:

TABLE 3.2   Human Diseases Treated by Gene Therapy

Single Gene Defect Diseases	
Diseases	**Targets**
Hemophilia A and B	Factor VIII and Factor IX
Cystic fibrosis	CFTR
Phenylketonuria	Phenylalanine hydroxylase
Pituitary dwarfism	hGH
Severe combined immunodeficiency (SCID)	Adenosine deaminase (ADA)
Hyperammonemia	Ornithine transcarbamylase
Duchenne muscular dystrophy	Dystrophin
Gaucher disease	Glucocerebrosidase
Emphysema	Alpha-1 antitrypsin
Multifactorial Diseases	
Diseases	Corrective Genes Used
Cardiovascular diseases	Myocardial infarction/heart attack (tPA)
Cancer	Interleukins and tumor suppressor
Alzheimer's disease	Nerve growth factor (NGF)
Rheumatoid arthritis	IL-1 antagonists
Acquired immunodeficiency syndrome (AIDS)	Cytokines, thymidine kinase (TK) gene, and cytomegalovirus infection

3.9.1   VIRAL VECTORS

Viruses have a tendency to encapsulate and deliver their gene in human cells to cause pathogenesis. This ability of the viruses has been exploited by scientists to deliver gene of interest in patient's cell. The disease causing genes of the virus are removed and replaced with desired gene. Once inside, the gene gets expressed by the cell's machinery, producing therapeutic protein that cures the disease. Viruses currently used as vector are as follows:

3.9.1.1   RETROVIRUS

It is the most commonly used gene delivery vehicle of human cells, as it can integrate therapeutic gene up to the size of 8 kb into the genome of the host cell. The inserted gene, therefore, becomes a permanent part of the host genome and can be expressed for a very long time. Target cells for retrovirus are generally dividing or proliferating cells. Lentiviruses and gammaretroviruses are the subclasses of retrovirus that are employed in gene therapy.

3.9.1.2   ADENOVIRUS

It is the most common virus that infects human respiratory tracts. It does not integrate its DNA into host genome. The insert size can be about 7–8 kb long. Its major advantage is that besides dividing cells, it can also infect in nondividing cells (Figure 3.16). Besides, majority of the patients have antibodies already present against this virus therefore, it gets cleared from the body very fast hence, ineffective for long-term therapy.

3.9.1.3   ADENO-ASSOCIATED VIRUS (AAV)

It is a single-stranded, small-sized human virus that requires helper adenovirus for its replication. It can infect both dividing and nondividing cells and can persist in an extrachromosomal state without integrating into the genome of the host cell. Due to its small size, not more than 4.5 kb of insert could only be accommodated.

3.9.1.4   HERPES SIMPLEX VIRUS (HSV)

This virus can introduce genes into cells of nervous system, hence called neurotropic virus. It is a double-stranded DNA virus and can accommodate a large insert.

3.9.2   NONVIRAL VECTORS

Most of the gene therapy attempts employ viral vectors due to their higher rate of transfection; however, they all have some safety issues associated with them. In recent times, nonviral vectors have proved to have better advantage over the viral vectors as they can be produced at larger scale and have low host immunogenicity. Furthermore, changes incorporated into these vectors have enhanced their transfection efficiencies. Some of these vectors are:

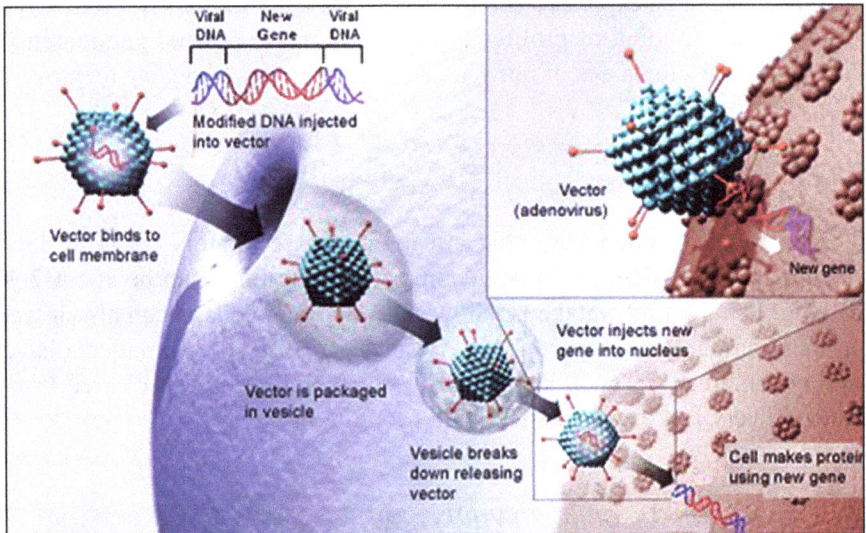

FIGURE 3.16   Gene therapy using an adenovirus
Source: https://commons.wikimedia.org/wiki/File:Figure_17_01_08.jpg). CNX OpenStax/ CC BY (https://creativecommons.org/licenses/by/4.0

3.9.2.1   DNA CONSTRUCT

This involves direct introduction of pure DNA constructs into target tissues. Though the efficiency of DNA uptake by cells and its further expression is much less, hence large amounts of DNA constructs are used for the purpose. Electroporation and gene gun are the methods employed to deliver DNA in such cases.

3.9.2.2   LIPOPLEXES AND DNA MOLECULAR CONJUGATES

These are artificial lipid-based DNA delivery system that employs lipid-DNA conjugates. There are three types of lipids: (1) anionic (negatively charged), (2) neutral, or (3) cationic (positively charged). Anionic and neutral lipids were initially used for the construction of lipoplexes for synthetic vectors. The delivery of such complexes was achieved by liposomes in human target cells. However, such lipoplexes were easily degraded by the host lysosomes. Henceforth, the cationic peptide poly-L-lysine (PLL) has been widely used that binds to the specific target receptor, forming DNA molecular conjugates and avoids lysosomal breakdown of DNA inside the cell.

3.9.2.3 HUMAN ARTIFICIAL CHROMOSOMES (HAC)

It is a microchromosome that can act as a new chromosome in a population of human cells. It is very small [6–10 megabases (Mb) in size compared to 50–250 Mb for natural chromosomes] and can accommodate large sequences (>100 kb) compared to other vectors. The advantages of using HAC vectors are that they remain autonomous and act as a normal chromosome thus, there is no integration of exogenous DNA in the host chromosome.

3.10   NONVIRAL GENE TRANSFECTION METHODS

Delivery of desired therapeutic gene can be achieved either by viral transduction as already discussed or by the use of certain "physical" or "chemical" methods. However, such methods have less efficiency as compared to viral transductions, as there is lower uptake across plasma membrane, inadequate DNA release, and inefficient nuclear targeting. These methods can be categorized as follows:

3.10.1   PHYSICAL METHODS

These methods use physical tools to achieve nucleic acid transfection. They are effective in transferring primary, progenitor, or stem cells; however, cells may sustain heavy trauma. The methods also require precision and accuracy for success.

3.10.1.1   GENE GUN/BIOLISTIC PARTICLE DELIVERY

The method employs high pressure delivery system to shoot tissues with gold or tungsten particles that are coated with DNA (Figure 3.17).

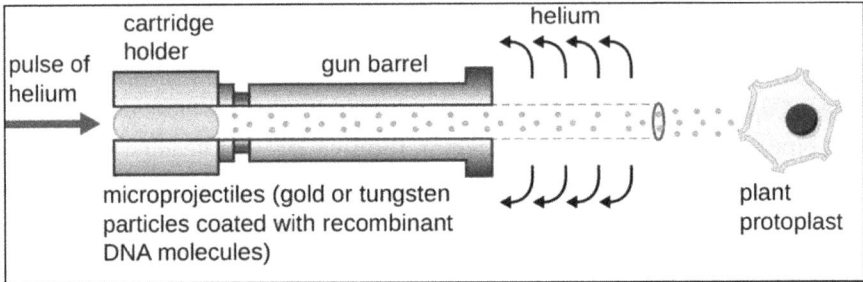

FIGURE 3.17   Gene gun.
Source: Image by CNX OpenStax. https://vi.wikipedia.org/wiki/T%E1%BA%ADp_tin:
OSC_Microbio_12_01_GeneGun.jpg (https://creativecommons.org/licenses/by/4.0/deed.en)

3.10.1.2   MICROINJECTION

This method uses a glass micropipette to insert microscopic substances including nucleic acids into living cells (Figure 3.18). The method requires an optical microscope commonly called micromanipulator. Generally, it is very precise but time-consuming and expensive.

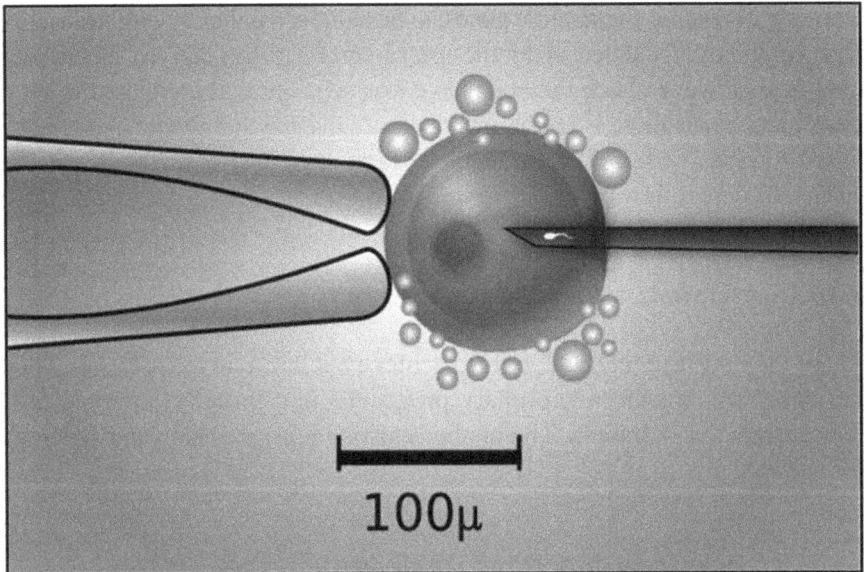

FIGURE 3.18   Microinjection of human egg.
Source: Image by KDS444. https://commons.wikimedia.org/wiki/File:Microinjection_of_a_
human_egg.svg) KDS444/CC BY-SA (https://creativecommons.org/licenses/by-sa/3.0

3.10.1.3 ELECTROPORATION

It is a convenient method for stable transfection of any cell type. However, it requires high cell number due to high rate of cell death during the procedure, hence not suitable for sensitive cells such as primary cells. During the process, mixture of cells and nucleic acid to be introduced are subjected to intense electric field (Figure 3.19). This leads to transient destabilization of cell membrane increasing its permeability to foreign nucleic acids. After removal of electric field, the membrane resumes its stability with the foreign nucleic acid in the cytoplasm of the cell. The method is easy but expensive.

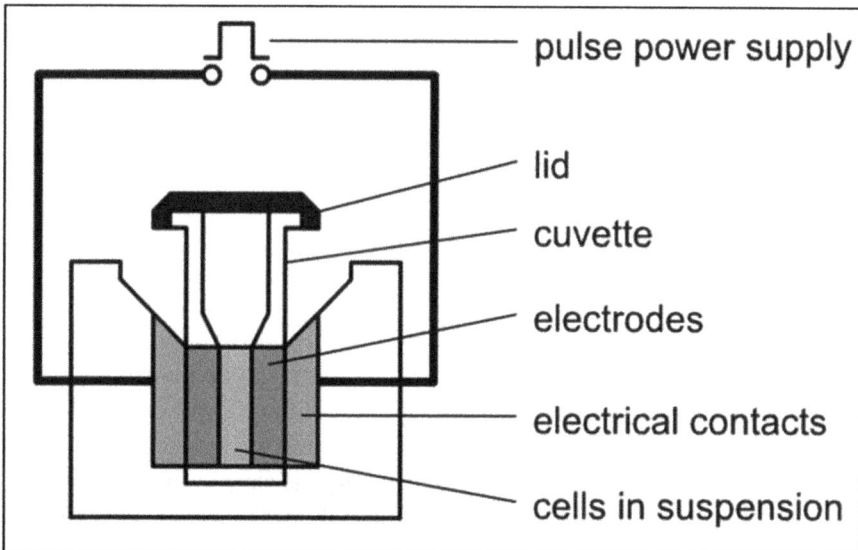

FIGURE 3.19 Electroporation.
Source: Image by Richard Wheeler. https://commons.wikimedia.org/wiki/File: Electroporation_Diagram.png (http://creativecommons.org/licenses/by-sa/3.0/

3.10.2 CHEMICAL-BASED DELIVERY

These methods make use of ligands that target delivery to precise cells. These methods are very effective in gene delivery in cancer cells; however, the dose of chemicals used can prove to be toxic for living cells. Such methods are, therefore, not suitable for primary progenitor or stem cells.

3.10.2.1   DETERGENT

Certain charged chemical compounds such as calcium phosphate are mixed with desired DNA (mostly cDNA). This mixture is used with the target cells. The detergent disturbs the target cell membrane making it porous, which allows the DNA to pass through it. The method is simple and inexpensive, but is dependent on cell constitution, pH, and purity and amount of nucleic acid used.

3.10.2.2   LIPOFECTION

This method makes use of liposomes. Liposome can be defined as artificial phospholipid vesicles that are used to deliver a variety of molecules including nucleic acids into the cells. They form a complex with therapeutic nucleic acid. These complexes pass through the cell membrane and releases foreign DNA into the cytoplasm. The method is inexpensive and reliable and yields stable transfections.

3.10.2.3   CATIONIC POLYMERS

Nucleic acids can form complex with certain cationic polymers such as diethylaminoethyl (DEAE) dextran. This complex can be picked up by the target cells by endocytosis. Once inside the cell, if the complex escapes lysosomal degradation, then the nucleic acids can reach the cytosol of the target cell leading to transgene expression. The method is simple and inexpensive, but efficiency is poor. Also, these cationic polymers tend to be toxic and hence not used with primary cells.

3.11   SUCCESS STORIES OF GENE THERAPY

Gene fixing by gene therapy has cured many patients, especially having single gene defects. It holds great promise for many other diseases such as cancer, heart disease, diabetes, and AIDS. Some of the most notable examples of gene therapy are:

1. *Adenosine deaminase-severe combined immunodeficiency*: Also called bubble boy disease. Tremendous work has been done to cure

this disease. *ADA* gene has been introduced in bone marrow of such patients who were born with obsolete immune system. The patients are currently leading normal lives without the need of any further treatments (Fischer et al., 2010; Gaspar et al., 2014; Otsu et al., 2015).

2. *Blindness*: Leber congenital amaurosis (LCA) is an inherited disease caused by an abnormality in a gene called RPE65. The disease appears just after birth and leads to severe vision loss and eventually total blindness. Using gene therapy, vision has been restored in many patients (Bainbridge et al., 2008).

3. *Parkinson's disease*: Gene therapy has significantly reduced the weakness of the symptoms associated with this neurodegenerative disease. AAV vector carrying glutamic acid decarboxylase gene was introduced in subthalamic nucleus of the patients. The cells gain the function of producing gamma-aminobutyric acid neurotransmitters and hence re-establish normal chemical balance (Le Witt et al., 2011).

4. *X-linked chronic granulomatus disorder*: The disease makes the person highly susceptible to microbial infections. As per the latest reports of the nine patients who received the therapy, six are currently in remission and no longer receiving other treatments (Kohn et al., 2020).

5. Multiple gene therapy has also been developed for diseases such as cancers and many of these trials are in phase III, hence raising our hopes to combat such dreaded disease (Zhang et al., 2018).

3.12 ADVANTAGES AND DISADVANTAGES OF GENE THERAPY

The advantages of gene therapy are much profound as compared to the difficulties that are faced by the scientists. These are as follows:

1. Gene therapy has the potential to cure certain hereditary diseases such as cystic fibrosis, ADA-SCID, and hemophilia.

2. Cure against certain diseases such as cancer is possible through gene therapy.

3. It provides a new chance to a person born with genetic defect to lead a normal life.

4. Gene therapy may be the only alternative to cure certain diseases for which we have been unsuccessful in finding any cure.

The gene therapy technology has the potential to revolutionize medical science; however, there are some hurdles that tend to slow the progress. These are as follows:

1. *Short-lived therapy*: The therapeutic gene that is introduced into dividing cells does not remain functional for a longer duration. The target cell also loses its stability, hence leading to multiple treatments.

2. *Triggers immune response*: The therapeutic gene containing viral vectors is often perceived as foreign bodies or antigens by the immune system that mounts an immune response making the whole process useless. Immune response is also triggered against foreign DNA, if inserted directly in host tissues.

3. *Difficulties associated with viral vectors*: Viral vectors used for the therapy can themselves lead to toxicity or inflammation in the host. Besides, there is a persistent danger of viruses turning virulent by acquiring new genes.

4. *Ineffective in multigene disorder*: Gene therapy has been found to be effective in single gene disorders. In certain diseases such as heart disease or arthritis, many genes are involved and this can be difficult to treat with this therapy.

5. *Mutation due to wrong insertions*: If the foreign DNA gets inserted at a position other than the expected place, it can lead to mutation in the gene that might express a harmful protein. For example, if the therapeutic gene gets inserted in tumor suppressing gene, it might lead to initiation of tumor in the host.

6. *Expensive*: It is an expensive therapy and most of the times the patient requires multiple cycles of gene therapy, for example, Alipogene tiparvovec is a gene therapy treatment against lipoprotein lipase deficiency that can cause severe pancreatitis and costs around at a cost of $1.6 million (approximately 12 crores in INR) per patient (Crasto, 2013; Gaudet et al., 2016).

3.13   ETHICAL ISSUES IN GENE THERAPY

Medical ethics become very important, especially when changes are leading to changes in the genomes. Some of the concerns are:

1. Can gene therapy be equated to "playing God", especially when germline changes are made and effects the future generations?

2. Is it right to use gene therapy at prenatal stage as it might increase the rate of abortions?
3. Should gene therapy be allowed to change basic human traits such as intelligence, height, or other physical appearances? Athletes might make use of the therapy to improve their performance and ability.
4. Will the therapy be used for rich and famous due to its high cost?

These are some of the concerns that have limited the use of gene therapy, especially the germline therapy, which is banned in almost all European countries.

3.14   FUTURE OF GENE THERAPY IN TISSUE ENGINEERING

Research in basic biology and medicine to repair, regenerate, and heal diseased and damaged tissues is propelled by the biomedical technology to apply in clinics for successful tissue regeneration and therapy. Tissue engineering is the new biomedical field that enables the stem cells to proliferate, differentiate, and model themselves to induce tissue regeneration, thus resulting in regenerative therapies for innumerable diseases. The recent advent of molecular biology techniques has revolutionized information about genome and gene manipulation, which had opened new horizons for gene therapy of several diseases and tissue engineering. Thus, gene therapy in tissue engineering is achieved for a huge range of different engineered tissues by combining various vectors, scaffolds, biomaterials, and the suitable gene of information and methodology. In tissue engineering, development of nonviral vectors of synthetic materials for enhanced transfection efficiency of gene both *in vivo* and *in vitro* has been obtained for future direction of gene delivery technology. Many gene therapies with genetically engineered cells were performed using viral as well as nonviral vectors wherein nonviral delivery is considered to be superior with developed concept on plasmid DNA release.

3.14.1   IN-VIVO TRANSFER

This approach pertains to the delivery of the targeted gene directly to the host's cell or tissue at a specific site. Thus, in-vivo gene therapy reduces risk of contamination due to only one procedural step. The disadvantages for this approach are that it does not remain specific for its gene expression as there are chances of low protein expression in the target cells and high expression of growth factors in the secondary tissues. It may also lead to inactivation or degradation of vectors and clearance from the injected site. These challenges associated with the delivery of direct injection that can be solved using suitable scaffolds with bioactive signal. The limitations of direct in-vivo delivery are being fostered by combining tissue engineering with gene therapy. A polymer scaffold is tagged along with the plasmid DNA for a sustained gene delivery and the extent for internalization. The scaffold helps in slow release of the DNA by delaying the clearance from targeted site and protects the DNA from degradation and immune responses. A scaffold can also hold a good number of transfected cells to reduce the use of viral as well as nonviral vectors. Adenovirus carrying the gene for PDGF (Jin et al., 2004) and *BMP7* gene (Dunn et al., 2005) was found useful in wound healing and stimulation of bone and collagen growth. These vectors are also incorporated into a scaffold to aid bone repair. In nonviral vector approach, gene-activated matrix (GAM) scaffolds are used to deliver plasmid DNA directly to the target cells. The gene gets automatically diffused due to high DNA catabolism in the bloodstream (Bonadio, 2000). Nonviral vectors, as GAM, were first used in bone repair for direct plasmid gene transfer (Fang et al., 1996). There are also known methods where delivery of the engineered gene directly to the target site in-vivo was performed without the use of any scaffolds. In such cases, viral vectors approach have remained the choice for gene delivery ex vivo due to their high efficiency in transfecting many cells and diminishing any toxic effects from transfection (Partridge and Oreffo, 2004). Adenoviruses carrying genes for bone and cartilage growth and differentiation, such as BMP13, growth differentiation factor 6 or cartilage-derived morphogenetic protein-2, recovered tendon and ligament tissues in animal experiments (Helm et al., 2001). Though they are reported to not elicit any surge of hypersensitivity, but one report on direct in-vivo introduction has shown that the viral vector was not entirely operative due to immune intrusion (Musgrave et al., 1999). Viral vectors in gene therapy raise serious safety concerns regarding generation of cancer due to repercussion of mutations, genetic modifications, and intercellular trafficking (Nathwani et al., 2004). Due to safety issues, nonviral approaches such as gene gun delivery, microinjection, and electroporation are preferred where a naked DNA can be directly delivered (Jaroszeski et al., 1999; Davidson et al., 2000). As no scaffold is used, plasmid DNA is condensed onto polymers or lipid formulations to increase transfection and uptake and protect it from degradation (Garnett et al., 1999; Agarwal et al., 2005). However, nonviral approach too has its demerits as it is less viable and unmethylated plasmid DNA is immunogenic (Partridge and Oreffo, 2004).

3.14.2 EX-VIVO TRANSFER

This approach pertains to genetic manipulation of the stem cell in culture and reintroducing the cells into the patient's body with or without a scaffold. Ex-vivo transfer is much safer as minimal immune responses are elicited against the viral particles or transfection agents. With the increase of procedural steps, there is a risk of contamination as the patient undergoes two invasive steps. The survival rate of transfected engineered cells *in vivo* is very low and there are chances of migrating to nonrelated sites via circulation; thus delivery of the therapeutic protein becomes difficult. To overcome this challenge, cells can be transplanted to porous polymer matrices scaffolds. The scaffolds can be selected depending upon the cell types, location, and the mode of vector vehicle. The use of scaffolds is mostly significant in repair of structural tissues such as bone and proposes a tremendous prospect for the assimilation of gene vectors. Adenoviruses seeded onto the matrix or a collagen sponge showed spine regeneration in rats (Wang et al., 2003). Adenovirus BMP2 vectors (adenovirus carrying human BMP2 cDNA) incorporated with different BMP genes are able to grow bone marrow, fibroblasts, mesenchymal stem cells, and chondrocytes (Lieberman et al., 1999). In case of nonviral approach, naked plasmid DNA or condensed DNA encoding BMP4 is incorporated on scaffolds made of hydroxyapatite, PGA, PLA, and collagen. This approach was particularly important in vascular and urothelial tissue engineering as well as in bone and cartilage regeneration (Jiang et al., 2005).

Finally, the ultimate aim of gene therapy is to deliver the gene of interest to the targeted site in a one-step approach. Scaffolds in tissue engineering help in providing a template for tissue formation, a physical support for cell adhesion for smooth delivery of gene or DNA, and induce specific cellular processes. Thus, the appropriate choice of scaffold is of prime importance and should consider the cell types, vector or gene, and the anatomical location it can support. Some studies have shown that wrong choice of scaffold may lead to nonspecific tissue response leading to activation and invasion of macrophages, neutrophils, and dendritic cells causing tissue damage (Weiler et al., 2000). Ono et al. (2004) have demonstrated that scaffolds of hydroxyapatite do not enable sufficient cells to enter and thus hindered osteogenesis. Regardless of these disadvantages, use of scaffolds is preferred as degradation of these polymers can be controlled for effective resorption, gene delivery, and tissue growth. Also, the delivery of more than one gene can be made possible, for example, GAM approaches can be harnessed for effective tissue engineering (Fang et al., 1996). Another study reported that a poly(lactic-*co*-glycolic acid) scaffold used for delivery of polyethylenimine-complexed DNA caused increased tissue regeneration (Huang et al., 2005b). Hence, most studies have indicated that use of scaffold definitely benefits gene therapy and FDA has approved the use of synthetic polymers as tools for gene delivery in tissue engineering. Nevertheless, gene therapy in tissue engineering is at research level and lots of improvement is still required in terms of vector, scaffolds, materials, level, and control of gene expression (Partridge and Oreffo, 2004). At present, clinical trials are mainly done using viral vectors but in the long run, nonviral vectors have to be improvised for safety and convenience.

3.15   CHALLENGES IN TISSUE ENGINEERING AND GENE THERAPY

As we come to the conclusion, this chapter lets us question our beliefs, present concerns, and past developments. Indeed a marriage of gene therapy to tissue engineering holds immense promise for future clinical prospects but at the same time, there are many challenges that are yet to be fulfilled. First challenge is to identify the disease characteristics as many susceptible genes prone to mutations are yet not known. Most of the prominent genetic diseases such as cystic fibrosis, muscular dystrophy, and Huntington's disease are caused by mutations in specific/single gene. There are certain other genetic disorders with hereditary disposition, such as cancer, dystonia, and Alzheimer's disease, which are controlled by not only several genes but epigenetic factors too have influence. Patients are usually screened before enrolling into any clinical trials for gene therapy as the same disease may be associated with several genes or a single gene may be responsible for cause of many diseases. Additionally, the mutation in one gene can affect many cell types such as, for example, cystic fibrosis affects both lungs and digestive system, so the gene therapy agent may need to replace the defective gene in more than one tissue or organ. Similarly, in diseases such as muscular dystrophy, innumerable cells throughout the body need correction which makes delivery of the genes a much challenging task. Sometimes, mutations are caused in multiple genes such as in cancer, thus making the choice of a single gene therapy more difficult. The diseased animal's models for clinical trials may not completely mimic the human system as the vectors may behave differently in terms of delivery and penetration into the tissue. A new gene inserted into patient's cellular system often affects the expression of surrounding sequences and vice versa. In such a scenario, short DNA segments are added with the gene of interest to insulate it from surrounding genes. Challenges are also seen in harvesting the appropriate number of cells and their expansion in culture for one or multiple patients. Often cells are harvested in more number and later transformed to iPSCs, thus allowing them to transform into a variety of cell types without the fear of immune rejection. Maintenance of such iPSCs in cultures and introducing them at the correct target site is a major challenge. Moreover, there is a risk that these new specialized cells may grow into tumors if not controlled for their growth and cell division. Also, there are chances of immune rejection as immune responses in human to vectors (as compared to animal models) may not be congenial.

The second most important challenge is in the expansion of genetically modified stem cells in culture before it is seeded into the scaffold for a desired duration of time. This may sounds simple; but it requires extensive studies for optimization. Postdelivery, there is a great deal of modalities that needs to be addressed regarding identification of promoter/control elements to ensure the production of the appropriate protein. This is basically achieved by introducing the "gene cassette" within the vector or the genome of the cells and by studying the vehicle properties in different tissue culture. If everything goes fine, then they are taken to the next level to be seeded into the scaffold for tissue engineering. This step may require further improvisation by adding new control elements to obtain results. Furthermore, introducing a bioengineered scaffold with desired genetically modified stem cells into humans needs much deliberation on understanding the immune responses; in some cases immune system needs to be boosted and in others suppressed.

Lastly, both tissue engineering and gene therapy are extremely costly endeavors. In USA, such funding is mostly provided by the NIH and private foundations for basic or applied research for gene and cell therapy as well as tissue engineering. Huge investment is doled for preclinical studies; mostly in laboratories, that may at the most suggest the potential benefit of a particular gene therapy in tissue engineering. Moving to the clinical trials still remains a huge challenge as it requires additional funding for extensive research on natural products as candidates for scaffolds in tissue engineering and manufacturing of clinical grade reagents. Last but not the least, a tremendous challenge is encountered for costs of clinical trials, ethical issues, and preparation of colossal regulatory documents. Despite all these, gene therapy and tissue engineering hold tremendous potential in treating fatal inherited diseases and can prove a blessing for afflicted patients.

KEYWORDS

- tissue engineering
- gene therapy
- regenerative medicine
- scaffold
- stem cells
- viral vectors

REFERENCES

Abbott, A. Gene therapy. Italians first to use stem cells. *Nature*. **1992**, 356(6369): 465.

Abedin, E., Lari, R., Shahri, N. M. and Fereidoni, M. Development of a demineralized and decellularized human epiphyseal bone scaffold for tissue engineering: A histological study. *Tissue Cell*. **2018**, 55: 46–52.

Agarwal, A., Unfer, R. and Mallapragada, S. K. Novel cationic copolymers as non-viral vectors for gene therapy. *J Control Release*. **2005,** 103: 245–258.

Aldana, A. A. and Abraham, G. A. Current advances in electrospun gelatin-based scaffolds for tissue engineering applications. *Int J Pharma*. **2017,** 523(2): 441–453.

Ananthaswamy, A. Undercover genes slip into the brain. *New Scientist*. **2003**, https://www.newscientist.com/article/dn3520-undercover-genes-slip-into-the-brain/?ignored=irrelevant (retrieved 17 August, 2010).

Asahara, T., Kalka, C. and Isner, J. M. Stem cell therapy and gene transfer for regeneration. *Gene Ther.* **2000,** 7: 451–457.

Ashammakhi, N., Hasan, A., Kaarela, O., Byambaa, B., Sheikhi, A., Gaharwar, A. K. et al. Advancing frontiers in bone bioprinting. *Adv Healthc Mater*. **2019**, 8(7): e1801048.

Atala, A., Bauer, S. B., Soker, S., Yoo, J. J. and Retik, A. B. Tissue-engineered autologous bladders for patients needing cystoplasty. *Lancet*. **2006,** 367(9518): 1241–1246.

Avanzi, M. P. and Brentjens, R. J. Emerging role of CAR T cells in non-Hodgkin's lymphoma. *J Nat Compr Canc Netw*. **2017**, 15(11): 1429–1437.

Bainbridge, J. W., Smith, A. J., Barker, S. S., Robbie, S., Henderson, R., Balaggan, K. et al. Effect of gene therapy on visual function in Leber's congenital amaurosis. *N Engl J Med*. **2008**, 358(21): 2231–2239.

Blaese, R. M., Culver, K. W., Miller, A. D., Carter, C. S., Fleisher, T., Clerici, M. et al. T lymphocyte-directed gene therapy for ADA-SCID: initial trial results after 4 year. *Science*. **1995,** 270(5235): 475–480.

Bonadio, J. Tissue engineering via local gene delivery. *J Mol Med.***2000**, 78: 303–311.

Bonadio, J. Tissue engineering via local gene delivery: update and future prospects for enhancing the technology. *Adv Drug Deliv Rev*. **2000**, 44: 185–194.

Boquest, A. C., Shahdadfar, A., Fronsdal, K., Sigurjonsson, O., Tunheim, S. H., Collas, P. et al. Isolation and transcription profiling of purified uncultured human stromal stem cells: alteration of gene expression after *in vitro* cell culture. *Mol Biol Cell.* **2005**, 16: 1131–1141.

Bruder, S. P., Kurth, A. A., Shea, M., Hayes, W. C., Jaiswal, N. and Kadiyala, S. Bone regeneration by implantation of purified, culture expanded human mesenchymal stem cells. *J Orthop Res*. **1998**, 16: 155–162.

Bryant, S. J. and Vernerey, F. J. Programmable hydrogels for cell encapsulation and neo-tissue growth to enable personalized tissue engineering. *Adv Healthc Mater.* **2018**, 7: 1700605.

Cavazzana-Calvo, M., Payen, E., Negre, O., Wang, G., Hehir, K., Fusil, F. et al. Transfusion independence and HMGA2 activation after gene therapy of human β-thalassaemia. *Nature*. **2010**, 467(7313): 318–322.

Cepko, C. L., Roberts, B. E. and Mulligan, R. C. Construction and applications of a highly transmissible murine retrovirus shuttle vector. *Cell*. **1984**, 37(3): 1053–1062.

Chaneton, B., Hillmann, P., Zheng, L., Martin, A. C., Maddocks, O. D., Chokkathukalam, A. et al. Serine is a natural ligand and allosteric activator of pyruvate kinase M2. *Nature*. **2012**, 491: 458–462.

Chang, K. H., Huang, A., Hirata, R. K., Wang, P. R., Russell, D. W. and Papayannopoulou, T. Globin phenotype of erythroid cells derived from human-induced pluripotent stem cells. *Blood.* **2010**, 115: 2553–2554.

Cho, A. N., Jin, Y., Kim, S., Kumar, S., Shin, H., Kang, H. C. et al. Aligned brain extracellular matrix promotes differentiation and myelination of human-induced pluripotent stem cell-derived oligodendrocytes. *ACS Appl Mater Interfaces.* **2019**, 11: 15344–15353.

Costa, J. B., Silva-Correia, J., Ribeiro, V. P., da Silva Morais, A., Oliveira, J. M. and Reis, R. L. Engineering patient-specific bioprinted constructs for treatment of degenerated intervertebral disc. *Mater Today Commun.* **2019**, 19: 506–512.

Crasto, A. M. Glybera—the most expensive drug in the world & first approved gene therapy in the West. All About Drugs. **2013**, http://www.allfordrugs.com/2013/07/16/glybera-the-most-expensive-drug-in-the-world-first-approved-gene-therapy-in-the-west/ (Retrieved 2 November, 2013).

Davidson, J. M., Krieg, T. and Eming, S. A. Particle-mediated gene therapy of wounds. *Wound Repair Regen.* **2000**, 8: 452–459.

Deev, R. V., Bozo, I. Y., Mzhavanadze, N. D., Voronov, D. A., Gavrilenko, A. V., Chervyakov, Y. V. et al. pCMV-vegf165 intramuscular gene transfer is an effective method of treatment for patients with chronic lower limb ischemia. *J Cardiovasc Pharmacol Ther*. **2015**, 20(5): 473–482.

Dellambra, E., Pellegrini, G., Guerra, L., Ferrari, G., Zambruno, G., Mavilio, F. et al. Toward epidermal stem cell-mediated ex-vivo gene therapy of junctional epidermolysis bullosa. *Hum Gene Ther*. **2000**, 11(16): 2283–2287.

Devarasetty, M., Mazzocchi, A. R. and Skardal, A. Applications of bioengineered 3D tissue and tumor organoids in drug development and precision medicine: current and future. *Biodrugs.* **2018**, 32: 53–68.

Dunn, C. A., Jin, Q., Taba, M., Franceschi, R. T., Rutherford, R. B. and Giannobile, W. VBMP gene delivery for alveolar bone engineering at dental implant defects. *Mol Ther.* **2005**, 11: 294–299.

Eltom, A., Zhong, G. and Muhammad, A. Scaffold techniques and designs in tissue engineering functions and purposes: a review. *Adv Mater Sci Eng.* **2019**, 2: 3429527.

Fang, J., Zhu, Y. Y., Smiley, E., Bonadio, J., Rouleau, J. P., Goldstein, S. A. et al. Stimulation of new bone formation by direct transfer of osteogenic plasmid genes. *Proc Natl Acad Sci USA.* **1996**, 93: 5753–5758.

Fischer, A., Hacein-Bey-Abina, S. and Cavazzana-Calvo, M. 20 years of gene therapy for SCID. *Nat Immunol.* **2010**, 11(6): 457–460.

Foong, C. Y. and Sultana, N. Fabrication of electrospun membranes based on poly(caprolactone) (PCL) and PCL/chitosan layer by layer for tissue engineering. *J Appl Membr Sci Technol.* **2015**, 17: 25–33.

Frazier, S. A., Embryo Gene Editing: Changing Life as We Know It. The Gist. May 31, 2019. Https://The-Gist.Org/2019/05/Embryo-Gene-Editing-Changing-Life-As-We-Know-It/

Friedmann, T. and Roblin, R. Gene therapy for human genetic disease? *Science.* **1972**, 175(4025): 949–955.

Garcia, J., Yang, Z., Mongrain, R., Leask, R. L. and Lachapelle, K. 3D printing materials and their use in medical education: a review of current technology and trends for the future. *BMJ Simul Technol Enhanc Learn.* **2018**, 4: 27–40.

Garnett, M. C. Gene-delivery systems using cationic polymers. *Crit Rev Ther Drug Carrier Syst.* **1999**, 16: 147–207.

Gaspar, H. B., Buckland, K., Rivat, C., Himoudi, N., Gilmour, K., Booth, C., Terrazs, D. et al. Immunological and metabolic correction after lentiviral vector mediated haematopoietic stem cell gene therapy for ADA deficiency. *Mol Ther.* **2014**, 22: S106.

Gaudet, D., Stroes, E. S., Méthot, J., Brisson, D., Tremblay, K., Bernelot-Moens, S. J. et al. Long-term retrospective analysis of gene therapy with alipogene tiparvovec and its effect on lipoprotein lipase deficiency-induced pancreatitis. *Hum Gene Ther.* **2016**, 27(11): 916–925.

Ghazanfari, S., Alberti, K. A., Xu, Q. B. and Khademhosseini, A. Evaluation of an elastic decellularized tendon-derived scaffold for the vascular tissue engineering application. *J Biomed Mater Res.* **2019**, 107: 1225–1234.

Ghosh, P. Gene therapy first for poor sight. BBC News. 1 May **2007**. http://news.bbc.co.uk/2/hi/health/6609205.stm (Retrieved 3 May, 2010).

Goodman, S. B., Yao, Z., Keeney, M. and Yang, F. The future of biologic coatings for orthopaedic implants. *Biomaterials.* **2013**, 34: 3174–3183.

Grant, R., Hallett, J., Forbes, S., Hay, D. and Callanan, A. Blended electrospinning with human liver extracellular matrix for engineering new hepatic microenvironments. *Sci Rep.* **2019**, 9: 6293.

Gregor, A., Filová, E., Novák, M., Kronek, J., Chlup, H., Buzgo, M. et al. Designing of PLA scaffolds for bone tissue replacement fabricated by ordinary commercial 3D printer. *J Biol Eng.* **2017**, 11(1): 31.

Haynesworth, S. E., Baber, M. A. and Caplan, A. I. Cell surface antigens on human marrow-derived mesenchymal cells are detected by monoclonal antibodies. *Bone.* **1992**, 13: 69–80.

Hill, K. L., Obrtlikova, P., Alvarez, D. F., King, J. A., Keirstead, S. A., Allred, J. R. et al. Human embryonic stem cell-derived vascular progenitor cells capable of endothelial and smooth muscle cell function. *Exp Hematol.* **2010**, 38: 246–257.

Howard, D., Partridge, K., Yang, X., Clarke, N. M., Okubo, Y., Bessho, K. et al. Immunoselection and adenoviral genetic modulation of human osteoprogenitors, *in vivo* bone formation on PLA scaffold. *Biochem Biophys Res Commun.* **2002,** 299: 208–215.

Huang, Y. C., Simmons, C., Kaigler, D., Rice, K. G. and Mooney, D. J. Bone regeneration in a rat cranial defect with delivery of PEI-condensed plasmid DNA encoding for bone morphogenetic protein-4 (BMP-4). *Gene Ther.* **2005b,** 12: 418–426.

Hutmacher, D. W. Scaffolds in tissue engineering bone and cartilage. *Biomaterials.* **2000,** 21(24): 2529–2543.

IANS. Army officer treated with new cell based therapy. http://indiatoday. intoday.in/story/army-officer-treated-with-new-cell-based therapy/. July 2, **2015**. Accessed 4 Sept, 2017.

Jang, J., Park, J. Y., Gao, G. and Cho, D. W. Biomaterials-based 3D cell printing for next-generation therapeutics and diagnostics. *Biomaterials.* **2018,** 156: 88–106.

Jaroszeski, M. J., Gilbert, R., Nicolau, C. and Heller, R. *In vivo* gene delivery by electroporation. *Adv Drug Deliv Rev.* **1999,** 35: 131–137.

Jiang, X. Q., Chen, J. G., Gittens, S., Chen, C. J., Zhang, X. L. and Zhang, Z. Y. The ectopic study of tissue-engineered bone with hBMP-4 gene modified bone marrow stromal cells in rabbit. *Chin Med J.* **2005,** 118: 281–288.

Jin, Q. M., Anusaksathien, O., Webb, S. A., Printz, M. A. and Giannobile, W. V. Engineering of tooth-supporting structures by delivery of PDGF gene therapy vectors. *Mol Ther.* **2004,** 9: 519–526.

Kehat, I., Kenyagin-Karsenti, D., Snir, M., Segev, H., Amit, M., Gepstein, A., Livne, E., Binah, O., Itskovitz-Eldor, J. and Gepstein, L. Human embryonic stem cells can differentiate into myocytes with structural and functional properties of cardiomyocytes. *J Clin Invest.* **2001,** 108: 407–414.

Knight, M. A. and Evans, G. R. Tissue engineering: progress and challenges. *Plast Reconstr Surg.* **2004,** 114: 26E–37E.

Kohn, D. B., Booth, C., Kang, E. M., Pai, S. Y., Shaw, K. L., Santilli, G. Net4CGD consortium et al. Lentiviral gene therapy for X-linked chronic granulomatous disease. *Nat Med.* **2020,** 26: 200–206.

Lanza, R., Langer, R. and Vacanti, J. P. *Principles of Tissue Engineering,* Academic Press, Cambridge, MA, USA, **2011**.

Lee, K. Y. and Mooney, D. J. Alginate: Properties and biomedical applications. *Prog Polym Sci.* **2012,** 37: 106–126.

Lee, T. H., Song, S. H., Kim, K. L., Yi, J. Y., Shin, G. H., Kim, J. Y. et al. Functional recapitulation of smooth muscle cells via induced pluripotent stem cells from human aortic smooth muscle cells. *Circ Res.* **2010,** 106: 120–128.

Levenberg, S., Rouwkema, J., Macdonald, M., Garfein, E. S., Kohane, D. S., Darland, D. C. et al. Engineering vascularized skeletal muscle tissue. *Nat Biotechnol.* **2005,** 23: 879–884.

Levine, B. L., Humeau, L. M., Boyer, J., MacGregor, R. R., Rebello, T., Lu, X. et al. Gene transfer in humans using a conditionally replicating lentiviral vector. *Proc Nat Acad Sci U S A.* **2006,** 103(46): 17372–17377.

LeWitt, P. A., Rezai, A. R., Leehey, M. A., Ojemann, S. G., Flaherty, A. W., Eskandar, E. N. et al. AAV2-GAD gene therapy for advanced Parkinson's disease: a double-blind, sham-surgery controlled, randomised trial. *Lancet Neurol.* **2011,** 10(4): 309–319.

Lian, Q., Zhang, Y., Zhang, J., Zhang, H. K., Wu, X., Lam, F. F. et al. Functional mesenchymal stem cells derived from human-induced pluripotent stem cells attenuate limb ischemia in mice. *Circulation.* **2010,** 121: 1113–1123.

Lieberman, J. R., Daluiski, A., Stevenson, S., Jolla, L., Wu, L., McAllister, P. et al. The effect of regional gene therapy with bone morphogenetic protein-2-producing bone marrow cells on the repair of segmental femoral defects in rats. *J Bone Joint Surg.* **1999**, 81: 905–917.

Maher B. Tissue engineering: How to build a heart? *Nat News.* **2013**, 499(7456): 20.

Majumdar, M. K., Banks, V., Peluso, D. P. and Morris, E. A. Isolation, characterization, and chondrogenic potential of human bone marrow-derived multipotential stromal cells. *J Cell Physiol.* **2000**, 185: 98–106.

Mavilio, F. and Ferrari, G. Genetic modification of somatic stem cells. The progress, problems and prospects of a new therapeutic technology. *EMBO Rep.* **2008**, 9(1): S64–S69.

Meyer, U., Meyer, T., Handschel, J. and Wiesmann, H. P. *Fundamentals of Tissue Engineering and Regenerative Medicine*, Springer, Berlin, Germany, **2009**.

Miri, A. K., Khalilpour, A., Cecen, B., Maharjan, S., Shin, S. R. and Khademhosseini, A. Multiscale bioprinting of vascularized models. *Biomaterials.* **2019**, 198: 204–216.

Murnaghan, I. Stem cells and radiation sickness. **2015**. http//www.explorestemcells.co.uk/ stem-cells-radiation-sickness.htlm (accessed 2 December 2016).

Musgrave, D. S., Bosch, P., Ghivizanni, S., Robbins, P. D., Evans, C. H. and Huard, J. Adenovirus-mediated direct gene therapy with bone morphogenetic protein-2 produces bone. *Bone.* **1999**, 24: 541–547.

Musgrave, D. S., Bosch, P., Lee, J. Y., Pelinkovic, D., Ghivizzani, S. C., Whalen, J. et al. Ex-vivo gene therapy to produce bone using different cell types. *Clin Orthop Relat Res.* **2000**, 378: 290–305.

Nathwani, A. C., Benjamin, R., Nienhuis, A. W. and Davidoff, A. M. Current status and prospects for gene therapy. *Vox Sanguinis.* **2004**, 87: 73–81.

Nathwani, A. C., Reiss, U. M., Tuddenham, E. G. D., Rosales, C., Chowdary, P. and Davidoff, A. M. Long-term safety and efficacy of factor IX gene therapy in hemophilia B. *N Engl J Med.* **2014**, 371(21): 1994.

Ono, I., Yamashita, T., Jin, H. J., Ito, Y., Hamada, H., Akasaka, Y. et al. Combination of porous hydroxyapatite and cationic liposomes as a vector for BMP-2 gene therapy. *Biomaterials.* **2004**, 25: 4709–4718.

Otsu, M., Yamada, M., Nakajima, S., Kida, M., Maeyama, Y., Hatano, N. et al. Outcomes in two Japanese adenosine deaminase-deficiency patients treated by stem cell gene therapy with no cytoreductive conditioning. *J Clin Immunol.* **2015**, 35(4): 384–398.

Ott, H. C., Matthiesen, T. S., Goh, S. K., Black, L. D., Kren, S. M., Netoff, T. I. et al. Perfusion-decellularized matrix: using nature's platform to engineer a bioartificial heart. *Nat Med.* **2008**, 14(2): 213–221.

Ott, M. G., Schmidt, M., Schwarzwaelder, K., Stein, S., Siler, U., Koehl, U. et al. Correction of X-linked chronic granulomatous disease by gene therapy, augmented by insertional activation of MDS1-EVI1, PRDM16 or SETBP1. *Nat Med.* **2006**, 12(4): 401–409.

Park, J., Lee, S. J., Lee, H., Park, S. A. and Lee, J. Y. Three-dimensional cell printing with sulfated alginate for improved bone morphogenetic protein-2 delivery and osteogenesis in bone tissue engineering. *Carbohydr Polym.* **2018**, 196: 217–224.

Parmaksiz, M., Elçin, A. E. and Elçin, Y. M. Decellularized bovine small intestinal submucosa-PCL/hydroxyapatite-based multilayer composite scaffold for hard tissue repair. *Mater Sci Eng C Mater Biol Appl.* **2019**, 94: 788–797.

Partridge, K. and Oreffo, R. O. C. Gene delivery in bone tissue engineering—progress and prospects using viral and non-viral strategies. *Tissue Eng.* **2004**, 10: 295–307.

Pina, S., Canadas, R. F., Jiménez, G., Perán, M., Marchal, J. A., Reis, R. L. et al. Biofunctional ionic-doped calcium phosphates—silk fibroin composites for bone tissue engineering scffolding. *Cells Tissues Organs.* **2017**, 204: 150–163.

Pollard, A. Stem cell research in India. https://www.ukibc.com/stem-cell-research-in-india/ 02 Jan **2013**. (Accessed 4 Sept, 2017).

Prasad, K., Sharma, A., Garg, A., Mohanty, S., Bhatnagar, S., Johri, S., InveST Study Group. Intravenous autologous bone marrow mononuclear stem cell therapy for ischemic stroke: a multicentric, randomized trial. *Stroke.* **2014**, 45(12): 3618–3624.

Puissant, B., Barreau, C., Bourin, P., Clavel, C., Corre, J., Bousquet, C. et al. Immunomodulatory effect of human adipose tissue-derived adult stem cells: comparison with bone marrow mesenchymal stem cells. *Br J Haematol.* **2005**, 129: 118–129.

Qasim, W., Zhan, H., Samarasinghe, S., Adams, S., Amrolia, P., Stafford, S. et al. Molecular remission of infant B-ALL after infusion of universal TALEN gene-edited CAR T cells. *Sci Transl Med.* **2017**, 9(374): eaaj2013.

Romero, Z., Urbinati, F., Geiger, S., Cooper, A. R., Wherley, J., Kaufman, M. L. et al. β-globin gene transfer to human bone marrow for sickle cell disease. *J Clin Invest.* **2013**, 123(8): 3317–3330.

Roseti, L., Parisi, V., Petretta, M., Cavallo, C., Desando, G., Bartolotti, I. et al. Scaffolds for bone tissue engineering: state of the art and new perspectives. *Mater Sci Eng C.* **2017**, 78: 1246–1262.

Sanzherrera, J., Garciaaznar, J. and Doblare, M. On scaffold designing for bone regeneration: a computational multiscale approach. *Acta Biomater.* **2009**, 5(1): 219–229.

Sestito, S., Falvo, F., Scozzafava, C., Apa, R., Pensabene, L., Bonapace, G. et al.Genetics and Gene Therapy in Hunter Disease. *Curr Gene Ther.* **2018**, 18(2): 90–95.

Simmons, P. J. and Torok-Storb, B. Identification of stromal cell precursors in human bone marrow by a novel monoclonal antibody, STRO-1. *Blood.* **1991**, 78: 55–62.

Stewart, K., Monk, P., Walsh, S., Jefferiss, C. M., Letchford, J. and Beresford, J. N. STRO-1, HOP-26 (CD63), CD49a and SB-10 (CD166) as markers of primitive human marrow stromal cells and their more differentiated progeny, a comparative investigation *in vitro*. *Cell Tissue Res.* **2003**, 313: 281–290.

Stolberg, S. G. The Biotech Death of Jesse Gelsinger. The New York Times Magazine. **1999**, https://www.nytimes.com/1999/11/28/magazine/the-biotech-death-of-jesse-gelsinger. html (Retrieved July 5, 2018).

Sultana, N. Scaffolds for tissue engineering. *MRS Bull.* **2003**, 28(4): 301–306.

Takahashi, K. and Yamanaka, S. Induction of pluripotent stem cells from mouse embryonic and adult fibroblast cultures by defined factors. *Cell.* **2006**, 126(4): 663–676.

Taylor, D. A., Sampaio, L. C., Ferdous, Z., Gobin, A. S. and Taite, L. J. Decellularized matrices in regenerative medicine. *Acta Biomater.* **2018**, 74: 74–89.

Thompson, L. *Correcting the Code: Inventing the Genetic Cure for the Human Body*, Simon & Schuster, **1994**.

Thomson, J. A., Itskovitz-Eldor, J., Shapiro, S. S., Waknitz, M. A., Swiergiel, J. J., Marshall, V. S. et al. Embryonic stem cell lines derived from human blastocysts. *Science.* **1998**, 282: 1145–1147.

Thorrez, L., Shansky, J., Wang, L., Fast, L., Vanden Driessche, T., Chuah, M. et al. Growth, differentiation, transplantation, and survival of human skeletal myofibers on biodegradable scaffolds. *Biomaterials.* **2008**, 29: 75–84.

Ude, C. C., Miskon, A., Idrus, R. B. H. and Abu Bakar, M. B. Application of stem cells in tissue engineering for defense medicine. *Military Med Res.* **2018**, 5(1): 7.

Ude, C. C., Miskon, A., Idrus, R. B. H. et al. Application of stem cells in tissue engineering for defense medicine. Military Med Res 5, 7 (2018). https://doi.org/10.1186/s40779-018-0154-9

Varma, D. M., Gold, G. T., Taub, P. J. and Nicoll, S. B. Injectable carboxymethylcellulose hydrogels for soft tissue filler applications. *Acta Biomater.* **2014**, 10: 4996–5004.

Vats, A., Tolley, N. S., Polak, J. M. and Buttery, L. D. Stem cells: sources and applications. *Clin Otolaryngol.* **2002**, 27: 227–232.

Velasco, D., Quílez, C., Garcia, M., del Cañizo, J. F. and Jorcano, J. L. 3D human skin bioprinting: a view from the bioside. *J 3D Print Med.* **2018**, 2: 141–162.

Wang, J. C., Kanim, L. E. A., Yoo, S., Campbell, P. A., Berk, A. J. and Lieberman, J. R. The effect of regional gene therapy with bone morphogenetic protein-2-producing bone marrow cells on spinal fusion in rats. *J Bone Joint Surg.* **2003**, 85: 905–911.

Wang, S., Lee, J. M. and Yeong, W. Y. Smart hydrogels for 3D bioprinting. *Int J Bioprinting.* **2015**, 1: 3–14.

Wang, Z. Z., Au, P., Chen, T., Shao, Y., Daheron, L. M., Bai, H. et al. Endothelial cells derived from human embryonic stem cells form durable blood vessels *in vivo*. *Nat Biotechnol.* **2007**, 25: 317–318.

Weiler, A., Hoffmann, R. F. G., Stähelin, A. C., Helling, H. J. and Südkamp, N. P. Biodegradable implants in sports medicine: the biological base. *Arthroscopy.* **2000**, 16: 305–321.

Wiles, M. V. and Johansson, B. M. Embryonic stem cell development in a chemically defined medium. *Exp Cell Res.* **1999**, 247: 241–248.

Wilson, J. F. Murine Gene Therapy Corrects Symptoms of Sickle Cell Disease. The Scientist – Magazine of the Life Sciences. **2002**. https://www.the-scientist.com/news/genetic-variation-illuminates-murky-human-history-55766 (Retrieved 17 August, 2010).

Xie, C. Q., Zhang, J., Villacorta, L., Cui, T., Huang, H. and Chen, Y. E. A highly efficient method to differentiate smooth muscle cells from human embryonic stem cells. *Arterioscler Thromb Vasc Biol.* **2007**, 27: e311–e312.

Yang, X., Lu, Z., Wu, H., Li, W., Zheng, L. and Zhao, J. Collagen-alginate as bioink for three-dimensional (3D) cell printing-based cartilage tissue engineering. *Mater Sci Eng C.* **2018**, 83: 195–201.

Yang, X. B., Roach H. I., Clarke N. M., Howdle, S. M., Quirk, R., Shakesheff, K. M. et al. Human osteoprogenitor growth and differentiation on synthetic biodegradable structures after surface modification. *Bone.* **2001**, 29: 523–531.

Yang, Y., Ritchie, A. C. and Everitt, N. M. Comparison of glutaraldehyde and procyanidin cross-linked scaffolds for soft tissue engineering. *Mater Sci Eng C Mater Biol Appl.* **2017**, 80: 263–273.

Yousefi, A. M., James, P. F., Akbarzadeh, R., Subramanian, A., Flavin, C. and Oudadesse, H. Prospect of stem cells in bone tissue engineering: a review. *Stem Cells Int.* **2016**, 2016: 1–13.

Zhang, P., Moudgill, N., Hager, E., Tarola, N., Dimatteo, C., McIlhenny, S. et al. Endothelial differentiation of adipose-derived stem cells from elderly patients with cardiovascular disease. *Stem Cells Dev.* **2011**, 20: 977–988.

Zhang, W. W., Li, L., Li, D., Liu, J., Li, X., Li, W. et al. The first approved gene therapy product for cancer ad-p53 (gendicine): 12 years in the clinic. *Hum Gene Ther.* **2018**, 29: 160–179.

Zhang, Y., Jiang, L. L., Zheng, T. Z., Sha, L., Wang, J. Z., Dong, H. C., et al. Development of decellularized meniscus extracellular matrix and gelatin/chitosan scaffolds for meniscus tissue engineering. *Biomed Mater Eng*. **2019,** 30: 125–132.

Zheng, C. X., Sui, B. D., Hu, C. H., Qiu, X. Y., Zhao, P. and Jin, Y. Reconstruction of structure and function in tissue engineering of solid organs: Toward simulation of natural development based on decellularization. *J Tissue Eng Regen Med*. 2018, 12(6): 1432–1447.

Zuk, P. A., Zhu, M., Mizuno, H., Huang, J., Futrell, J. W., Katz, A. J., et al. Multilineage cells from human adipose tissue: implications for cell-based therapies. *Tissue Eng*. **2001,** 7: 211–228.

WEBLINKS

https://tercit.wordpress.com/

https://www.springer.com/journal/13770

https://home.liebertpub.com/publications/tissue-engineering-parts-a-b-and-c/595/overview

https://www.open.edu/openlearn/science-maths-technology/science/biology/gene-therapy/content-section-5

https://ghr.nlm.nih.gov/primer/therapy/genetherapy

http://www.genetherapynet.com/JoomlaTest2/index.php?option=com_content&view=article&id=164:diseases-treated-with-gene-therapy-&catid=97:patient-information&Itemid=14

https://www.yourgenome.org/facts/what-is-gene-therapy

https://www.genengnews.com/news/gene-therapy-trial-helps-six-x-cgd-patients/

CHAPTER 4

Tissue Engineering and Application in Tropical Medicine

SORA YASRI[1*] and VIROJ WIWANITKIT[2]

[1]Private Academic Practice, Bangkok, Thailand

[2] Department of Community Medicine, Dr DY Patil University, Pune, India

*Corresponding author. E-mail: sorayasri@outlook.co.th

ABSTRACT

The modeling of the natural tissue growth and development is the basic concept and process of the novel tissue engineering. Following the model, the artificial tissue is the desired product of the tissue engineering process that can be applied in therapeutic management of medical problems, especially for those diseases that require tissue replacement of tissue loss. To introduce the new technology such as tissue engineering for management of tropical diseases, it becomes a new challenging issue in tropical medicine. There are many reports on the possible advantages of applications of tissue engineering technology for management of many tropical diseases (such as tropical infections, cancers, and anemias). Focusing on tropical cancers, the possible usefulness is reported in liver and urinary bladder cancers. For tropical anemias, the advantage is mentioned for management of inherited hemoglobin disorder. Furthermore, it is the main question how can we successful introduce the new tissue engineering technology to the resourced-limited tropical countries where the tropical diseases actually exist. The international collaboration for improvement of the tissue engineering technology in developing tropical countries where the problems actually exist is required.

4.1 INTRODUCTION

Anatomically, cell is the basic smallest functional compartment of living things. The groups of cell in our body will form a larger functional unit that is called tissue. Tissue is an important basic part of the body, since it is the main component of the organ in our body. There are various tissues in human body and different tissues have different characteristics and functions. In medicine, the study of tissue is the basic practice requirement for any undergraduate medical students. The histology and histopathology are the main medical subjects that cover the knowledge on normal and pathological tissue. The study on the tissue can help in diagnosis of underlying pathology for several medical disorders. The histopathology is the basic diagnostic investigation for many diseases such as infectious diseases and malignancies. Basically, if there is any defect in tissue, there will be the abnormality in its basic physiological function that will further result in anatomical abnormality. The microanatomical abnormality in tissue can be detected by means of clinical microscopy. The use of microscope with specific special staining technique is the basic principle in histopathology examination.

Nevertheless, the dealing with tissue is not limited to only diagnosis purpose. Application of tissue engineering for therapeutic purpose is also possible. New advent in biotechnology helps the medical scientist to success in manipulation of tissue and use the tissue for management of medical problem. The tissue engineering is the specific biomedical technology aiming creation of functional tissues (Zheng et al., 2018). The engineering of the tissue is usually aimed at management of existed pathologies. The main aim of using engineered constructed tissue is to replace the old impaired tissue. This is the process that is called artificial regeneration or tissue repairing. The important fact that should be known is the limitation of the human adult tissue for self-repairing. The complete adult tissue is usually in its final form and might not possible for regeneration or reconstruction. The main structural tissues in human beings such as bone, cartilage, dental, and cardiac or nervous tissues are in their final forms without change for regeneration. Only a few tissues that might be self-regenerate such as skin tissue.

The concept of tissue engineering is finding for the cells with potential for further growth and development into tissue. The use of artificial materials and external biochemical factors to promote and support the formation of the tissue is the main step in tissue engineering (Urry and Pattanaik, 1997). To achieve this purpose, the basic knowledge on cytology, cytobiomaterial science, and biochemical engineering is needed. Selection and designing of new biomaterial that compatible with *in vivo* condition are the hallmark for successful engineering of tissue. The biomaterials have to be well prepared and construct. The selected biomaterials will be the supportive structure for cell growth, development, and formation of tissue. Those required biomaterials are termed as scaffold (Takezawa, 2003). At present, the scaffold is usually designed based on natural materials (such as gelatin or collagen). Step by step, the construction of scaffold must be primarily done then the growing of cell plus induction of development has to be further performed (Sachlos and Czernuszka, 2003). The induction of differentiation of cell to finalize formation of tissue becomes the critical step of tissue engineering. The induction is usually by the use of biological inducer. This needs the good control, which might be done in bioreactor or in-vivo regeneration. Without good control and standards, the unwanted adverse effects might occur.

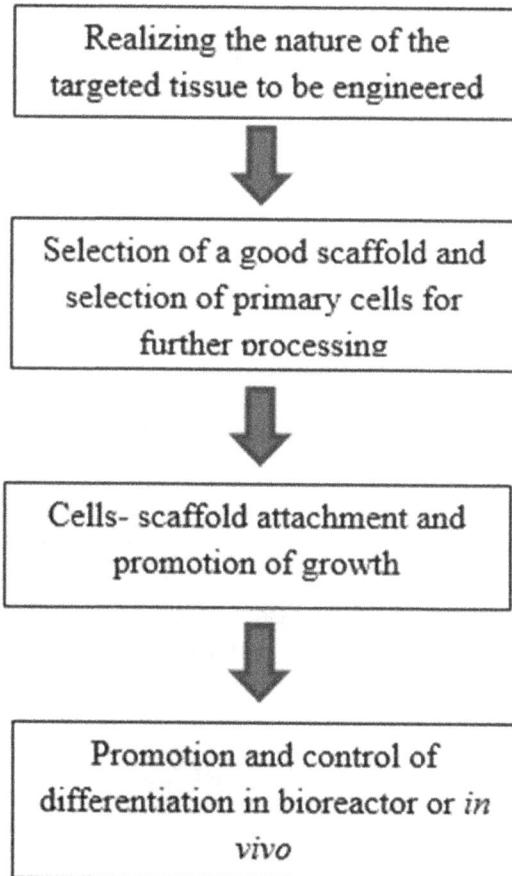

FIGURE 4.1 Brief diagram showing important concepts and steps for tissue engineering.

The overall process is the copying of the natural process of tissue formation that starts from the primary progenitor cells (Figure 4.1). The overall process is a natural-like process; hence, the effectiveness and safety are expected. With the environment of in-vivo biochemical stimulation, growth and development of cells naturally occur. This is the process for growth and development of cells that can finalize in the functional tissues. The biotechnology process of tissue engineering walks following this pathway of natural wisdom.

The applications can be seen in several fields of medicine. The good examples are application in neurology for artificial nerve regeneration, the application in orthopedics in management of bone and cartilage loss, and the application in dermatology for caring skin disorders such as psoriasis. Also, there are many allied researches that help support the success of tissue engineering such as researches on biomaterials for finding new effective and safe scaffolds and the researches on the natural products and herbal products for using as growth stimulators in tissue engineering process. Based on many new data on tissue engineering technology, there is a new hope for management of many medical disorders.

4.2 APPLICATIONS OF TISSUE ENGINEERING IN TROPICAL MEDICINE

As already mentioned, the tissue engineering becomes an important new technology that can be very useful in several medical purposes. In medicine, the applied tissue engineering technology can be seen in several fields including tropical medicine. Basically, tropical medicine is a specific branch of medicine that deals with the tropical diseases. Since most people in our world live in the tropical area, the tropical medicine becomes an important subject globally. The tropical medicine usually deals with many important diseases that are still the present global problem. The emerging and re-emerging of many tropical diseases occur within the past few years. In this chapter, we have summarized and discussed on the applied tissue engineering technology in some important tropical diseases.

4.2.1 TROPICAL INFECTION

In tropical countries, many infections are very common. The specific infections that frequently occur in the tropical zone are called tropical infection.

With the appropriate temperature in the tropical area, several pathogens grow well and become the problematic threatens to the local people living in tropical countries. Many tropical infections are still the global public health threat. Due to the heavy populated nature in several countries, any outbreak of tropical infection usually affects a large group of population and this becomes the global concern. In addition, due to the good transportation and globalization, the chance that a tropical infection will be transferred to the nontropical setting is possible and this can be the starting point of worldwide pandemic of tropical infection. At present, many tropical infections such as dengue and malaria already exist in nontropical zone. This phenomenon is due to the serious global warming and climate change. Therefore, the issue on tropical infection is important knowledge for practitioners in not only tropical zone but also nontropical zone.

Basically, the pathological process of tropical infection is similar to the general process of pathological infection. The effect on cell and tissue can be seen. This might be the direct invasion by the pathogen or the result from reaction of human body (such as immunopathology). The destruction of cells and tissues can be seen. Hence, the loss of tissues in tropical infection is possible. The role of tissue engineering in those cases is very interesting.

4.2.1.1 MALARIA

Malaria is a tropical mosquito-borne infection. It is one of the most problematic mosquito-borne infections. The infection is caused by blood protozoa in *Plasmodium* species. The infection occurs at red blood cell and considered as an important tropical blood infection. The infected people might have acute febrile illness. The patient usually presents with high fever and usually required hospitalization for antimalarial drug treatment. In serious case, fatality can occur. The pathological conditions in malaria can be seen in several organ systems including kidney and brain. There are some few reports regarding the use of tissue engineering technology for management of malaria. The brain sequelae can be seen in the case of cerebral malaria (Lackner et al., 2011) and the use of tissue engineering might be the solution for this problem (Behjati, 2012). Nevertheless, until present, there is still no report on the successful usage of tissue engineering technology for management of cerebral malaria.

4.2.1.2 DENGUE

Dengue is another important tropical mosquito-borne infection. The mosquito vector is *Aedes* mosquito. It is one of another problematic mosquito-borne infection. The infected people might have acute febrile illness with important triad of hemoconcentration, thrombocytopenia, and atypical lymphocytosis. The standard management of the patient is the fluid replacement therapy. Although the disease can be self-limited, there might be a serious clinical problem. The most severe form is called dengue hemorrhagic shock. The patient with dengue hemorrhagic shock will develop severe hemorrhage and shock. In serious case, fatality can occur. The pathological conditions in dengue can be seen in several organ systems including eye, kidney, and brain. Different from malaria, there is still no report regarding the use of tissue engineering technology for management of dengue. This might be due to the fact that dengue is considered a self-limited infection and there are usually no tissue sequelae after infection.

However, the tissue engineering technology is proposed for usefulness in vaccine development against dengue. In recent report, developed a new vaccine candidate based on highly immunogenic polyimmunoglobulin G scaffold (PIGS) fused to the consensus dengue envelope protein domain III (cEDIII) (Kim et al., 2018). Kim et al. (2018) found that the purified polymeric fraction of dengue PIGS (D-PIGS) induced stronger immune activation than the monomeric form, suggesting a more efficient interaction with the low-affinity Fcγ receptors on antigen-presenting cells.

4.2.1.3 YELLOW FEVER

Yellow fever is another important tropical mosquito-borne infection. It is one of another problematic mosquito-borne infection. The infection is caused by arbovirus and can cause serious illness. The infection is endemic in several tropical African and South American countries. The management of infection is usually difficult and it is recommended for primary prevention by yellow fever vaccination. The role of tissue engineering in management of yellow fever is rarely mentioned.

4.2.1.4 LEISHMANIASIS

Leishmaniasis is an important tropical vector-borne disease. The infection can be seen in several forms including visceral forms. It is classified as a fly-borne disease and is endemic in several tropical countries. Severe tissue destroy can be seen in cases of visceral leishmaniasis. Focusing on application on tissue engineering, some ongoing studies are presently done. Gutiérrez et al. reported the study on using chitosan-based tissue engineering technique for management of skin problem due to leishmaniasis (Gutiérrez et al., 2013). The aim is regeneration of the dermatological lesions in leishmaniasis.

The SADS cell, isolated from human adipose tissue, is mentioned for its advantage in tissue management for leishmaniasis (Fesharaki et al., 2018). Fesharaki et al. (2018) reported that SADS cells had potential to differentiate into early and mature progenitor neurons *in vitro*. There are many newly developed biomaterials that are proposed for usefulness in management of leishmaniasis. The good example is hybrid chitosan-ß-glycerol phosphate-gelatin nano-/microfibrous scaffolds (Lotfi et al., 2016) and polycaprolactone nanofibers (PCL/gelatin nanofibrous scaffolds) (Saburi et al., 2020; Soleimanifar et al., 2019). Lotfi et al. (2016) proposed that hybrid chitosan-ß-glycerol phosphate-gelatin nano-/microfibrous scaffolds with keratinocyte seeding were a promising treatment for wound healing in leishmaniasis. Fesharaki et al. (2018) found that gelatin and platelet-rich plasma coated into the structure of nanofibrous scaffolds have a significant positive influence on the bioactivity of scaffolds.

Additionally, there are also some reports on supplementary substance for promoting of scaffolds for management of leishmaniasis. For example, liposomal amphotericin B (AmBisome®) is a new therapeutic agent that is useful for promoting scaffolds. Forrester et al. (2019) found that the tissue response to AmBisome® treatment varied between target organs. Forrester et al. (2019) concluded that full restoration of homeostasis was not associated with parasitological cure.

Lahiry et al. (2020) reported on the use of *Saraca asoca*, an important plant species of India, for promoting of scaffolds. In their animal model study, the scaffold for management of leishmaniasis was good based on using *Saraca asoca* extract (Lahiry et al., 2020). The bromine and copper components in the extract are proposed as the basic elements that help promote scaffolds (Lahiry et al., 2020).

4.2.1.5 TRYPANOSOMIASIS

Trypanosomiasis is another important tropical vector-borne protozoon infection. It is a well-known tropical blood infection seen in several tropical

South American and African countries. Severe tissue destroy can be seen
in cases of severe trypanosomiasis, Chagas disease. Focusing on application on tissue engineering, some ongoing studies are presently done (Soares
and Santos, 2009). Tissue engineering and cell therapy are presently widely
investigated for its feasibility as a new mean of recovering the heart function lost due to chronic pathology in trypanosomiasis (Soares and Santos,
2009). The main possible advantage of using tissue engineering technology
in Chagas disease is for management of cardiac pathology (Soares and
Santos, 2009). Chachques (2009) noted that the tissue engineering is the
possible new effective way for management of Chagas heart disease, which
was previously noncurable. Clinically, the tissue engineering might be useful
in cardiac regenerative therapy in American trypanosomiasis (Chachques,
2009). Some new biosubstances are developed for management of Chagas
disease (Rodrigues et al., 2014). Design, synthesis, and evaluation of the new
derivatives are reported (Kashif et al., 2017). de Menezes et al. (2015) noted
that hydroxamic acid derivatives containing *o*-ethoxy (HAD1) and *p*-ethoxy
(HAD2) as substituent in the aromatic ring linked to the isoxazoline ring
were promising scaffolds for rational compound optimization in Chagas
disease.

4.2.1.6   FILARIASIS

Filarial parasite is a pathogenic parasite worm that can be transmitted by
mosquito bite. It is one of another problematic mosquito-borne infection seen
in several tropical countries. The infection can induce lymphatic obstruction
and can result in disability. Elephantiasis is the most important infectious-
induced disability. The elephantiasis is still common several developing
countries and considered the big local public health burden. Nevertheless,
filariasis does not widely spread and gets less interest from medical scientist
comparing to other famous tropical vector-borne infection. At present, there
is still no report on using tissue engineering for management of filariasis. In
fact, the tissue engineering technology might be useful for management of
cases with elephantiasis.

4.2.1.7   ZIKA VIRUS INFECTION

Zika virus is an important arbovirus infection. The infection has been
reported for many years, but it comes the well-known problem when there

is a big outbreak in South American tropical countries. This viral infection has a similar clinical presentation to other arbovirus infection, but there might be a wider clinical spectrum. This arbovirus infection becomes the problem worldwide due to multimodal transmission of the pathogenic virus. The infection is usually asymptomatic, but there are some reports on the relationship between maternal Zika infection during pregnancy and microcephaly in the offspring. For management of Zika virus infection, there are some reports on using tissue engineering technology. The possibility of regeneration of brain pathology by tissue engineering in cases with congenital Zika virus disease has been proposed (Kostic, 2016; Chakradhar, 2017).

4.2.1.8 JAPANESE ENCEPHALITIS

Japanese encephalitis is another important tropical mosquito-borne infection. The infection is caused by arbovirus namely Japanese encephalitis virus. The disease might be usually asymptomatic, but it can sometimes result in fatality. In symptomatic cases, the neurological impairment due to brain involvement is observable. The tissue engineering technology might be useful in management of those cases with neurological sequelae. In animal model, it is proven that stem cell therapy can be helpful in management of neurological problem in Japanese encephalitis (Bian et al., 2016).

4.2.1.9 LEPROSY

Leprosy is an important *Mycobacterium* infection. It is common in several poor tropical countries. In severe cases, the neuropathy can be seen. The permanent destroy of nerve becomes the important pathology in leprosy. The problem is noncurable by standard management. The use of tissue engineering might be the new hope for management of leprosy-related neuropathy (Illarramendi et al., 2012). In leprosy, chronic ulcers are a common sequelae and the delayed healing of chronic plantar ulcers due to leprosy is the lack of growth factors and cytokines (Natallya et al., 2019). The tissue engineering is the new hope for management of this problem (Dickinson and Gerecht, 2015). Sivasubramanian et al. (2018) reported using new human amnion (Amn)-derived biomaterial scaffolds in healing chronic wounds in leprosy-cured, but deformed, persons. Natallya et al. (2019) reported using human amniotic membrane stem cell secretome gel for healing of leprosy chronic plantar ulcers. Natallya et al. (2019) noted that this new therapeutic approach was effective.

Additionally, there are also some reports on supplementary substance for promoting of scaffolds for management of leprosy. For example, Jagati et al. (2019) reported using platelet-rich fibrin membrane over scaffold of collagen sheet as a new effective alternative. Aghamohamadi et al. (2019) reported preparation of Aloe vera acetate and electrospinning is useful in promoting regeneration and the new biomaterial also had antimicrobial property.

4.2.1.10   SCHISTOSOMIASIS

Schistosomiasis is the parasitic disease that is caused by the fluke in *Schistosoma* species. The causative agent is known as blood fluke. The species namely *Schistosoma mansoni* is an important blood fluke that can result in chronic liver disease and fibrosis. In case with severe liver dysfunction, the patient might die. The use of tissue engineering technology for management of the chronic liver problem due to *Schistosoma mansoni* is mentioned. In an animal model study, Hegab et al. (2018) reported that bone marrow-derived mesenchymal stem cell therapy was effective for management of chronic liver disease in murine *Schistosoma mansoni*. For *Schistosoma haematobium*, the chronic parasitic infection in urinary bladder might occur and it can result in cancer. To management of *Schistosoma*-related urinary bladder cancer, surgical treatment is indicated. Tissue engineering can play role as regenerative medicine in the management of invasive bladder cancer in this case (Hyndman et al., 2012).

4.2.1.11   LEPTOSPIROSIS

Leptospirosis is leptospiral bacterial infection. The pathogen can cause virulent disease. The patient might have acute febrile illness and can have jaundice and renal problem. The mortality in leptospirosis is high in cases with renal failure problem. The pathogen is usually transmitted during the rainy season and common in several developing tropical countries. The role of tissue engineering in management of leptospirosis is limited mentioned. In fact, it might have the role in management of acute renal failure which is an important complication of leptospirosis. The good example is the use of mesenchymal stem cell in management of ischemia in acute renal failure (Hu and Zou, 2017). Hu and Zou (2017) reported that mesenchymal stem cell-based tissue engineering technology is useful for renal ischemia-reperfusion injury in leptospirosis.

4.2.1.12   VIRAL HEPATITIS

Viral hepatitis is an important group of infection. The main affected organ in this viral infection is liver. Several hepatitis viruses can cause hepatitis. The good examples are hepatitis A virus, hepatitis B virus, and hepatitis C virus. In tropical developing countries, the hepatitis virus infection is common and becomes the big local public health problem. Some specific kinds of viral hepatitis, especially for hepatitis B and hepatitis C, it can result in chronic liver pathology. The impairment of liver cells can be seen and this can further result in hepatitis failure, cirrhosis, or malignant transformation. The liver fibrosis is common in chronic hepatitis viral infection. The deterioration of liver function in chronic viral hepatitis is common and becomes important problem in infected patients. To manage the chronic viral hepatitis, it is usually difficult and requires good investigation. Similar to the case of using tissue engineering for regenerative therapy for brain pathology in Japanese encephalitis, the role of tissue engineering in regeneration of liver tissue problems, especially for fibrosis, in chronic viral hepatitis can be expected (Köhn-Gaone et al., 2016). In addition, engineered liver model can be useful in novel drug discovery (Lin et al., 2015).

4.2.1.13   TUBERCULOSIS

Tuberculosis is an important respiratory tract infection. This infection is considered as a common chronic respiratory disease. The patient might have chronic cough and can develop hemoptysis. Weight loss is also a common clinical presentation. The tuberculosis is caused by *Mycobacterium* pathogen. The infection is detectable in several tropical developing countries and the infection is considered the big public health problem globally. The standard management of tuberculosis is the antituberculosis drug treatment. The role of tissue engineering for management of tuberculosis is interesting. The use of mesenchymal stromal cell therapy for management of multidrug-resistant tuberculosis is the good example of applied tissue engineering for tuberculosis management (Joshi et al., 2015). In a recent study by Skrahin et al. (2014), it is proven that autologous mesenchymal stromal cell infusion is an effective adjunct treatment in patient with multidrug- and extensively drug-resistant tuberculosis. In this alternative therapeutic approach, there are some observable adverse effects of stem cell therapy including nausea and diarrhea (Skrahin et al., 2014).

Regarding regenerative therapy for tuberculosis, the tissue engineering might play role in patient with bone tuberculosis. The role of tissue engineering is proposed in regenerative treatment in patient with bone tuberculosis. Huang et al. (2015) found that isoniazid (INH)-conjugated poly(lactide-*co*-glycolide) was a long-term controlled drug release that could promote tissue regeneration for bone tuberculosis therapy (Garg and Goyal, 2014). Zhou et al. (2018) reported that hydrophilic INH and hydrophobic rifampicin (RFP) molecularly dispersed into polyvinyl alcohol that could induce obvious bone regeneration and fusion due to the inhibition of tuberculosis-associated inflammatory changes in animal model. Zhu et al. (2015) reported using fabricated three-dimensional (3D)-printed macro-/mesoporous composite scaffolds loading with high dosages of INH)/RFP antituberculosis drugs. Zhu et al. (2015) proposed that the newly developed composite scaffolds were useful in bone regeneration and local therapy after osteoarticular tuberculosis debridement surgery. Li et al. (2017) reported that dopamine-assisted fixation of drug-loaded polymeric multilayers was useful in management of osteoarticular implants for tuberculosis therapy. Li et al. (2017) noted that the technique is safe and the implant has a long-term efficacy against tuberculosis. The thermoresponsive and self-healing liposome-in-hydrogel system is an antitubercular drug carrier for localized bone tuberculosis therapy. Liu et al. (2019) concluded that the system could rapidly release drug into synovial fluid to reach effective inhibitory concentrations against pathogen after localized injection.

4.2.1.14 CHOLERA

Cholera is an important gastrointestinal tract infection. It is a bacterial infection that is transmitted by contaminated food and drink. This infection is considered as serious infection. The patient might have severe watery diarrhea and require good fluid replacement therapy. In serious case, the patient might end up with death. The role of tissue engineering for management of cholera is limited, but there are many tissue engineering-related researches based on cholera toxin. Immunologically, cholera toxin adjuvant is proven effective for promoting antigen priming of T cells (Hörnquist and Lycke, 1993).

4.2.1.15   BABESIOSIS

Babesiosis is an important tropical blood infection. The infection can be seen in red blood cell similar to malaria. However, the infection is usually seen in animal and it is not common in human beings. For human case, the role of tissue engineering technology is not proposed.

4.2.2   TROPICAL CANCER

4.2.2.1   CHOLANGIOCARCINOMA

Cholangiocarcinoma is an important cancer of the biliary tract. This infection is related to an important tropical trematode infection, opisthorchiasis. The highest incidence of this infection is seen in Indochina, where the liver fluke is highly incidence. The high incidence of liver fluke infestation in Indochina is believed to due to the rooted behavior of ingestion of raw fish. The chronic liver fluke infection can result in cholangiocarcinogenesis. In endemic countries, the patient usually presents with advanced disease and the treatment is usually hopeless (Wiwanitkit, 2003). The surgery is usually not successful in getting rid of tumor mass and the chemotherapy is usually not effective. Similar to other cancers, tissue engineering and regenerative therapy are a hope for management of cholangiocarcinoma at present (Hibi et al., 2014).

4.2.2.2   HEPATOCELLULAR CARCINOMA

The hepatocellular carcinoma is related to many hepatitis viruses, especially for hepatitis B and hepatitis C viruses, which are common in tropical countries. Also, the cancer is related to heavy alcoholic drinking which is a common bad health behavior. The management of hepatocellular carcinoma is usually difficult. The liver transplantation might be the hope for management, but the availability of the donated liver is usually limited. Zheng et al. (2010) noted that liver tissue engineering was the new hope for possible management of advanced hepatocellular carcinoma. The application of the tissue engineering technology for management of hepatocellular carcinoma is the same way as that already described in chronic viral hepatitis. Scaffolds are proposed for usefulness in hepatic regeneration. Bruni et al. (2003) noted that specific scaffold attachment region was located in a locus targeted by hepadnavirus integration in hepatocellular carcinomas.

4.2.2.3 STOMACH CARCINOMA

Stomach carcinoma is an important cancer of gastrointestinal tract. This cancer is related to *Helicobacter pylori* infection, which is a common bacterial infection in tropical countries. The management of this cancer is usually difficult. The surgical management is the general standard therapy at present. The use of tissue engineering and stem cell therapy is the new hope for management of stomach carcinoma (Maemura et al., 2013). The tissue-engineered neostomach is the good example. The aim of using neostomach is for increasing the capacity for food intake by acting as a new food reservoir and restoration of mucosa and smooth muscle layers in the stomach tissue (Maemura et al., 2003).

4.2.2.4 URINARY BLADDER CARCINOMA

Urinary bladder carcinoma is another important cancer in urinary tract. The tropical infection, blood fluke, *Schistosoma haematobium*, is confirmed as a carcinogenic factor for urinary bladder carcinoma. The management of urinary bladder cancer usually requires surgical management. The use of tissue engineering and stem cell therapy in management of urinary bladder carcinoma is the new approach (Singh et al., 2018). The neourinary conduit is the good example of tissue engineering application. The neourinary conduit is constructed by novel tissue engineering technology and grafting implantation is needed for therapeutic application. The aim of implantation of neourinary conduit is to regain appropriate biological and mechanical properties for storage and transportation of urine (Singh et al., 2018). Nevertheless, there are still many present problems in using graft from tissue engineering technology. Graft ischemia is a big problem and if the ischemia occurs, it might result in fibrosis or perforation (Alberti, 2016).

4.2.3 TROPICAL ANEMIA

4.2.3.1 THALASSEMIA

Thalassemia is an important hemoglobin disorder. The basic pathophysiology is the genetic defect that results in abnormal globin synthesis. At present, thalassemia is common in several tropical countries, especially for tropical Southeast Asia. The bone defect and hepatosplenomegaly are common sequel in thalassemia. Many patients require transfusion therapy for correction of anemic problem. The risk of this transfusion treatment is well known. The iron overload is a common complication in the patient with polytransfusion and requires iron chelation therapy. At present, the gold standard for the effective treatment of thalassemia is stem cell therapy. Hence, the role of tissue engineering for management of thalassemia is confirmed (Felfly and Haddad, 2014). Many studies are in development and trial phases. The good examples are on the management of thalassemia-related wound. Afradi et al. (2017) reported on the use of tissue engineering technology in treatment of 100 chronic thalassemic leg wounds by plasma-rich platelets. Afradi et al. (2017) reported using new platelet-rich plasma (PRP) gel consisting of cytokines, growth factors, chemokines, and a fibrin scaffold derived from a patient's blood and noted that the technique was useful in wound management in thalassemic patient.

4.2.3.2   SICKLE CELL ANEMIA

Sickle cell anemia or hemoglobin S disorder is an important well-known tropical anemia. This anemic disorder is a genetic defect due to a single mutation. The beta-globin chain of hemoglobin is defective in this hemoglobinopathy. The abnormal banana-shaped red cell is the hallmark in blood film. The patients usually have the anemic problem and might be complicated by thrombohemostatic disorder. Similar to thalassemia, the stem cell therapy becomes the new therapeutic modality for management of sickle cell anemia (Sadelain et al., 2008).

4.2.3.3   HEMOGLOBIN E DISORDER

Hemoglobin E disorder is a genetic defect due to a single mutation. The beta-globin chain of hemoglobin is defective in this hemoglobinopathy. The patients usually have the anemic problem and might be serious, if it coexists with thalassemia. In tropical Indochina countries, the hemoglobin E disorder is highly prevalent and some patients require transfusion therapy. As already mentioned, the complication in the patient with hemoglobin E disorder who receives multiple transfusions can be expected. The use of tissue engineering and stem cell therapy becomes the new approach for management of hemoglobin E disorder (Sadelain et al., 2008).

4.3   CURRENT AND FUTURE SITUATIONS OF TISSUE ENGINEERING RESEARCH IN TROPICAL MEDICINE

As already mentioned, the tissue engineering technology can be applied for management of several tropical diseases. Hence, the tissue engineering technology is expected to be the new hope for management of difficult-to-manage pathologies in several tropical disorders. Nevertheless, it can be seen that there are not many researches on this area. Indeed, tropical medicine usually deals with the neglected important diseases existed in poor developing countries. Due to the nature of limited infrastructure in tropical developing countries, the local fund for research and development on tissue engineering for management of tropical disease is usually not available and most of the researches are usually by the investigator teams from nontropical developed Western countries.

4.3.1   SITUATION IN TROPICAL ASIA

At present, there are some research teams on tissue engineering in tropical Asia. The tropical medicine research centers locate in several tropical Asian countries and those places are the hubs for tropical medicine research in tropical Asia. For example, in Singapore, a rich tropical Asian country, the good tissue engineering researches are ongoing at present. Nevertheless, there is no research from poor countries in Indochina.

4.3.2   SITUATION IN TROPICAL SOUTH AMERICA

The tropical medicine research centers locate in several tropical South American countries and those places are the hubs for tropical medicine research in South America. The well-known center is at Brazil. Several ongoing tropical medicine researches are presently performed in Brazil. There are also some researches on tissue engineering for management of both tropical diseases and nontropical diseases such as Parkinson's disease (Mendes Filho et al., 2018). The famous research team in Brazil is on stem cell research for management of Chagas cardiomyopathy (Tanowitz et al., 2015).

4.3.3 SITUATION IN TROPICAL AFRICA

Similar to tropical South America, there are some research teams on tissue engineering in tropical Africa. Research teams on tissue engineering perform researches in some countries such as Nigeria. Similar to the situation in tropical South America, the fund for researching is usually not available.

The research can benefit from the easy available cases for trails. Nevertheless, the main obstacle is the lack of expertise and fund for generation of a good research. The international collaboration for improvement of the tissue engineering technology in developing tropical countries where the problems actually exist is required. For future perspective, due to the chance of expansion of the endemic areas of tropical diseases, there should be increased consideration of several neglected tropical diseases. The integration between tissue engineering technique and other novel biomedical technologies such as nanotechnology and bioinformatic approach will help to increase the effectiveness of applied tissue engineering for management of tropical diseases. The possibility of application is usually mentioned in many tropical diseases (Table 4.1).

TABLE 4.1 Current Situations of Using Tissue Engineering for Management of Tropical Diseases in Tropical Medicine

Diseases	Details
Tropical infection	There are some ongoing researches on using tissue engineering for management of some tropical infections. The disease that gets most assessed is the Chagas disease that the tissue engineering treatment is proposed to be a possible effective regenerative therapy for cardiomyopathy
Tropical cancer	Similar to general cancer, the tissue engineering is the new hope for effective management of patients with advanced tropical cancers. The engineered tissue is proposed for usefulness in regeneration and functional restoration
Tropical anemia	The role of tissue engineering for tropical anemia is observable in genetic hemoglobinopathy. The stem cell therapy becomes the present curative management of several genetic tropical anemic disorders

4.4   CONCLUSION

In tropical medicine, there are many ongoing researches for using tissue engineering technology for management of tropical diseases and there are already some reports on this issue. Generally, the main aim of the tissue engineering technology application is for restoration of function and regeneration of the lost tissue due to the pathological disorder. The good examples of widely studied tropical diseases are tropical infections and tropical malignancies. The tropical infection that the tissue engineering for treatment is much studied is the Chagas disease, which is a common infection in tropical America. Another infection that is much studied is leishmaniasis. However, there are several considerations on how to apply the tissue engineering for management of tropical diseases. Several underlying problems in the tropical zone such as poverty and limited resources might be the main barrier to successful implementation of the new tissue engineering in the tropical countries where the endemic areas of tropical diseases area. It is necessary that the specific research on tissue engineering technology for management of tropical diseases should be promoted and supported.

KEYWORDS

- **tissue**
- **engineering**
- **tropical medicine**
- **infection**
- **cancer**
- **anemia**

REFERENCES

Afradi, H., Saghaei, Y., Kachoei, Z. A., Babaei, V. and Teimourian, S. Treatment of 100 chronic thalassemic leg wounds by plasma-rich platelets. *Int J Dermatol.* **2017,** 56(2): 171–175.

Aghamohamadi, N., Sanjani, N. S., Majidi, R. F. and Nasrollahi, S. A. Preparation and characterization of Aloe vera acetate and electrospinning fibers as promising antibacterial properties materials. *Mater Sci Eng C Mater Biol Appl.* **2019,** 94: 445–452.

Alberti, C. Why ever bladder tissue engineering clinical applications still remain unusual even though many intriguing technological advances have been reached? *G Chir.* **2016**, 37: 6–12.

Behjati, M. Letter: chronic non-healing wounds and cerebral malaria—for better or for worse? *Int Wound J.* **2012**, 9(4): 456–458.

Bian, P., Ye, C., Zheng, X., Yang, J., Ye, W., Wang, Y., Zhou, Y., Ma, Z., Han, P., Zhang, H., Zhang, Y., Zhang, F., Lei, Y. and Jia, Z. Mesenchymal stem cells alleviate Japanese encephalitis virus-induced neuroinflammation and mortality. *Stem Cell Res Ther.* **2017**, 8(1): 38.

Bruni, R., D'Ugo, E., Argentini, C., Giuseppetti, R. and Rapicetta, M. Scaffold attachment region located in a locus targeted by hepadnavirus integration in hepatocellular carcinomas. *Cancer Detect Prev.* **2003**, 27: 175–181.

Chakradhar, S. Disease in three dimensions: Tissue engineering takes on infectious disease. *Nat Med.* **2017**, 23(1): 2–4.

Chachques, J. C. Cellular cardiac regenerative therapy in which patients? *Exp Rev Cardiovasc Ther.* **2009**, 7(8): 911–919.

de Menezes Dda, R., Calvet, C. M., Rodrigues, G. C., de Souza Pereira, M. C., Almeida, I. R., de Aguiar, A. P. et al. Hydroxamic acid derivatives: a promising scaffold for rational compound optimization in Chagas disease. *J Enzyme Inhib Med Chem.* **2016**, 31(6): 964–973.

Dickinson, L. E. and Gerecht, S. Engineered biopolymeric scaffolds for chronic wound healing. *Front Physiol.* **2016**, 7: 341.

Felfly, H. and Haddad, G. G. Hematopoietic stem cells: potential new applications for translational medicine. *J Stem Cells.* **2014**, 9(3): 163–197.

Fesharaki, M., Razavi, S., Ghasemi-Mobarakeh, L., Behjati, M., Yarahmadian, R., Kazemi, M. et al. Differentiation of human scalp adipose-derived mesenchymal stem cells into mature neural cells on electrospun nanofibrous scaffolds for nerve tissue engineering applications. *Cell J.* **2018**, 20(2): 168–176.

Forrester, S., Siefert, K., Ashwin, H., Brown, N., Zelmar, A., James, S. et al. Tissue-specific transcriptomic changes associated with AmBisome® treatment of BALB/c mice with experimental visceral leishmaniasis. *Wellcome Open Res.* **2019**, 4: 198.

Garg, T. and Goyal, A. K. Biomaterial-based scaffolds—current status and future directions. *Expert Opin Drug Deliv.* **2014**, 11(5): 767–789.

Gutiérrez, J., Vallejo, B., Barbosa, H., Pinzón, J. and Delgado, G. *In vitro* analysis regarding the safety of components used in a film-based therapeutic system loaded with meglumine antimoniate and its activity toward Leishmania major experimental infections: a preliminary study. *Immunopharmacol Immunotoxicol.* **2013**, 35: 321–328.

Hegab, M. H., Abd-Allah, S. H., Badawey, M. S., Saleh, A. A., Metwally, A. S., Fathy, G. M. et al. Therapeutic potential effect of bone marrow-derived mesenchymal stem cells on chronic liver disease in murine *Schistosomia mansoni*. *J Parasit Dis.* **2018**, 42(2): 277–286.

Hibi, T., Shinoda, M., Itano, O. and Kitagawa, Y. Current status of the organ replacement approach for malignancies and an overture for organ bioengineering and regenerative medicine. *Organogenesis.* **2014**, 10(2): 241–249.

Hörnquist, E. and Lycke, N. Cholera toxin adjuvant greatly promotes antigen priming of T cells. *Eur J Immunol.* **1993**, 23(9): 2136–2143.

Hu, H. and Zou, C. Mesenchymal Stem Cells in Renal Ischemia-Reperfusion Injury: Biological and Therapeutic Perspectives. *Curr Stem Cell Res Ther.* **2017**, 12(3): 183–187.

Huang, D., Li, D., Wang, T., Shen, H., Zhao, P., Liu, B. et al. Isoniazid conjugated poly(lactide-co-glycolide): long-term controlled drug release and tissue regeneration for bone tuberculosis therapy. *Biomaterials.* **2015,** 52: 417–425.

Hyndman, M. E., Kaye, D., Field, N. C., Lawson, K. A., Smith, N. D., Steinberg, G. D. et al. The use of regenerative medicine in the management of invasive bladder cancer. *Adv Urol.* **2012,** 2012: 653–652.

Illarramendi, X., Rangel, E., Miranda, A. M., Castro, A. C., Magalhães-Gde, O. and Antunes, S. L. Cutaneous lesions sensory impairment recovery and nerve regeneration in leprosy patients. *Mem Inst Oswaldo Cruz.* **2012,** 107 Suppl 1: 68–73.

Jagati, A., Chaudhary, R. G., Rathod, S. P., Madke, B., Baxi, K. D. and Kasundra, D. Preparation of platelet-rich fibrin membrane over scaffold of collagen sheet, its advantages ver compression method: a novel and simple technique. *J Cutan Aesthet Surg.* **2019,** 12(3): 174–178.

Joshi, L., Chelluri, L. K. and Gaddam, S. Mesenchymal Stromal Cell Therapy in MDR/XDR Tuberculosis: A Concise Review. *Arch Immunol Ther Exp (Warsz).* **2015,** 63: 427–433.

Kashif, M., Moreno-Herrera, A., Lara-Ramirez, E. E., Ramírez-Moreno, E., Bocanegra-García, V., Ashfaq, M. et al. Recent developments in trans-sialidase inhibitors of *Trypanosoma cruzi. J Drug Target.* **2017,** 25(6): 485–498.

Kim, M. Y., Copland, A., Nayak, K., Chandele, A., Ahmed, M. S., Zhang, O. et al. Plant-expressed Fc-fusion protein tetravalent dengue vaccine with inherent adjuvant properties. *Plant Biotechnol J.* **2018,** 16(7): 1283–1294.

Köhn-Gaone, J., Gogoi-Tiwari, J., Ramm, G. A., Olynyk, J. K. and Tirnitz-Parker, J. E. The role of liver progenitor cells during liver regeneration, fibrogenesis, and carcinogenesis. *Am J Physiol Gastrointest Liver Physiol.* **2016,** 310(3): G143–154.

Kostic, M. Stem cell hydrogel, jump-starting zika drug discovery, and engineering RNA recognition. *Cell Chem Biol.* **2016,** 23(8): 885–886.

Lackner, P., Beer, R., Broessner, G., Helbok, R., Dallago, K., Hess, M. W., Pfaller, K., Bandtlow, C. and Schmutzhard, E. Nogo-A expression in the brain of mice with cerebral malaria. *PLoS One.* **2011,** 6(9): e25728.

Lahiry, S., Bhattacharyya, D., Chakraborty, A., Sudarshan, M. and Manna, M. Saraca asoca seed extract treatment recovers the trace elements imbalances in experimental murine visceral leishmaniasis. *J Parasit Dis.* **2020,** 44(1): 131–136.

Li, D., Li, L., Ma, Y., Zhuang, Y., Li, D., Shen, H. et al. Dopamine-assisted fixation of drug-loaded polymeric multilayers to osteoarticular implants for tuberculosis therapy. *Biomater Sci.* **2017,** 5(4): 730–740.

Lin, C., Ballinger, K. R. and Khetani S. R. The application of engineered liver tissues for novel drug discovery. *Expert Opin Drug Discov.* **2015,** 10(5): 519–540.

Liu, P., Guo, B., Wang, S., Ding, J. and Zhou, W. A thermo-responsive and self-healing liposome-in-hydrogel system as an antitubercular drug carrier for localized bone tuberculosis therapy. *Int J Pharm.* **2019,** 558: 101–109.

Lotfi, M., Bagherzadeh, R., Naderi-Meshkin, H., Mahdipour, E., Mafinezhad, A., Sadeghnia, H. R. et al. Hybrid chitosan-ß-glycerol phosphate-gelatin nano-/microfibrous scaffolds with suitable mechanical and biological properties for tissue engineering. *Biopolymers.* **2016,** 105(3): 163–175.

Maemura, T., Shin, M. and Kinoshita, M. Tissue engineering of the stomach. *J Surg Res.* **2013,** 183(1): 285–295.

Maemura, T., Shin, M., Sato, M., Mochizuki, H. and Vacanti, J. P. A tissue-engineered stomach as a replacement of the native stomach. *Transplantation*. **2003**, 76(1): 61–65.

Mendes-Filho, D., Ribeiro, P. D. C., Oliveira, L. F., de Paula, D. R. M., Capuano, V., de Assunção, T. S. F. et al. Therapy with mesenchymal stem cells in Parkinson disease: history and perspectives. *Neurologist*. **2018**, 23(4): 141–147.

Natallya, F. R., Herwanto, N., Prakoeswa, C., Indramaya, D. M. and Rantam, F. A. Effective healing of leprosy chronic plantar ulcers by application of human amniotic membrane stem cell secretome gel. *Indian J Dermatol*. **2019**, 64(3): 250.

Rodrigues, G. C., Feijó, D. F., Bozza, M. T., Pan, P., Vullo, D., Parkkila, S. et al. Design, synthesis, and evaluation of hydroxamic acid derivatives as promising agents for the management of Chagas disease. *J Med Chem*. **2014**, 57(2): 298–308.

Saburi, E., Atabati, H., Kabiri, L., Behdari, A., Azizi, M., Ardeshirylajimi, A., Enderami, S. E. et al. Bone morphogenetic protein-7 incorporated polycaprolactone scaffold has a great potential to improve survival and proliferation rate of the human embryonic kidney cells. *J Cell Biochem*. **2019**, 120(6): 9859–9868.

Sachlos, E. and Czernuszka, J. T. Making tissue engineering scaffolds work. Review: the application of solid freeform fabrication technology to the production of tissue engineering scaffolds. *Eur Cell Mater*. **2003**, 5: 29–39.

Sadelain, M., Boulad, F., Lisowki, L., Moi P. and Riviere, I. Stem cell engineering for the treatment of severe hemoglobinopathies. *Curr Mol Med*. **2008**, 8(7): 690–697.

Singh, A., Bivalacqua, T. J. and Sopko, N. Urinary tissue engineering: challenges and opportunities. *Sex Med Rev*. **2018**, 6(1): 35–44.

Sivasubramanian, S., Mohana, S., Maheswari, P., Victoria, V., Thangam, R., Mahalingam, J., Chandrasekar-Janebjer, G. et al. Leprosy-associated chronic wound management using biomaterials. *J Glob Infect Dis*. **2018**, 10(2): 99–107.

Skrahin, A., Ahmed, R. K., Ferrara, G., Rane, L., Poiret, T., Isaikina, Y. et al. Autologous mesenchymal stromal cell infusion as adjunct treatment in patients with multidrug and extensively drug-resistant tuberculosis: an open-label phase 1 safety trial. *Lancet Respir Med*. **2014**, 2(2): 108–122.

Soares, M. B. and Santos, R. R. Current status and perspectives of cell therapy in Chagas disease. *Mem Inst Oswaldo Cruz*. **2009**, 104 Suppl 1: 325–332.

Soleimanifar, F., Hosseini, F. S., Atabati, H., Behdari, A., Kabiri, L., Enderami, S. E. et al. Adipose-derived stem cells-conditioned medium improved osteogenic differentiation of induced pluripotent stem cells when grown on polycaprolactone nanofibers. *J Cell Physiol*. **2019**, 234(7): 10315–10323.

Takezawa, T. A strategy for the development of tissue engineering scaffolds that regulate cell behavior. *Biomaterials*. **2003**, 24(13): 2267–2275.

Tanowitz, H. B., Machado, F. S., Spray, D. C., Friedman, J. M., Weiss, O. S., Lora, J. N., et al. Developments in the management of Chagas cardiomyopathy. *Exp Rev Cardiovasc Ther*. **2015**, 13(12): 1393–1409.

Urry, D. W. and Pattanaik, A. Elastic protein-based materials in tissue reconstruction. *Ann N Y Acad Sci*. **1997**, 831: 32–46.

Wiwanitkit, V. Clinical findings among 62 Thais with cholangiocarcinoma. *Trop Med Int Health*. **2003**, 8(3): 28–30.

Zheng, M. H., Ye, C., Braddock, M. and Chen, Y. P. Liver tissue engineering: promises and prospects of new technology. *Cytotherapy*. **2010**, 12(3): 349–360.

Zheng, C. X., Sui, B. D., Hu, C. H., Qiu, X. Y., Zhao, P. and Jin, Y. Reconstruction of structure and function in tissue engineering of solid organs: Toward simulation of natural development based on decellularization. *J Tissue Eng Regen Med.* **2018,** 12(6): 1432–1447.

Zhou, C. X., Li, L., Ma, Y. G., Li, B. N., Li, G., Zhou, Z. et al. A bioactive implant in situ and long-term releases combined drugs for treatment of osteoarticular tuberculosis. *Biomaterials.* **2018,** 176: 50–59.

Zhu, M., Li, K., Zhu, Y., Zhang, J. and Ye, X. 3D-printed hierarchical scaffold for localized isoniazid/rifampin drug delivery and osteoarticular tuberculosis therapy. *Acta Biomater.* **2015,** 16: 145–155.

CHAPTER 5

Skin Tissue Engineering: Past, Present, and Perspectives

SINEM SELVIN SELVI, MERVE ERGINER HASKÖYLÜ, and
EBRU TOKSOY ÖNER*

*IBSB, Department of Bioengineering, Marmara University, 34722,
İstanbul, Turkey*

Corresponding author. E-mail: ebru.toksoy@marmara.edu.tr

ABSTRACT

Since skin is the outermost layer of human body and protects it from external hazards, any damage of this tissue such as wounds and burns may result in serious health problems. Skin tissue engineering applications are found to be one of the first ones in history because of its importance and urge. Skin tissue engineering field tries to develop skin substitutes, which are cheap, easy to handle, nontoxic, biodegradable, biocompatible together with fast healing, and vascularization activities. There are several application methods and substitutes present in literature including commercially used clinical ones and laboratory-scale created and in-vitro tested ones. Here, in this chapter, we discuss history of tissue engineering, wound healing methods, skin substitutes, and materials used for it with the current and promising applications.

5.1 INTRODUCTION

5.1.1 SKIN TISSUE ENGINEERING AND HISTORY

Acute injuries and traumas affect tissue, cell, and organ function (Iqbal et al., 2018). Tissue engineering and regenerative medicine seek for alternative ways to restore and repair injured or malfunctioned tissue of human body in the light of biology, material science, medicine, engineering, mechanics, and become a significant area for past three decades (Rahmani Del Bakhshayesh et al., 2018; Zhang et al., 2017). This field tries to develop biocompatible tissue constructs that come in contact with present cells or tissues and provides three-dimensional matrix while supporting cell–cell signaling, production of growth factors, extracellular matrix (ECM), proliferation, and differentiation of cells in the implanted area to regenerate damaged tissue. Natural- or synthetic-based scaffolds such as hydrogels, micro-/nanofibrous scaffolds, porous matrices, fibers, sponges, foams, and so on are highly used to provide similar ECM environment to native one and help cells to grow, proliferate, and differentiate to replace damaged tissue function and shape (Iqbal et al., 2018). Since skin is an organ with largest surface area and outermost layer, engineering of this tissue is popular because of clinical and academic needs. Skin tissue engineering seeks alternative ways to traditional wound healing applications with natural or synthetic polymers that include cellular or acellular therapies to develop scaffolds and skin substitutes that promote wound healing. Biocompatibility, nonimmunogenicity, nontoxicity, mechanical stability, water vapor transmission rate, protection from microorganisms, porosity that supports gas and nutrient exchange together with fast healing, minimized pain, and reduced scarring are basic requirements of tissue-engineered skin (Bhardwaj et al., 2018; Groeber et al., 2011; Iqbal et al., 2018; Vig et al., 2017).

First tissue-based treatments were skin grafting techniques. Concept is basically grafting and transferring of the skin and transplantation to another location of the patient's body. In 3000 BC, Hindu tilemaker caste members described first skin grafting method where amputated noses result from the judicial punishment were reconstructed (Adigbli et al., 2016). In 1794, first autologous skin grafting was reported by Bunger, Reverdin, and Baronio in Europe. In 1881, cadaveric skin allograft was stated by Girdner. In following years, cell and tissue preservation techniques were developed and under favor of this development, cells could be stored for a long time. After this progress, cell cryopreservation at subzero temperatures then in following years, skin cryopreservation was developed by Polge (1949) and Billingham (1952), respectively. First synthetic skin product was reported in 1962, but the very first successful skin products were developed in the late 1970s. Howard Green and his colleagues carried out skin biopsy from the patient and grow epidermis tissue in 1975. Autologous cultured epithelium cells were the first commercialized skin product and named as Epicel® (Genzyme, USA) in 1979. Sheets of autologous keratinocytes were collected from recipient and used to cover the burned tissue; however, Epicel® did not have dermis tissue and, therefore, product was intensely sensitive and had practical difficulties. In 1980s, genuine skin tissue engineering started with composite living skin equivalent by Bell in 1981 and later these composites were commercialized as Apligraf® (Organogenesis, USA). In 1987, these methods were firstly entitled as "tissue engineering" (Figure 5.1). More of these skin tissue-engineered products were commercialized together with mostly cartilage during the 1990s. Simple products and technology served the purpose for skin (epidermis) and cartilage tissue because vascularization and other complicated tissue processes are not necessary in these systems. For other kind of tissues, vascular supply, complex combinations of different cells in three-dimensional (3D), and identified cell sources are necessary. During 2000s, due to bubble burst in high technology products, funding of tissue-engineering companies was decreased instantly. By 2004, skin, cartilage, and other tissue-engineered applications were decreased by more than 50% and almost 800 employees lost their job. This market slump was compensated by stem cell companies and nearly 300 employees tend toward the field. However, startup financing was very limited till 2008. Skin tissue engineering technologies have been developing by scientists and engineers to overcome the basic problems, but generally not focusing on the clinical problems. Nontherapeutic applications of skin tissue engineering are opening new fields and helping the development of new therapeutic products but today, clinically acceptable solutions for blood vessels, heart, liver, cornea, and bladder still could not be offered, despite significant researches and efforts (Berthiaume et al., 2011; Dhasmana et al., 2018b; Herman, 2002).

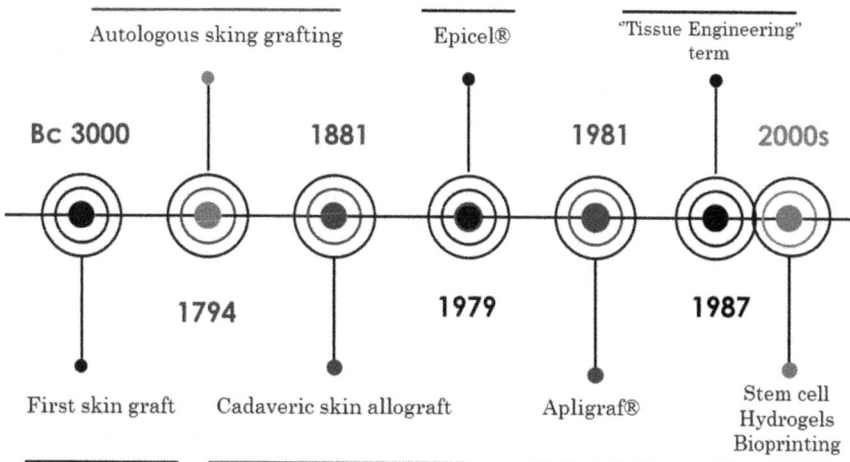

FIGURE 5.1   Significant landmarks of skin tissue engineering.

"Skin tissue engineering" search was performed on Google scholar between 2000 and 2018 September and 911,000 results were found. In 2000, there were 11,900 publications in search and 35,700 publications in 2017. The results show the increase in results of skin tissue engineering publications. In order to create effective skin scaffolds similar to native one, anatomy and physiology of the skin need to be understood in detail.

5.2   ANATOMY OF SKIN

Skin is evolved to act as a protective barrier against penetration of pathogens, toxins, and any other external damage together with perceptual, neural, cosmetic, and regulatory properties (Figure 5.2). It maintains body hydration and electrolyte balance. Self-renewal activity of skin results in new skin layers forming every 2–3 weeks. Skin mainly consists of three layers called epidermis, dermis, and hypodermis. Epidermis contains squamous epithelium, melanocyte cells (pigment containing), Langerhans cells and Merkel cells (pressure-sensing), and keratinocytes, which act as a protective barrier. Stratum basale, stratum spinosum, stratum granulosum, stratum lucidum, and stratum corneum are five different layers of epidermis. Cells in the basement layer (stratum basale) proliferate, differentiate, and migrate to upper layers, reach stratum corneum, the outermost layer that comes in contact with cosmetics, toxins, pathogens, textiles, and many other surfaces. Corneocytes in the stratum corneum covered with thin hydrophobic lipid layer that protect water loss from skin. Dermis, beneath epidermis, is mainly responsible for mechanical properties of skin and consists of fibroblasts, ECM, fibronectin, proteoglycans, elastin, collagen, blood vessels, lymphatic vessels, sebaceous glands, sweat glands, hair follicles, and nerve endings. It is separated from epidermis with basement layer and collagen, integrins, and laminins in its structure are responsible for epithelial-mesenchymal crosstalk. Hypodermis separates dermis from muscles (muscular fascia) and mainly consists of adipose tissue (Bhushan, 2017; Vig et al., 2017; Wong and Chang, 2009; Yildirimer et al., 2012). Collagen and elastin are structural proteins that support this tissue. Collagen binds cells together and is responsible for shape and function of animal body while elastin maintains extensibility to those collagenous tissues and is crucial for characteristic functions (Bailey, 2001). Hyaluronic acid (HA) is a high-molecular weight linear glycosaminoglycan synthesized by fibroblasts and keratinocytes and plays important roles in skin hydration and barrier function (Adrien et al., 2017).

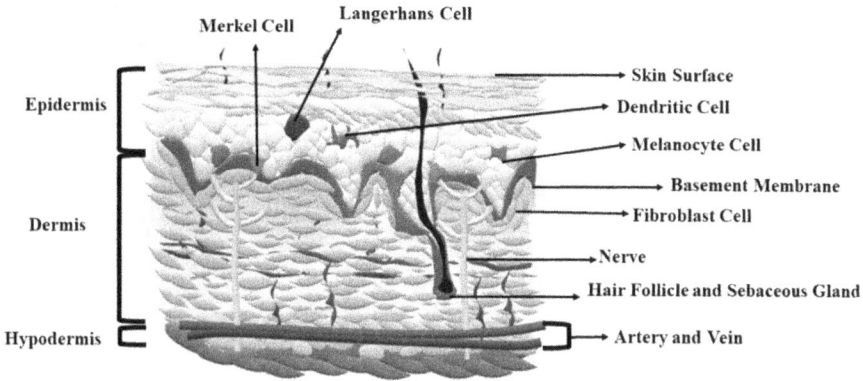

FIGURE 5.2   Anatomy of skin.

5.3   CHARACTERIZATION OF WOUND TYPES AND HEALING PROCESS

Skin can be damaged in several ways such as trauma (accidental, cut), burns (chemical, electrical, fire), UV radiation, ulcers (genetic, cancer, diabetes, venous, surgical, etc.), or infection (chronic and acute). Those damages can result in infection, loss of skin function, increased morbidity, and even death (Dhasmana et al., 2018a). Therefore, any wound occurring in this tissue affects human health dangerously. The treatment of those wounds might be expensive. 6.5 million people are suffering from 25 billion dollar treatment costs of those wounds in worldwide and low cost methods with fast healing procedure are in need (Chouhan et al., 2018). Wound types are classified in three main titles by rank, type, and thickness. Wounds are divided into two as tidy and untidy wounds by rank; into five main sections as clean, lacerating, hematoma, bruising, and abrasion by type; and again into five main groups as epidermal loss only, superficial, deep, and full by thickness.

Only epidermal loss wounds heal well with basic dressings and full re-epithelialization is expected with minimal scar tissue. Superficial wounds have partial thickness and good re-epithelialization is expected where epidermis and some papillary dermis are lost. In this type of wounds, tissue engineering aimed to help wound healing with little scar tissue. Deep wounds have long healing process and wound proceeds into epidermis, papillary, and also into deeper reticular dermis. Temporary or semipermanent tissue engineering skin dressings are preferred in this wound type. Healthy dermal wound beds are applied before skin grafts and also stem cell and/or growth factors can be used to decrease the healing time. Final wound type is full thickness where epidermis and all dermis tissues are lost sometimes with subdermal fat structures. In this type of wounds, there is complete skin tissue loss and underlying tissue should be covered with complex skin layers including epidermis and dermis. Permanent/semipermanent tissue-engineered scaffolds with full composites should be applied and also stem cells, growth factors, and vascular supply are needed in most cases. Skin grafts are still advanced methods for full-thickness wounds, if there is adequate autologous skin available on patient. Wound types and healing progresses are given in Table 5.1 and specified according to wound thickness (Adigbli et al., 2016; Ho et al., 2017; Madaghiele et al., 2014).

TABLE 5.1   Wound Types With Healing Progress According to Wound Thickness

	Location	Healing Time	Wound Closure/Scar
Epidermal loss	Epidermis	~5–7 days	Epidermal regeneration/ possible small scar formation
Partial thickness	Epidermis and papillary dermis	~2–4 weeks	Epithelial tissue regeneration/ possible small scar formation
Superficial	Epidermis, papillary, and reticular dermis	~3–5 weeks	Epithelial tissue regeneration/ scar formation
Deep			
Full thickness	Epidermis, dermis, and subdermal tissue	Months	No complete tissue regeneration/scar formation

Burn wounds can be classified according to hot sources as dry (fire and flame) and wet (scald). Burn shock occurs when 20% or more patient body surface is burned. Enhancement in capillary permeability causes hydrostatic pressure across protein and fluid transport from intravascular to interstitial space and decreased cardiac output causes shock. Basically, there are three zones on burn wounds: zone of coagulation, statis (or ischemia), and hyperemia. Coagulation zone is center of the burn, which is exposed to highest heat degree and maximum damage occurs in this area. Protein denaturation starts above 40 °C, so tissue necrosis is observed due to degradation and coagulation. Out of this zone, zone of statis is the least understood part of burn where perfusion is decreased and at the outmost area there is hyperemia where blood flow is increased by inflammatory vasodilation (widening of blood vessels) and likely to heal. Burns have high systemic inflammation unlike other wounds but wound healing phases are similar with other wounds such as inflammatory, proliferative, and remodeling. At the beginning of inflammation, neutrophils and monocytes are active in burn site and start the immune response. In this phase, infection is inhibited with necrotic tissue degradation and signal activation starts for healing. Same with other wounds in burns, keratinocytes and fibroblasts are involved to process in proliferative phase and scar maturation is observed as collagen and elastin reformation continue in remodeling stage (Monstrey et al., 2008; Rowan et al., 2015; Ter Horst et al., 2018; Wang et al., 2018). Superficial burns heal fast and epidermal tissue is regenerated rapidly but in more critical burn wounds, hair bulge is damaged so tissue regeneration is slow and scarred.

5.3.1   WOUND HEALING

Wound healing is the response of the body to restore the injury and gain the normal structure of tissue and its function. Wound healing involves four main stages named hemostasis, inflammation, proliferation, and remodeling. Hemostasis stage is started when keratinocytes respond to epidermal violation. This response is followed by clotting and vasoconstriction (narrowing of blood vessels) with secretion of growth factors and proinflammatory cytokines. Second stage is inflammation where neutrophils react to debride the wound area and lasts around 4–6 days. Secreted transforming growth factor-β (TGF-β) transforms monocyte cells into macrophages and by this transformation, inflammatory response occurs. Macrophages secrete fibroblastic growth factors and start the angiogenesis. Proliferative stage starts with granulation tissue formation and lasts around 2 weeks. Granulated tissue formation is induced by vascular endothelial growth factor (VEGF) and fibroblast growth factor (FGF) and starts in ECM with endothelial cell reproduction and angiogenesis. Fibroblasts are the most significant cells in this stage and wound shrinkage is executed by myofibroblasts. Fibroblasts secrete important ECM components such as collagen and glucosamine, which promote the skin healing. Final wound healing stage is remodeling phase and can last from months to years. First secreted collagen type is type III collagen and is replaced by type I collagen in second week. Collagen accumulation peaks at around third week and is balanced by degradation. Abnormal ECM function, diminishing level of growth factors, insufficient blood supply, and increasing of inflammatory interleukins and tumor necrosis factor (TNF) prevent proliferation stage and remodeling phase. These kinds of wounds are called chronic wounds. Significant cells and growth factors responsible in wound healing are given in Table 5.2 (Barrientos et al., 2008; Barrientos et al., 2014; Ho et al., 2017).

TABLE 5.2 Cells and Significant Growth Factors Responsible in Wound Healing Phases (Barrientos et al., 2008, 2014; Ho et al., 2017)

	Hemostasis	**Inflammation**	**Proliferation**	**Remodeling**
Process	Clotting (formation of platelet fibrin) Vasoconstriction	Macrophage secretion Inflammatory	Collagen and glycosamine production Granulation tissue formation Endothelial cell reproduction Angiogenesis	Collagen maturation Scar formation
Duration	Hours	4–6 days	~2 weeks	12–18 months
Predominant cell	Keratinocytes Platelets Endothelial cells	Neutrophils Monocytes Macrophages Endothelial cells Fibroblasts	Macrophages Fibroblasts Myofibroblasts T lymphocytes	T lymphocytes Fibroblasts Myofibroblasts
Cytokines	IL-1, TGF-α, TGF-β, PDGF, EGF, VEGF, and FGF	EGF, PDGF, TGF-β, FGF, IFN-α, TNF-α, and IL-1, -8, -10	EGF, VEGF, TGF-β, FGF, and IL-6	TGF-β, PDGF, and IGF-1

5.3.2 WOUND CARE

Wound survival rates are increased up to 97% over in last decades due to improved burn wound care and skin tissue engineering techniques. As in the skin tissue engineering publications, burn publications have been increased in recent years due to technological progresses. Commercial wound care products and clinical settings have been significantly increased over past few decades. It is important to make wound care preference according to wound type, pathophysiologic, and wound healing stage. The most common and complicated wounds are diabetic, surgical, ulcers, traumatic wounds, and deep severe burns.

Excision and grafting have been common and standard burn wound care for decades. Blood loss, infection risk, and death rate are decreased with excision method for patients without inhalation problems. To prevent infection, wound covering is necessary as soon as possible. Autografts are very common in permanent wound closure therapy, especially for full-thickness burns. They are favorable for reducing infection and tissue rejection but on the other hand remain pain on the own donor site. In 1979, cultured epithelial autografts (CEAs) were started to be used on burn treatments (Green and Elisseeff, 2016). It was thought to enhance the stem cell numbers and to increase burn wound healing. Somehow, with applying CEA alone, complete healing is not achieved and patients were faced to wound contractures even months after. Therefore, CEA with delivery system and matrix surface was developed and burn wound healings were improved. Besides, skin grafts are used as traditional burn dressing and xenografts are an outstanding choice for safety and cost-effectiveness. Also, Epicel® is still applied to burns as cellular therapy. Commercially available dermal components for burn closure include acellular surface generally from human such as Alloderm® and GraftJacket™ to decrease bacterial contamination and silver-containing dressings were introduced. Major commercially available burn dressings contain different polymers and substrates, for example, Aquacell®, Comfeel®, Biobrane®, Silverlon® (with antimicrobial activity), Fibracol®, Puracol®, Dermagel®, and SilvaSorb® (as hydrogel) are some of the commercially available ones. Presence of infection, fluid accumulation, and cleanness are important factors for choosing suitable wound dressings. Most of these dressings contain silver for antimicrobial and pain-reducing properties, but recent researches show that healing time is extended when applied on the infected wound and it needs to be replaced immediately after infection (Aziz et al., 2012; Nikkhah et al., 2013; Qian et al., 2017). Alternatively, methylene blue, honey, and polyhexamethylene biguanide are commonly used as antimicrobial agents. Recently, cell treatments have been developed. For example, in ReCell® (Avita, USA), small unit of biopsy is obtained and keratinocytes, melanocytes, and stem cell mixture are prepared for spraying technique. This method is highly favorable due to small unit need and decreased healing time for donor and patient. Wound healing processes and time can depend on characteristics of patient such as smoking, nutrition, obesity, age, and stress. Also, infection, diseases, and oxygenation can affect the healing. Temporary substitutes adhere on fresh wounds and are replaced after healing. Semipermanent substitutes are left on sanitized wound and in long run, autologous skin grafts are applied where epidermal,

dermal, or both analogs integrate onto the skin as permanent substitutes. Skin tissue engineering provides replica of skin tissue as cell layers, scaffolds, and growth factors and improves 3D structures. These scaffolds contain native matrix and/or polymeric tissue (Dhasmana et al., 2018b). Synthetic and natural biomaterials and their application will be discussed next in this chapter.

5.4   MATERIALS USED IN SKIN TISSUE ENGINEERING

Wound and burn dresses protect the injury zone and are developed to decrease the scar formation and healing time. Materials that used to produce these dresses are very important due to biocompatibility, biodegradability, nontoxicity, tissue-mimicking properties, and stability. Natural, synthetic, and biosynthetic (composite) polymers are being utilized for this purpose. Polysaccharides such as alginates, chitin, chitosan, heparin, proteoglycans, and proteins such as collagen, gelatin, fibrin, silk fibroin, and keratin are excessively preferred for wound tissue dressings.

5.4.1   NATURAL POLYMERS

Natural polymers are recognized by human body and are used in stem cell culture and regenerative medicine. They are highly preferred in the form of hydrogels and different types of polysaccharides such as β-glucans, dextran, cellulose (neutral), alginic acid, HA (acidic), chitin, chitosan (basic), heparin, chondroitin sulfate, dermatan sulfate, and keratan sulfate (sulfated) are being used widely (Bedian et al., 2017; Bhardwaj et al., 2018; Mogoşanu and Grumezescu, 2014). Alginate consists of β-D-mannuronic acid and α-L-glucunoric acid residues and can be found in cell wall of seaweed. Alginate is used to form sphere-like hydrogel in general whereby carboxyl and hydroxyl groups of glucunoric acid are blocked. These hydrogels are mimicking the ECM, so fibers and foams in skin tissue engineering can be replaced with alginate hydrogels (Koehler et al., 2017; Venkatesan et al., 2015). Pullulan is an $\alpha(1\rightarrow4)$, $\alpha(1\rightarrow6)$-D-glucan generally synthesized by fungus *Aureobasidium pullulans* from starch. Pullulan is used as antibacterial hydrogel wound dressing and water absorption is remarkable and can swell up to 4000%. Dextran is used in carboxymethyl benzyl amide sulfonate form in general to obtain heparin-mimetic and biomedical properties (Nahain et al., 2018). Dextran is being used to control *Staphylococcus aureus* proliferation and lipophilic odor molecule captures with longer activation time (Logeart-Avramoglou and Jozefonvicz, 1999). Cellulose is preferred as scaffold for chronic wounds and shows pain reducing and healing time-shortening properties. Granulation and epithelialization of the partial- and full-thickness wounded tissue are increased with cellulose dressings. Bacterial cellulose (BC) is now used for wound dressings and skin tissue engineering and has unique properties such as being a never-drying membrane. BC displays well mechanical strength and high physicochemical properties. Cellulose is used as regenerative medicine based on its ECM similarity and applied to injured skin for small-diameter blood vessel replacement (Kirdponpattara et al., 2017; Zmejkoski et al., 2018; Zulkifli et al., 2017). Chitin is an amino polysaccharide and the major component of crustaceans, insects, invertebrates, and wall of fungi. Chitosan is the deacetylated and soluble form of chitin and obtained by treating shells with sodium hydroxide. Levan is β-(2,6)-linked fructan-type homopolysaccharide and widely distributed in nature. Levan has a unique nature with biocompatible, water-soluble, adhesive, and heparin-mimetic properties for medicine, food, and cosmetic industries (Avsar et al., 2018; Erginer et al., 2016; Oner et al., 2016). Polyhydroxy-alkanoates (PHAs) are the member of aliphatic polyesters and synthesized by many of the bacteria and there are more than 150 different monomers of PHAs. They are suitable for skin tissue applications due to their biodegradable, biocompatible, and piezoelectric properties. In addition, scaffolds that formed with PHA have well cell adherence and suitable for cell growing and communication (Bedian et al., 2017; Getachew et al., 2016). HA is the most important ECM component and used for skin regeneration (Hussain et al., 2017). HA consists of N-acetyl-D-glucosamine and glucuronic acid and helps tissue to heal with scar free and enhances angiogenesis.

Proteins and peptides are significant for ECM and are used for skin tissue engineering applications extensively. Collagen is present in human body and especially skin which generated by fibroblasts is the most frequently used polymer in skin tissue engineering. Collagen has a major role in wound healing and new tissue formation with cell proliferation (Ramanathan et al., 2017; Sharif et al., 2018; Tangsadthakun et al., 2017). Partial- and full-thickness wounds are suitable for collagen dressings. Collagen is also used in third-degree burns and is favorable for allergic people (Oryan et al., 2018; Prabhu et al., 2018). Another important and underrated polymer is fibrin, which is also responsible for wound healing process similar with collagen. When skin barrier is damaged, fibrin network is developed rapidly. Fibrin scaffolds are used as cell transplant, hemostatic, and anti-inflammatory agent (Bencherif et al., 2017; Heher et al., 2018). Silk fibroin is also used for its adherent property, especially as skin grafts (Farokhi et al., 2018). Silk fibroin is a natural biopolymer and produced by *Bombyx mori* silkworms and contains both hydrophilic and hydrophobic domains. It has biocompatibility, controlled biodegradability, and easy fabrication characteristics. Biologically active functional silk fibroin is also used for its adherent property, especially as skin grafts in wound healing (Farokhi et al., 2018).

5.4.2 SYNTHETIC POLYMERS

Synthetic polymers are nonbiological component that have advantage of stability and controlled production, but they sometimes might be bioinert or lack of bioactivity. Synthetic polymers should not cause toxicity in living tissues when they degrade to their component. Their cost-effective production and availability make them popular in skin tissue engineering. Synthetic polymers consisting of nanobiomaterials with small pores and large surface area is used for wound and burn dressings (Gupta et al., 2010, Keservani et al., 2016). Today, many of these dressings are formed with electrospining techniques and main synthetic polymers are polyvinylpyrrolidone (PVP), polyvinyl alcohol (PVA), polyethylene glycol (PEG), and polyethylene oxide (PEO). In general, synthetic biomaterials are combined to form strong matrices.

One of the most known synthetic polymers is PVA and prepared by polymerizing vinyl acetate and polyvinyl acetate is converted to PVA. PVA-hydrogel membranes are significantly used for wound dressings and covers. PVA is not used only for cover, but also for healing efficiency (Kamoun et al., 2017). PVA-chitosan membranes showed rapid healing on full-thickness wound and nontoxicity (Yang et al., 2010). PEG is a biocompatible hydrophilic polymer and can interact with growth factors and ECM materials in skin tissue applications. PEG scaffolds are the most significant skin regeneration matrices in synthetic polymers. Similar with PVA, PEG can be cross-linked or blended with other polymers to improve mechanical properties and show antimicrobial activity, which is very important for wound dressings. PEG shows good cell adherence and growth under *in vitro* conditions (Chen et al., 2013; Jeong et al., 2017). PVP containing proton-accepting carbonyl moiety in pyrrolidone rings and its interaction with collagen polymer is wanted. In this interaction, collagen is hydrogen donor and generates hydrogen linkage with carbonyl group of PVP. PVP provides matrix support and protects the skin wound extensively and increases biostability with combination of other polymers (Moghaddam et al., 2018; Olmos-Zuñiga et al., 2017).

5.4.3 BIOSYNTHETIC POLYMERS

Stability and mechanical properties of natural polymers can be improved with synthetic ones and make biologically active, strong, and stable scaffolds with desired parameters. Combinations of bio- and synthetic materials have been extensively used as wound matrices and act as temporary epidermis to protect wound zone mechanically. Skin tissue engineering needs bio-/synthetic polymer scaffolds with high mechanical properties and new synthetic materials with new blends are being researched for skin tissue regeneration (Sionkowska, 2011). Combinations of bio- and synthetic materials have been extensively used as wound matrices and act as temporary epidermis to protect wound zone mechanically. TransCyte® (Shire, Switzerland) is one of the significant matrices that are composites of neonatal fibroblasts in nylon mesh. In that system, mesh supports for tissue growth and fibroblasts help in production of new ECM (Noordenbos et al., 1999). Skin tissue engineering needs bio-/synthetic polymer scaffolds with high mechanical properties and new synthetic materials with new blends are being researched for skin tissue regeneration (Sionkowska, 2011).

5.5 TREATMENT METHODS

5.5.1 SKIN GRAFTING

Skin grafting techniques such as autografting, allografting, and xenografting are used widely for wound healing studies. Autologous skin grafting technique is a treatment method of wounds by patient's own skin tissue that includes full epidermis and partial dermis shaved from donor site (generally inner tights or buttocks) using dermatome and placed on damaged site (Akan et al., 2003). This method is recommended for the deep dermal wounds that heal slowly and is called as clinical gold standard for full-thickness recovery (Groeber et al., 2011; Janeway et al., 2001). Even though no immune rejection risk occurs in this method, donor site is also another wound and comprises infection risk and extends hospital stay and recovery. Wound healing also depends on the thickness of dermis shaved. In conclusion, this method fails to satisfy treatment on deeper and larger wounds (Iqbal et al., 2018; Vig et al., 2017). Allografts are in use since World War II and this method includes cadaveric or viable tissue transfer from donors among same species and commonly used for burn treatment worldwide. Cadavers are stored frozen to use in need, thus suitable for skin banking.

Allografts act as a barrier besides promoting angiogenesis, preventing fluid loss, supplying growth factors, and cytokine for wound healing, but host immune rejection makes those grafts act as a temporary cover. Viral transfer risk of hepatitis B, C, and human immunodeficiency virus limits their usage (Dhasmana et al., 2018a; Groeber et al., 2011; Vig et al., 2017). Xenografts transfer tissues between different species and used as temporary grafts to promote dermal regeneration with collagen in their structure and overcome larger surface wound dressing problems with availability of tissues in large scale. Bovine and porcine dermal tissues are highly preferred on production of acellular scaffolds and are FDA approved while cadaveric goat tissue is also gaining importance with its cheaply availability, less immunogenicity, and reduced susceptibility to viruses and prions (Dhasmana et al., 2018a; Vig et al., 2017).

5.5.2 COMMERCIALLY AVAILABLE SKIN SUBSTITUTES

Skin substitutes are used to cover wounds that are deeper than epidermis and refer to biologic, synthetic, or mixed materials. Composition, targeted layer, permanence time, and the presence of cellular components vary between scaffolds that are available for skin regeneration applications. A substitute can be classified according to their material (biological, synthetic, combination), cellularity (cellular, acellular), layering (single layer, bilayer), replaced region (epidermis, dermis, both), and permanence (biodegradable, permanent) (Davison-Kotler et al., 2018). A functional skin substitute: (1) should protect fluid loss; (2) should be stable and degradable; (3) should allow vascularization, cellular proliferation inside scaffolds, and reduce scarring; and (4) should be user friendly, flexible, resistant to tearing, and inexpensive. Epidermal and dermal layer containing components are known to retain much more water than those single-layered ones. Fast degrading scaffolds reduce cellular migration inside scaffold while slow degrading ones are mechanically and biologically inert. Those substitutes can activate immune response and reduce dermal tissue formation success (Davison-Kotler et al., 2018; Van der Veen et al., 2010). Biological skin substitutes act as skin and promote natural ECM synthesis, re-epithelialization, and cheaper while synthetic ones can be synthesized in controlled condition suitable to demand but their bioactivity might be lower and can have toxicity (Farhadi-hosseinabadi et al., 2018).

In current tissue engineering strategies, skin substitutes can be applied alone or adhere to skin grafting as wound patch. These skin substitutes can be classified as temporary, semipermanent, and permanent (Horch et al., 2005). Tissue-engineered skin substitutes with cellular or acellular content gained popularity and solve drawbacks of traditional grafting techniques used in clinic. Advantages of living cellular substitutes over acellular scaffolds are secretion of cytokines, chemokines, and growth factors that promote re-epithelialization, and angiogenesis (Boink et al., 2018). On the other hand, those substitutes are complex and have risk of host immune rejection unless cells are autologous (Davison-Kotler et al., 2018).

5.5.2.1 EPIDERMAL SUBSTITUTES

Cultured epithelial autografts are used to treat burns. Keratinocytes from donor site biopsy are harvested enzymatically after separation of epidermis from dermis and cultured on mitotically inactivated mouse fibroblasts under xenogenic-free conditions. Epithelial cell cultures have limitations due to isolation difficulties and high costs (Leigh and Watt, 1994; Supp and Boyce, 2005a,). Both keratinocyte and epithelial culturing take time to construct sheets because of high cell number need and might be ineffective on large surface wounds. Commercially available allogenic products instead of autologous ones save money and time, but they both have risk of poor attachment and blister formations (Groeber et al., 2011; Woodley et al., 1988). Bioseed®-S, Epicel®, LaserSkin®, and Myskin® are autogenic keratinocyte-based single-layered epidermal substitutes (Davison-Kotler et al., 2018; Groeber et al., 2011; Vig et al., 2017) (Table 5.3). Bioseed®-S is a cost-effective (0.5 \$/cm^2) substitute, mainly used in leg ulcers or burns. Autologous keratinocyte cells are cultured in laboratory and applied to wound in a natural gel-like fibrin sealant, which fixes dividing cells on wound. Clinical studies on venous leg ulcers showed 50% increase in wound healing when compared to traditional therapies, but it is ineffective in infectious chronic wounds (Dhasmana et al., 2018b; Hüsing et al., 2003). Epicel® is an autologous keratinocyte sheet on petrolatum gauze used for full-thickness burns more than 30% of body surface and congenital nevus with low risk of rejection. High cost (15.15 \$/cm^2), 1-day shelf-life, 2–3 weeks of cell culturing, risk of infection, and lack of dermal component are general drawbacks of Epicel® (Carsin et al., 2000; Dhasmana et al., 2018b).

TABLE 5.3 Classification of Skin Substitutes Clinically Used and Found in Market

	Product	Company	Replaced Region	Materials	Permanence
Cellular skin substitutes	Epibase®	Genverier Lab, Sophia Antipolis, France	Epidermis	None/autologous keratinocyte	Temporary
	ReCell®	Avita, USA	Epidermis	Autologous keratinocyte and melanocyte	Temporary
Noncellular skin substitutes	Biobrane®	Bertek Pharmaceuticals, Morgantown, WV, US	Epidermis-dermis	Biosynthetic	Permanent
	Integra®	Integra Life Sciences, Plainsboro, NJ, US	Epidermis-dermis	Biosynthetic	Temporary
	Suprathel®	BioMed Sciences, Allentown, PA, USA	Epidermis	Synthetic	Temporary
	Hyalomatrix®	Anika Therapeutics, Inc., Bedford, MA, USA	Epidermis-dermis	Biosynthetic	Temporary
	Smart Matrix®	Smart Matrix Limited, Northwood, UK	Dermis	Natural	Temporary
	Silverlon®	Argentum, USA	Epidermis	Synthetic	–
	Comfeel®	Coloplast, USA	Epidermis	Natural	-
	Opsite®	Smith & Nephew, Massachusetts	Epidermis	Synthetic	–
	Fibracol®	Johnson & Johnson, NJ	Epidermis	Biosynthetic	–
	Aquacell®	ConvaTec, USA	Epidermis	Natural	–
Decellularized skin substitutes	Alloderm®	LifeCell Corporation, Branchburg, NJ	Dermis	Natural	Temporary
	Cadaveric Skin Dermagraft®	Intercytex Ltd., Manchester, UK	Dermis	Natural	Temporary
	GraftJacket®	Wright Medical Technology, Inc., USA	Dermis	Natural	–
	Apligraf®	Organogenesis/Novartis, Canton, MA, US	Epidermis-dermis	Natural	Temporary
	Orcel®	Ortec International, New York, USA	Epidermis-dermis	Natural	Temporary

TABLE 5.3 (Continued)

	Product	Company	Replaced Region	Materials	Permanence
	LaserSkin®	Fidia Advanced Biopolymers, Padua, Italy	Epidermis	Natural	Temporary
	Bioseed®-S	BioTissue Technologies GmbH, Freiburg, Germany	Epidermis	Natural	Temporary
	Hyalograft 3D®	Fidia Advanced Biopolymers, Italy	Epidermis-dermis	Natural	Permanent
	PermaDerm™	Regenicin, Inc., NJ, US	Epidermis-dermis	Natural	Temporary
	PolyActive®	Holland Composite Implants B.V., The Netherlands	Epidermis-dermis	Synthetic	Temporary
	MySkin®	Regenerys Ltd., Sheffield, UK	Epidermis	Synthetic	Temporary
	Trancyte®	Advanced BioHealing, Inc., USA	Epidermis-dermis	Biosynthetic	Permanent
Xenogenic skin substitutes	Permacol™	Tissue Science Laboratories plc, UK	Dermis	Natural	Temporary
	OASIS®	Cook Biotech, Inc., West Lafayette, US	Dermis	Natural	Temporary
	Matriderm®	Medskin solutions, Dr Suwelack AG, Billerbeck, Germany	Dermis	Natural	Temporary
	Puracol®	Medline, USA	Epidermis-dermis	Natural	

LaserSkin® is a temporary skin substitute that keratinocytes and fibroblasts are grown on microperforated HA membranes and used for diabetic ulcers with features such as cell migration, biocompatibility, less immunogenicity, and reduced scarring, but it is high cost (129 $/cm²), short lifespan, and could only be applied on partial-thickness epidermal wounds restrict its usage (Caravaggi et al., 2003; Dhasmana et al., 2018b). Myskin® is a keratinocyte subconfluent culture on synthetic plasma polymerized silicone film and used for neopatic pressure, diabetic foot ulcers, or superficial burns (Shevchenko et al., 2009). Cell spraying is another method used for deep dermal injuries or correction of pigment disorders to create an epidermal cover where proliferative keratinocytes from donors are sprayed to wound but risk of infection and donor rejection are limitations of this method. Epibase® overcomes this problem with using autologous confluent keratinocytes to spray over wound to make an outer layer, but it is expensive (53 $/cm²), requires long cultivation period, has short shelf-life, and difficult to handle (Dhasmana et al., 2018b; Gravante et al., 2007; Kirsner et al., 2012). Suprathel® is an acellular, synthetic (poly-D,L-lactide) absorbable epidermal wound adhesive used for partial-thickness burns or acute surgical wounds with low cost (1 $/cm²), long shelf-life, and reduced bleeding features while treatment time in deeper wounds increases (Dhasmana et al., 2018b; Rashaan et al., 2017). Silverlon®, Aquacell®, Fibracol®, Dermagel®, Comfeel®, and Opsite® are other epithelial substitutes used for burns and wounds.

5.5.2.2   DERMAL SUBSTITUTES

On deep wounds, partial or complete damage occurs in epidermis and dermis layers and cannot be healed completely or adequately due to lack of keratinocytes to restore epithelium and those kind of wounds require full-thickness skin substitutes that maintain skin function and restoration (Dhasmana et al., 2018a; Janewa et al., 2005,). In full-thickness burns, epidermal and dermal layers need to be replaced both. Usage of dermal constructs provides mechanical stability to the wounds (Groeber et al., 2011). There are several commercially available dermal substitutes present in market including autograft, allograft, and xenograft ones. Alloderm®, Matriderm®, Cadaveric Skin Dermagraft®, OASIS Wound Matrix®, Permacol®, and Smart Matrix® are some of them (Davison-Kotler et al., 2018) (Table 5.3). Alloderm® is a lyophilized cadaveric human acellular dermis that is used for burns and full-thickness wounds from surgeries but it is expensive (6.45 $/cm²) (Dhasmana et al., 2018b; Gordley et al., 2009; Varkey et al., 2015). Matriderm®

is a xenogenic highly porous bovine lyophilized acellular dermal substitute that consists of collagen I, III, and V and is coated with elastin hydrolysate used for full-thickness burns with ECM deposition, neovascularization, and great cellular infiltration abilities (Límová, 2010; Vilela et al., 2018). Cadaveric Skin Dermagraft® is an allogenic bioabsorbable, human neonatal foreskin fibroblast seeded on a polygalactin mesh matrix coated with porcine dermal collagen. It is used to cover chronic wounds and diabetic ulcers and second- and third-degree burns. It has long shelf-life but allogenity-derived immune rejection risk and lack of strong ECM result in infections and cellulitis are disadvantages (Dhasmana et al., 2018b; Varkey et al., 2015; Vig et al., 2017). OASIS Wound Matrix® is a porcine small intestine submucosa acellular ECM-derived natural sheet used for burns, trauma, chronic lower limbs, postoncological resections, and diabetic foot ulcers. It is effective in full-thickness wounds and highly costly (11.2 $/cm^2) (Agostini et al., 2018; Dhasmana et al., 2018b; Scarritt et al., 2019). Permacol® is a porcine dermis cross-linked sheet used for soft-tissue repairs, abdominal wall reconstruction, and has good esthetic functionality but it is expensive (17 $/cm^2), have risk of infection, hematoma and seroma generation, and lack of vascularization (Dhasmana et al., 2018b; Scarritt et al., 2019; Vig et al., 2017). Smart Matrix® is a human fibrin and alginate matrix used to treat wounds (Davison-Kotler et al., 2018). Cultured autologous dermal fibroblasts are seeded on a 3D HA-derived scaffold, Hyalograft® 3D, to treat deep burns and diabetic ulcers with growth factors and cytokines from fibroblasts and enhanced basement membrane formation (Dhasmana et al., 2018b; Límová, 2010; Shevchenko et al., 2009). Dermal constructs are important for healing with reduced scar tissue formation. Using keratinocyte sheets alone, it may result in inadequate healing and before usage of epidermal sheets (natural or commercially available), dermal vascularization needs to be achieved (Groeber et al., 2011). Dermal scaffold Lando® is shown to have vascularization effect on full-thickness skin defect porcine model that resulted in reduced infection, smoother and granulated tissues, dryer wound, and increased microvessel (CD31$^+$, α-SMA$^+$) VEGF expression in 14 days (Qiu et al., 2018).

5.5.2.3   EPIDERMAL AND DERMAL SUBSTITUTES

Epidermal and dermal substitutes are sophisticated and advanced ones that contain both autologous and allogenic cells (keratinocytes and fibroblasts) together with scaffolds that mimic epidermal and dermal layers of skin and provide cytokine, ECM, or growth factors for host cells. Allogenic fibroblasts used in substitutes carry immune rejection risk (Groeber et al., 2011; Supp and Boyce, 2005a). Apligraf®, Biobrane®, Hyalomatrix®, Integra®, Orcel®, PolyActive®, TranCyte®, PermaDerm™, and denovoSkin™ are examples for commercially available ones (Table 5.3). Apligraf® is a bilayer constructed sheet of human allogenic neonatal cultured fibroblasts and keratinocytes together with bovine type I collagen and used for treatment of epidermolysis bullosa, chronic venous insufficiency ulcers, and diabetic foot ulcers. Usages of this substitute have limitations such as repeated application requirement, reduced in-vivo cell survival, disease transfer risk, short shelf-life, and difficulties in handling (Allie et al., 2018; Davison-Kotler et al., 2018; Dhasmana et al., 2018b). Biobrane® consists of silicone membrane to mimic epidermis and nylon mesh for dermis mimicry implanted in porcine collagen. It is used for treatment of carcinogenic surgery wounds and surface burns. It has low pain and morbidity risk, cheap (1.30 $/cm^2) while intolerant to contaminated wound bed, requires immediate coverage and infection, or toxic shock syndrome generation risks limits its usage (Agostini et al., 2018; Dhasmana et al., 2018b; Vig et al., 2017). Hyalomatrix® is another acellular HA- and silicon membrane-derived 3D scaffold with cellular invasion and capillary growth abilities used for partial-thickness wound, but causes infection in wound site (Dhasmana et al., 2018b; Mohebichamkhorami and Alizadeh, 2018). Integra® is a silicone membrane (epidermal layer), shark chondroitin-6-sulfate glycosaminoglycan, and bovine type I collagen (dermal layer) containing substitute and deep partial-thickness or full-thickness burns are treated with it. Although it has good esthetic function and neodermis formation ability, it has poor adhesion, requires two-stage application process, has infection risk, and expensive (6.15 $/cm^2) (Dhasmana et al., 2018b; Vig et al., 2017). Orcel® is a bilayer substitute where allogenic neonatal foreskin fibroblasts are cultured on type I collagen matrix as dermal side and keratinocytes are cultured in air-liquid interface (epidermal side) and used for partial-thickness burns. Even it is recurred scarring and favors cell migration, it is expensive (6.32 $/cm^2), have rejection and contamination risks, and can be used as biological dressing instead of permanent one (Dhasmana et al., 2018b; Mohebichamkhorami and Alizadeh, 2018). PolyActive® is a cellular synthetic bilayer scaffold that fibroblasts and keratinocytes are cultured on PEO terephthalate/polybutylene terephthalate and serves as temporary substitute (Mohebichamkhorami and Alizadeh, 2018). PermaDerm™ is autologous human fibroblast and keratinocyte seeded bilayer bovine collagen matrix. Inexpensiveness (1 $/cm^2), reduced mortality and morbidity rate in deep burns, and shorter wound closure time are advantages while induced immunogenic response and frequent regrafting requirement are limitations of this matrices (Dhasmana et al., 2018b; Mohebichamk-horami and Alizadeh, 2018). TranCyte® is one of the significant matrices that composite of neonatal fibroblasts in nylon mesh. In that system, mesh supports for tissue growth and fibroblasts help in production of new ECM (Noordenbos et al., 1999).

Several skin grafts and substitutes are produced by researchers, but there is no ideal skin substitute has been placed in market up to now. Skin grafting is a time-consuming and expensive process to produce grafts (2–3 weeks culturing) and covering 1% of body with Epicel® is known to cost more than $13,000. Commercially available skin substitutes have drawbacks such as poor mechanical integrity, scarring, immune rejection, and poor revascular-ization ability-related cellular death. Substitutes also known to have short lifespan such as fibrin-containing dermal substitutes that can be cultured 12 weeks and storage of those cells is another problem. Thus, economi-cally friendly and large scale productions are in need. Currently available cellular substitutes contain fibroblasts and keratinocytes; thus, they do not have ability to generate hair follicles and sweat glands. To overcome these problems, endothelial cells, stem cells, and other types of cells need to be integrated with grafting technique (Groeber et al., 2011; Vig et al., 2017).

5.5.3 SCAFFOLDS

Various strategies are developed for production of skin tissue supporting scaffolds, which can be cellular/acellular, synthetic, biosynthetic, or natural. Nanofibers, sponges, 3D-printed scaffolds, foams, cryogels, and decel-lularized matrices are highly used in skin tissue engineering applications. Biological activity of cells and tissues can be regulated via biochemical factors such as hormones and growth factors; biophysical features of scaf-fold have important effects on biological response in the concept of "mate-riobiology." This concept considers properties of biomaterials that effect biological response, functionality, and seek to improve biological behaviors of those materials with multidisciplinary approach (Qian et al., 2017). Proliferation, differentiation, migration, and other functionalities of cells are affected by pore size, mechanical properties such as Young's modulus (stiffness), elasticity, topography [two-dimensional (2D)], geometry (3D), chemical, and temporal properties such as degradation rate and biocompat-ibility of scaffolds. Smaller pore sizes are known to limit extension of stem cells. Stiffness of a material affects cellular adhesion and most cells prefer to adhere surfaces that have similar stiffness of themselves (McCarthy et al.,

2018; Qian et al., 2017). Cells prefer to adhere stiffer 2D surfaces instead of soft ones. Adhesion of cells is important but understanding 3D environment and cellular behavior is important for designing full-thickness scaffolds, disease models, and biomimetic materials. 3D scaffolds instead of 2D ones provide variable of geometric parameters, porous structure, special degradability, and stiffness (Qian et al., 2017). Cellular migration and proliferation can be manipulated by material elasticity, contact angle, surface wettability, surface roughness, decoration with functional groups, ECM proteins, and special motifs (Arima and Iwata, 2007; Dubin-Thaler et al., 2004; Petrie and Yamada, 2012; Smith et al., 2015). ECM provides microenvironment for cells and supports their growth and proliferation, plays role in cell–cell interaction, and stimulates fibroblasts to control cellular phenotype, function, adhesion, genetic, or protein expression with biochemical information. ECM-mimicking skin substitute designs with essential growth factors, cytokines, integrins, motifs such as arginine-glycine-asparagine (RGD) for cell-ECM, cadherins for cell–cell adhesion, and tripeptides for improved cellular migration, proliferation, and protein synthesis are gained popularity in postinjury applications (Bhardwaj et al., 2018; Iqbal et al., 2018; Qian et al., 2017). Restrata wound matrix (RWM) is a sterile single-use novel synthetic nanofabricated scaffold and used for wound defects coverage. These synthetic polymers are polyglactin 910 poly(lactic-co-glycolic acid) (PLGA) and polydioxanone and used as resorbable sutures. High mechanical properties such as durability, conformable, nonfriable, and absorbable made it a good candidate for skin tissue engineering applications (Kumbar et al., 2008; Zhong et al., 2011). Cellular scaffolds used in treatment are illustrated in Figure 5.3.

5.5.3.1 HYDROGELS

Hydrogels are highly hydrated polymeric networks that consist of chemically or physically cross-linked 3D structures. They have huge water holding capacity due to their hydrogen bonding. Their water content can reach up to 90% by weight (Jeong et al., 2017). Due to their low foreign body response, flexible, sensitive, and water content characteristics, they have been becoming focus of tissue dressings. First hydrogel application was performed by Wichterle and Lim (1960) and cross-linked poly(2-hydroxyethyl methacrylate) to use as contact lens material. First developed polymeric materials were hydrogels and in 1980s, hydrogels have been already used for cell encapsulation (Lim and Sun, 1980). Today, hydrogels are mainly used for

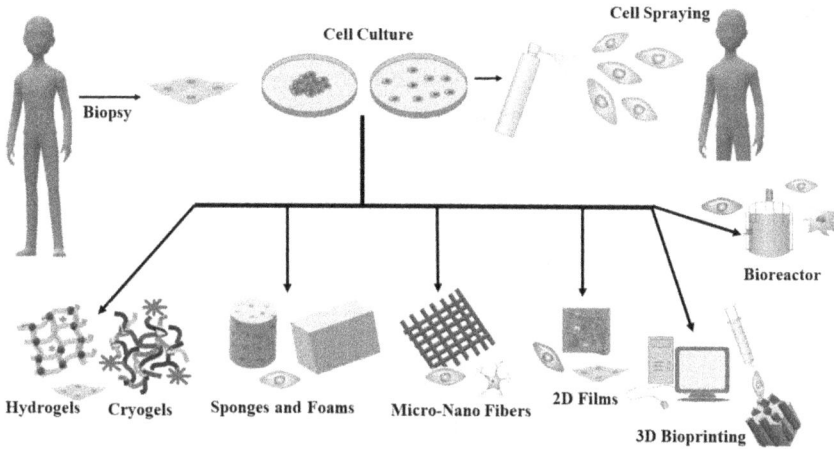

FIGURE 5.3   Scaffolds used in cell-based treatment.

wound healing in clinical applications for their 3D ECM biomimetic properties and there are numerous types of hydrogels based on their response,
origin, and structure composition (Bhardwaj et al., 2018; El-Sherbiny and
Yacoub, 2013; Naahidi et al., 2017; Sorg et al., 2017). Hydrogels are not only
used as primary wound dressings, but also as skin regenerative matrices.
These materials are easily modified and engineered to manage cell attachment, integrity, biocompatibility, biodegradability, and molecular response.
Beside these beneficial properties, conjugation methods and/or ionic charges
could cause poor biocompatibility (Naahidi et al., 2017; Silva-Correia et al.,
2013). As burn and wound care applications, hydrogels can be used in first
aid treatment, as primary wound dressings, and also as skin regenerative
scaffolds. They can absorb and hold the wound exudate, which promote the
fibroblast proliferation and also migration of keratinocyte. Hydrogels have
been using for decreasing the temperature of wound area and to reduce the
pain in first aid treatments. When clean water is not available, hydrogels are
very good source to cool the wound zone under favor of high water capacity.
As primary wound dress, hydrogels are used to increase wound closure and
to reduce scar and contracture in partial-thickness wounds. In full-thickness
wounds, hydrogels are used as skin regenerative matrices for normal dermis
with vessels and nerves (Caló et al., 2018; Madaghiele et al., 2014). Hydrogels, with pore size below 100 nm (in the swollen state), prevent microorganisms, but allow transportation of significant bioactive materials such as
pharmaceuticals. These molecules can be trapped in hydrogel network and
drug release can be provided by drug delivery system on the wound bed

(Chakavala et al., 2012; Hamedi et al., 2018). Hydrogels also can adapt their structure to wound bed due to flexible and elastic features. Dressing changes are less painful with hydrogels because of not sticky form of the network surface and also transparent hydrogels are providing significant advantages to observe wound area without disassemble the dressing. There are several commercially available gel-type treatments for wound care such as amorphous gels, gel gauze, and sheets. Amorphous gel can be injected into cavity wounds and gauze and sheets are suitable for generally superficial wounds. One of the examples for commercially available hydrogel product is MySkin® and it is a direct wound dressing with easy application (Mishra et al., 2018). Hydrogel products are already in the market for skin care; on the other hand, researches on hydrogel to increase skin healing have been increasing since the beginning of the century. For this cause, natural and synthetic polymers are commonly used to form hydrogels. Natural polymers such as collagen, chitin/chitosan, HA, keratin, fibrin, and decellularized ECM have been processed from organisms due to low cytotoxicity. For partial-thickness wounds, chitin hydrogel and zinc oxide nanoparticles were blended to form antimicrobial product with microporous structure. This wound dresses have antimicrobial activity, nontoxic, and blood clotting properties (Kumar et al., 2012). Another important and attractive polymer in skin tissue engineering is keratin due to its biocompatibility and wound repair effects. In one study, keratin hydrogel was used as chemical burn dressing in mice model and thermal burn in swine model. In both studies, keratin hydrogel improved the wound closure and promoted cell proliferation (Poranki et al., 2014). Wang et al. (2017) used feather keratin from chicken to form hydrogel and investigated wound healing abilities *in vivo*. Keratin hydrogels show high compatibility and decrease immunogenicity with toxicity and suggested good wound dress. Combinations of natural polymers are also commonly used in hydrogel form. Wu et al. (2017) combined HA and gelatin with cross-linker such as 1-ethyl-3-(3-dimethylamineopropyl)carbodiimide hydrochloride. This hydrogel showed excellent fluid uptake with good moisture environment support for wound zone. *In vivo* test results indicated cell proliferation effect and wound closure. Development of levan hydrogels is also significantly increasing due to unique properties of levan polysaccharide such as biocompatibility, low intrinsic viscosity and adherence, and decreasing of production costs are making levan an important polysaccharide in skin tissue engineering applications (Choi et al., 2018; Oner et al., 2016; Osman et al., 2017). Same with the other biomaterials, HA hydrogels are favorable with its healing properties and cell proliferation effects. HA is a component molecule of skin, so provides healing with minimum scar tissue and moisture (Collins and Birkinshaw, 2013; Murphy et al., 2017). Collagen hydrogels are also universally used in burn and wound healing and Apligraf® is the significant commercially available collagen hydrogels product and viable cells (Supp and Boyce, 2005b). For full-thickness burn, tissue treatments such as dextran-based hydrogel promoted migration of angiogenic cells and tissues over 7 days. By day 21, wounds with hydrogels developed epithelial structure and hair follicles (Sun et al., 2011). As a synthetic material, PVA hydrogels are commonly used as wound dressings. Oliveira et al. (2014) reported PVA hydrogels with silver nanoparticles as antimicrobial agents and when burn conditions were provided, PVA hydrogels take up wound's fluid and swell. Other important polymer is PEG and in general PEG is blended with natural polymers such as cellulose. In one study, carboxymethyl cellulose (CMC) was used for wound dressing and as skin repair material. In hydrogel system, PEG played a significant role in hybrid polymeric network formation and favorable for biocompatibility (Capanema et al., 2018). In beginning of the 21st century, 3D bioprinting technology has been a significant method to develop new materials for skin tissue applications after first bioprinting of viable cells by Dr Thomas Boland (Su and Al'Aref, 2018). In order to obtain highly viscous with high mechanical strength, hydrogels are started to be substitutes in bioprinters. A bioprinter company (PrintAlive Bioprinter, Canada) has developed a method for creating fibroblast and keratinocyte bilayered hydrogels to form suitable matrix for skin transplantation (Mearian, 2015; Yoon, 2014). HA hydrogel studies increased recently due to healing efficiency of the hydrogels. Solubilized amnion membrane and HA hydrogel were applied to the full-thickness wound model *in vivo* and remarkable wound closure with re-epithelialization occurred (Murphy et al., 2017). Choi et al. (2018) prepared injectable levan-based hydrogel as a dermal filler with combination of CMC. Cell proliferation and collagen synthesis in human dermal fibroblasts are increased and levan hydrogel showed enhanced anti-wrinkle properties when compared to HA in mouse. So, results showed that levan is favorable for dermal fillers for skin tissue and wound healing. Pullulan hydrogels prevent dehydration of wound zone and exudate accumulation. Not only wound dress but also antibacterial drugs can be loaded into pullulan hydrogels to prevent microbial biofilm formation (Gurtner et al., 2011; Xu et al., 2018). All these findings are remarkable and exciting developments for skin tissue engineering achieved by hydrogels. Fluid intake capacity, antimicrobial and pain reduction properties with enhanced cell proliferation, and skin regeneration make hydrogels a special significant medical skin care product.

5.5.3.2 CRYOGELS

Cryogels are generated via controlled freeze thaw of polymer solutions. Those scaffolds are ECM analog with highly porous structures that promote cellular migration, encourage healing, prevent infection, and their sponge-like structure prevents fluid deposition in wounds. They are also good carriers to protect adhesive cells from excess compression forces of injection with minimally invasive delivery abilities and good candidates for skin tissue engineering applications (Béduer et al., 2018; Hixon et al., 2017). Hixon et al. (2017) investigated effect of 3D-printed, collagen I-coated CMC-free formed centrimetric scale cryogels on human foreskin fibroblasts (*in vitro*) and CD1 mice (*in vivo*). Highly porous, elastic cryogels are found to be biocompatible and remained encapsulation free for 3 months without any sign of inflammation and controlled cell seeding density, tissue infiltration, and vascularization are observed. Shape memorizing 3D-printed injectable methacrylated hyaluronic acid (MA-HA) cryogels are shown good candidates for skin sculpting and soft-tissue reconstructions on mice experiments and angiogenicity, tissue compatibility, shape predictability and retention abilities, and without any inflammatory response (Cheng et al., 2017).

Collagen-chondroitin-6-sulfate (glycosaminoglycan) scaffolds for wound healing are generated via freeze-drying process by Ansari et al. (2018) and amniotic fluid-derived stem cells are preferred due to their proliferation capability, multipotency, cytokine secretion [VEGF, epidermal growth factor (EGF), and TGF-β], and lack of immunogenicity. Great cellular expansion, spreading, and growth on scaffolds are shown after 14 days.

5.5.3.3 SPONGES

Sponge scaffolds are used as dermal substitutes, which provide ECM for fibroblast proliferation in controlled conditions with reduced scarring and wound contraction. Integra®, Terudermis®, and Pelnac® are commercial version of collagen-based scaffolds that aimed fibroblast infiltration and collagen durability (Maver et al., 2015). Choi et al. (2018) generated oxygen-releasing hydrogel sponge scaffolds by hydrogen peroxide (H_2O_2) containing PLGA microspheres engrafted into alginate-based hydrogels and their wound healing activity is tested *in vitro* and *in vivo*. Induced neovascularization, cell proliferation, and facilitated wound healing are observed and authors concluded that oxygen-releasing sponges are strong candidate in application of oxygen-requiring tissues. In one study, cross-linked succinyl pullulan and carboxymethyl chitosan composites were used to form wound dressing sponges. Sponge dress indicated the reducing effect on releasing of wound exudates with no cytotoxicity. Pullulan-containing dress healed full layer of skin wound in *in vivo* experiments. Also, this material complex accelerated the fibroblast proliferation with increase of epithelial migration and indicated the importance of using biomaterials together (Wang et al., 2017).

5.5.3.4   NANOFIBERS

Nanofibers are great wound dressing for skin tissue engineering applications with their natural ECM mimetic activity, large surface area, reproducibility, and fabrication easiness that improve cell adhesion, differentiation and proliferation, high porosity, wound tissue fluid absorption, ideal wettability, and good drug or growth factor carrier abilities (Bhardwaj et al., 2018; Lin et al., 2018). Gelatin/chitosan electrospun scaffolds are shown to improve proliferation and attachment of human dermal fibroblast cells with the content of 30% chitosan (Pezeshki-Modaress et al., 2018). Functionalized citrus pectin and silk fibroin 3D scaffold are proposed as a candidate of dermal skin substrate by Türkkan et al. (2018) with high porosity, water uptake, stability, similar elastic modulus with skin, and increased adhesion, penetration, and proliferation of L929 (murine fibroblast) cells. Bioactive glass (BG) is used in soft tissue engineering because of its angiogenic activity and biocompatibility. BG microfibers are shown to stimulate VEGF secretion, tube formation, endothelial growth, and angiogenic gene expression of fibroblasts in full-thickness skin-defected rats (Zhao et al., 2015). Lin et al. (2018) proposed poly(ε-caprolactone) (PCL) electrospun nanofibers with BG nanoparticles on it as candidates for skin tissue engineering applications. Improved hydrophilicity, elastic modulus, stability, cellular adhesion, and proliferation were observed in presence of BG.

5.5.3.5   DECELLULARIZED SCAFFOLDS

Acellular scaffolds can be created with decellularization of allograft of xenograft tissues (cadaveric tissues, goat, porcine, or bovine tissues) and provide environment for cells with their ECM architecture to attach and proliferate and chemical–structural information for cellular and vascular growth. Contamination risk of immunogens such as DNA, prions, and alpha-gal needs to be tested prior to implantation and limits their usage (Bhardwaj et al., 2018; Dhasmana et al., 2018a). Effect of connective tissue growth factor-loaded mouse decellularized dermal matrix investigated on streptozotocin (STZ)-induced type 2 diabetes mice and improved wound closure, enhanced fibronectin, TGF-β, and alpha-smooth muscle actin expression are observed (Yan et al., 2018b).

5.5.3.6 FOAMS AND FILMS

Moon Lee et al. (2016) investigated wound healing performance of Medifoam®N over other polyurethane foam dressings on rat wound models. Medifoam®N showed improved wound healing with smallest pore size, moderate thickness, density, tensile strength, fluid absorption and retention, good angiogenesis, and collagen deposition capacities. HA foams with silver component decreased the wound size up to 77% on the rat skin without inflammation after 1 week (Cho et al., 2002). 3D-layered artificial skin from skin fibroin is developed due its biocompatible and ECM-mimicry properties (Gholipourmalekabadi et al., 2018). Levan-based thin films are developed for healing the injured tissue due to its metalloproteinase activation, which is a significant key process in tissue healing (Sturzoiu et al., 2011). Costa et al. (2013) integrated phosphonated levan and chitosan layer-by-layer and observed good cell adherence when compared to only chitosan (110 cells per mm^2 with levan and 20 cells per mm^2 for only chitosan). Also, levan with PEO revealed good stability, flexibility, and biocompatibility that suits for skin tissue engineering. Gomes et al. (2018) report the use of chitosan, alginate, and sulfated levan for free-standing films and films with sulfated levan indicate high tensile and shear stress with four times higher adhesion than chitosan-alginate control films. In general, antibacterial chitin-/chitosan-based films with silver nanoparticles were produced for wound healing (Archana et al., 2015; Cremar et al., 2018; Ghannam et al., 2018; Madhumathi et al., 2010; Mehrabani et al., 2018). Summa et al. (2018) combined alginate and povidone-iodine (PVPI) complex films and treated on mouse model wounds. Designed-material treatment has shown complete wound closure in only 12 days with excellent wound healing capacities of alginate and antiseptic release from PVPI. Films also reduced the inflammatory response on human fibroblast after infection (Summa et al., 2018). In 2017, 2D transition metal dichalcogenides thin-layered nanosheets were developed using aqueous silk fibroin by Huang et al. (2017). Due to peroxidase-like activity of nanosheets, silk fibroin-based films provided disinfection on wound area and enhanced healing.

5.6 RECENT AND FUTURE PROMISING TECHNIQUES FOR SKIN EQUIVALENT DESIGNING

5.6.1 CELL CO-CULTURES

Cellular co-culturing method is generally used for development of 3D full-thickness skin substitutes that are similar to natural skin. Human dermal fibroblasts (Thangapazham et al., 2014), keratinocytes (foreskin) (Li et al., 2004), angiogenic endothelial progenitor cells (King et al., 2014), hair follicle stem cells (Dong et al., 2007), keratinocyte stem cells (Fortunel et al., 2010), bone marrow-derived stem cells (Dabiri et al., 2013), adipose-derived mesenchymal stem cells (Jackson et al., 2012), differentiated embryonic stem cells, or induced pluripotent stem cells are used for development of skin substitutes for cell-based treatments (Thangapazham et al., 2014; Vig et al., 2017). Culturing human dermal fibroblast or epithelial cells together with keratinocytes are known to effect keratinocyte growth positively via growth factors or cell–cell interactions (Vig et al., 2017). To overcome hypopigmentation problems, keratinocytes, melanocytes, and Langerhans cells are cocultured together with dermal fibroblasts to help in natural pigmentation and immunologic reaction observation of cultured skin equivalents (Vig et al., 2017). Coculturing cells with 3D-printed scaffolds and bioreactor system allow designing skin substitutes that match with hosts own skin and may help to treat pigmentation-based diseases.

5.6.2 STEM CELL THERAPY

Stem cells are self-renewal cells and have ability to differentiate to different cell types (multipotency). Bone marrow-derived mesenchymal stem cells (MSCs) are adult stem cells and can differentiate to bone, cartilage, fat, and skin tissues and are good candidates for cell-based therapies used in bone marrow transplantation (Pittenger et al., 1999). Difficulties of MSCs isolation from bone marrow made MSCs-derived adipose stem cells (ASCs) alternative because of harvesting easiness in large numbers from fat tissues (McCarthy et al., 2018). ASCs are shown to reduce inflammation and promote chronic wound healing and neovascularization in animal studies. Those abilities made ASCs strong candidates for skin tissue regeneration applications. Healing mechanism is followed by: (1) ASCs differentiation to keratinocyte, pericyte, or other cells to normalize wound bed and (2) cytokine and chemokine secretion for tissue regeneration (Bertozzi et al., 2017; Frykberg and Banks, 2015; McCarthy et al., 2018; Toyserkani et al., 2015; van den Broek et al., 2013). ASCs cytokines help in angiogenesis with the secretion of vascular endothelial growth factor-A (VEGF-A), Angiotensin-I (Ang-I), Basic fibroblast growth factor, fibroblast growth factor-2 (FGF-2), and transforming growth factor-β1 (TGF-β1) (Cerqueira et al., 2016; Ucuzian et al., 2010), decreased inflammation [interleukin-6 (IL-6)] (Blaber et al., 2012), granulation of tissue formation with IL-8 (CXCL8) (van den Broek et al., 2013), re-epithelialization (EGF) (Cerqueira et al., 2016), and increased type I to type III collagen formation (Hu et al., 2016). Exosomes secreted by ASCs metabolized by fibroblasts in cytoplasm and effect fibroblast proliferation, migration, and secretion of collagen (Hu et al., 2016). Wang et al. (2017) found that ASCs exosomes increased collagen production by fibroblasts at the early stages of wound healing while collagen production in late stages is decreased. Thus, wound healed with reduced scar formation. Pre-subjecting ASCs to hypoxia is known to improve paracrine secretion of those cells, which promote angiogenesis through VEGF. Cell survival is increased both *in vivo* and *in vitro* with the activation of transcription factor hypoxia inducible factor-1α in hypoxia treatment (McCarthy et al., 2018). Mouse pressure ulcer model is treated with subcutaneous injection of ASCs at the level of dermis, subcutaneous adipose tissue, and muscle layers by Strong et al. (2015). Kuo et al. (2016) subcutaneously injected ASCs to STZ-induced diabetic dorsal rodent model and via paracrine and autocrine affected enhanced wound healing is observed. Although human ASCs are good candidates for skin tissue engineering, they are eliminated by immune system and suspension of those cells in injectable gels increased retention and function in murine wound models (full thickness) (Feng et al., 2017; Park et al., 2014). Enzymatically digested, lipoaspirated, and centrifuged adipose tissue containing ASCs mixture is called stromal vascular fraction (SVF). SVF cells together with cell-assisted lipotransfer is reported to improve survival and retention of cells (Zielins et al., 2016). Wounds with complex structure or larger surface area are treated with noninjectable forms of ASCs such as cultured cell sheets and artificial skins. (McCarthy et al., 2018). Kato et al. (2015) showed improved wound healing and paracrine activity supported angiogenesis when they used allogenic rat ASCs cultured sheets combined with artificial skin on type 2 diabetic and obese rats. Scaffolds support cellular growth by providing microenvironment for cells to attach and grow. ASCs seeded onto those scaffolds increased vascularization, healing, ASCs survival, and reduced inflammation in animal models (McCarthy et al., 2018). 3D scaffolds provide structural support and microenvironment to ASCs allowing specific differentiation, prolonged survival, improved cytokine secretion, and vascularization (McCarthy et al., 2018). When combined with materiobiology, skin tissue engineering can create biologically active surfaces for rapid wound closure and healing with reduced side effects. Hair follicle development on murine full-thickness wound model treated with ASCs-seeded human amniotic membranes is shown by Minjuan et al. (2016). Bayati et al. (2017) investigated effect of PCL nanofibers as a dermal substitute cultured with ASCs on keratinocyte differentiation and wound healing model in albino Wistar rats. Increased cellular proliferation and expression of cytokeratin 14, filaggrin, and involucrin are observed in in-vitro cultured cells on scaffolds while increased epithelialization and fastened wound closure rate are shown in rat models. Human adipose-derived mesenchymal stem cells (hASCs) containing injectable HA-alginate cross-linked hydrogels are investigated for the regenerative efficacy on vocal fold wound healing in White New Zealand rabbits by Kim et al. (2014). Combination of hydrogels with hASCs showed increased ECM production, type I collagen production, and fibroblast differentiation and regeneration. Design of stem cell fate deciding scaffolds in 3D environment with the use of 3D printers and bioreactors or organ-on-chip techniques may help for stem cell differentiation and creation of full-thickness skin tissues including hair and vascular system.

5.6.3   3D BIOPRINTING

Three-dimensional-bioprinted biomimetic skin equivalents are good alternative to existing grafting techniques allowing controlled complex 3D skin construction with desired biomaterials and cells in precise location with flexibility and repeatability via computer control and have potential for drug screening, clinical transplantation, disease model studying, cosmetic, and chemical testing. This technique is good for deep burns and full-thickness wounds offering decreased pain, shortened healing time, and improved cosmetic appearance (He et al., 2018; Yan et al., 2018a). Cubo et al. (2016) bioprinted scaffold-free 100 cm² 3D human bilayered skin that contain human plasma, primary human fibroblasts, and keratinocytes from skin biopsies below 35 minutes and immunodeficient mice used for *in vivo* tests while *in vitro* analyses performed with human keratinocytes (hKCs). No morphological and viability change was observed in hKCs after printing method and no difference is observed between bilayer dermoepidermal equivalents and generated skin and human skin. In another study, human skin is bioprinted via bovine gelatin, alginate, and fibrin containing bioink together with human dermal fibroblasts and epidermal keratinocytes and similar characteristics with native human skin is observed and printability of large skin area is shown by printing adult size human ear with same ingredients (Pourchet et al., 2017). Koch et al. (2012) used laser-assisted bioprinting technique to create an example of human skin tissue (epidermis and dermis) with mouse NIH-3T3 fibroblasts, human keratinocyte (HaCaT) cell lines embedded in collagen type I seeded onto Matriderm™ sheet. After 10 days of cultivation, cellular proliferation, fibroblast and collagen penetration into Matriderm™ sheet, and basement layer formation between fibroblasts and keratinocytes are observed. 3D-layered artificial skin from skin fibroin is developed due to its biocompatible and ECM-mimicry properties (Gholipourmalekabadi et al., 2018). Rimann et al. (2016) produced layer-by-layer 3D-printed dermal equivalents with primary human dermal fibroblasts in photocross-linked (365 nm) PEG-based bioink. Cells were cultured for 7 weeks but fully stratified epidermis could not be observed. Skin-derived extracellular matrix is used as bioink for 3D-printed full-thickness human skin model with improved epidermal organization, dermal ECM secretion, wound closure, and re-epithelialization and neovascularization abilities are shown with *in vivo* and *in vitro* tests by Kim et al. (2018). 3D-printed scaffolds are promising in skin tissue engineering applications with their enhanced bioactivity with different cells when used in proper place and have advantage over other scaffolds due to its similarity with native skin.

5.6.4   *IN VITRO SKIN MODELS*

Rat and pig skins are highly preferred as human alternative models but using real human skin or these models are expensive and have limitations such as ethical issues, individual-dependent result difference, and difficulties in obtaining. Use of immortalized cell lines that lack 3D structure or primary lines from several donors also limits reproducibility due to genetic variety. Usage of animals is prohibited in EU for cosmeceutical testing since 2009 (Almeida et al., 2017; Bhushan, 2017). Minimizing the stress for animals via adequate healthcare, use of narcosis and housing (Refine), decreasing number of animals used in tests (Reduce), and replacement of tests with *in vitro* models (Replace) are achieved with 3R principles (Replace, Reproduce, and Refine) (Groeber et al., 2011). *In vitro* skin models are created as an alternative to animal models and are used to test toxicity, drug delivery, wound healing, skin irritations, cosmetics, or diseases and give most probable *in vivo-/in vitro*-related results. To achieve natural skin mimicry, synthetic skins should have barrier function, permeability, and give reaction to environmental inputs. Epskin™ (L'OREAL, France), SkinEthic™ (SkinEthic, France), and Epiderm™ (MatTek Corporation, USA) are commonly used for testing skin irritation, sensitization, skin microbiome, penetration, and corrosion (Almeida et al., 2017; Bhushan, 2017; Pellevoisin et al., 2018). Those models together with specific disease models will provide information about response of skin to created biomaterials or ingredients used before implantation and will help to understand complex reactions that occur in skin due to its complex structure. When combined with materiobiology, material science, and 3D printing technologies, new skin models can be created to use clinically or academic studies for know-how.

5.6.5 BIOREACTOR IN SKIN TISSUE ENGINEERING

Bioreactors for skin tissue engineering application give ability to create *in vivo* cell niche and study the molecular and cellular changes in physiology and pathophysiology and help to create disease models (Selden and Fuller, 2018). Perfused vascular network with vascularized porcine decellularized jejunum scaffold (BioVaSc) and tailored bioreactor system is proposed as a first vascularized skin alternative to animal models as shown by Groeber et al. (2016). Human fibroblasts, keratinocytes, and microvascular endothelial cells are seeded to BioVaSc and cultured for 14 days at the air-liquid interface. Presence of complex *in vivo* such as vasculature and skin barrier formation made this substitute a sophisticated *in vitro* model for dermatological research.

5.6.6 ORGAN-ON-CHIP SYSTEM

Culturing cells under tissue such as physiologically relevant microenvironment is performed with the use of organ-on-chip systems (microphysiological systems), which are perfusion chamber containing microfluidic cell culture devices. Culturing of skin cells in relevant 3D environment to create a 3D skin equivalent can be achieved with the use of microfluidics and 3D skin models (Alexander et al., 2018; Song et al., 2018). This system allows us to develop high throughput, low cost animal model alternatives. Sriram et al. (2018) combined fibrin-based dermal matrix with biomimetic organ-on-chip to develop a human skin equivalent. Epidermal morphogenesis, differentiation, and barrier function are enabled with dynamic perfusion and controlled microenvironment. Authors proposed this system as a promising equivalent to overcome limitations of collagen-based skin equivalents.

5.7 CONCLUSION AND FUTURE PROSPECTS

Over the last two decades, important developments in skin tissue engineering have been maintained. Ultimate goal for this field is the high quality wound repair with minimum scar formation and due to this goal fabrication of engineered scaffolds and cellular therapies have been increasing. There are numerous commercially available skin care products including cellularized/noncellularized hydrogels, electrospun fibers, and other skin substitutes. However, there are significant limitations in development of tissue-like 3D scaffolds due to lack of skin appendages formation such as hair follicle and sweat glands, so real skin formation could not be achieved. Up to now, products in the market could only replace the skin partially with maintaining a protective barrier and only a few of them are under the clinical trial. There is no ideal skin tissue substitute to come through these problems. Despite the success of some researches on stem cell therapies, there are still significant problems, for example, there is still no standard for which stem cell is suitable for that wound type. It would seem that for next step in skin tissue-engineered products should be using stem cells and scaffolds together properly to obtain full regeneration of the wound zone. One of the major problems is large-sized skin loss (up to 50%) burn patients. In general, wound healing studies were performed on small-sized animal models, so large-sized wounds are still uncharted area. Another challenge is their low applicability in clinic treatments due to high cost production of these skin substitutes. To overcome this problem, biomedical procedures should be improved and more technically advanced medical facilities are needed to produce low-cost products with high yields.

Today, most of the scientists focus on biosensors to obtain soft, compatible, and functional devices to analyze the healing time and microorganism of the wound zone. So, in the future, these biosensors will provide high rate of tissue regeneration and monitor the effects of substitutes and scaffolds through the tissue healing. On the other hand, 3D bioprinting technology, skin models, bioreactors, and skin-chip technologies are believed to overcome the hurdles with the formation of ECM-like substances, vascularization, and cell fate with electrical stimuli and will provide skin appendages fully vascularized and mimicked.

In conclusion, there are numerous different treatments for different types of wounds and other skin problems nowadays. Researches and publications have been increasing very fast; therefore, real and functional artificial skin may be developed in the future with association of all of the skin tissue engineering knowledge.

ACKNOWLEDGMENT

Special thanks to TUBITAK "116M838" project, TUBITAK "2211C" scholarship, FEN-C-YLP-120917–0549, and FEN-C-DRP-170118–0014 BAP projects for financial support.

KEYWORDS

- **skin tissue engineering**
- **wound healing**
- **burn dressing**
- **wound treatment methods**

REFERENCES

Adigbli, G., Alshomer, F., Maksimcuka, J. and Ghali, S. *Principles of Plastic Surgery, Wound Healing, Skin Grafts and Flaps,* 1st edition. UCL Press: London, **2016**.

Adrien, A., Bonnet, A., Dufour, D., Baudouin, S., Maugard, T. and Bridiau, N. Pilot production of ulvans from Ulva spp. and their effects on hyaluronan and collagen production in cultured dermal fibroblasts. *Carbohyd Polym.* **2017,** 157: 1306–1314.

Agostini, T., Pascone, C., Perello, R. and Di Lonardo, A. An Approach to Keloid Reconstruction with Dermal Substitute and Epidermal Skin Grafting. Recent Clinical Techniques, Results, and Research in Wounds. Springer (Cham). **2018,** 2: 1–12.

Akan, M., Yildirim, S., Misirlioglu, A., Ulusoy, G., Aköz, T. and Avc, G. An alternative method to minimize pain in the split-thickness skin graft donor site. *Plast Reconstr Surg.* **2003,** 111: 2243–2249.

Alexander, F. A., Eggert, S. and Wiest, J. Skin-on-a-Chip: Transepithelial electrical resistance and extracellular acidification measurements through an automated air–liquid interface. *Genes.* **2018,** 9: 114.

Allie, D. E., Hebert, C. J., Lirtzman, M. D., Wyatt, C. H., Keller, V. A., Vivekananthan, K., et al. Adjunctive Bioengineered Bi-layered Cell Therapy (Apligraf®) With excimer laser revascularization improves wound healing and lim. *Sign.* **2018,** 3.

Almeida, A., Sarmento, B. and Rodrigues, F. Insights on *in vitro* models for safety and toxicity assessment of cosmetic ingredients. *Int J Pharm.* **2017,** 519: 178–185.

Ansari, M., Kordestani, S. S., Nazralizadeh, S. and Eslami, H. Biodegradable cell-seeded collagen-based polymer scaffolds for wound healing and skin reconstruction. *J Macromol Sci B.* **2018,** 57: 100–109.

Archana, D., Singh, B. K., Dutta, J. and Dutta, P. Chitosan-PVP-nanosilver oxide wound dressing: *in vitro* and *in vivo* evaluation. *Int J Biol Macromol.* **2015,** 73: 49–57.

Arima, Y. and Iwata, H. Effect of wettability and surface functional groups on protein adsorption and cell adhesion using well-defined mixed self-assembled monolayers. *Biomaterials.* **2007,** 28: 3074–3082.

Avsar, G., Agirbasli, D., Agirbasli, M. A., Gunduz, O. and Oner, E. T. Levan-based fibrous scaffolds electrospun via co-axial and single-needle techniques for tissue engineering applications. *Carbohyd Polym.* **2018,** 193: 316–325.

Aziz, Z., Abu, S. F. and Chong, N. J. A systematic review of silver-containing dressings and topical silver agents (used with dressings) for burn wounds. *Burns.* **2012,** 38: 307–318.

Bailey, A. J. Molecular mechanisms of ageing in connective tissues. *Mech Ageing Dev.*2001, 122: 735–755.

Barrientos, S., Brem, H., Stojadinovic, O. and Tomic-Canic, M. Clinical application of growth factors and cytokines in wound healing. *Wound Repair Regen.* **2014,** 22: 569–578.

Barrientos, S., Stojadinovic, O., Golinko, M. S., Brem, H. and Tomic-Canic, M. Growth factors and cytokines in wound healing. *Wound Repair Regen.* **2008,** 16: 585–601.

Bedian, L., Villalba-Rodríguez, A. M., Hernández-Vargas, G., Parra-Saldivar, R. and Iqbal, H. M. Bio-based materials with novel characteristics for tissue engineering applications–A review. *Int J Biol Macromol.*2017, 98: 837–846.

Béduer, A., Piacentini, N., Aeberli, L., Da Silva, A., Verheyen, C., Bonini, F. et al. Additive manufacturing of hierarchical injectable scaffolds for tissue engineering. *Acta Biomater.* **2018,** 76: 71–79.

Barrientos, S., Stojadınovic, O., Golinko, M. S., Brem, H. and Tomic-Canic, M. Growth factors and cytokines in wound healing. *Wound Repair Regen.* **2008,** 16: 585–601.

Barrıentos, S., Brem, H., Stojadınovıc, O. and Tomic, C. M. Clinical application of growth factors and cytokines in wound healing. *Wound Repair Regen.* **2014,** 22: 569–578.

Berthiaume, F., Maguire, T. J. and Yarmush, M. L. Tissue engineering and regenerative medicine: history, progress, and challenges. *Annu Rev Chem Biomol Eng.*2011, 2: 403–430.

Bertozzi, N., Simonacci, F., Grieco, M. P., Grignaffini, E. and Raposio, E. The biological and clinical basis for the use of adipose-derived stem cells in the field of wound healing. *Ann Med Surg.* **2017,** 20: 41–48.

Bhardwaj, N., Chouhan, D. and Mandal, B. B. *Functional 3D Tissue Engineering Scaffolds: 3D Functional Scaffolds for Skin Tissue Engineering.* Woodhead Publishing: Cambridge, **2018.**

Bhushan, B. Skin and Skin Cream. *Biophysics of Skin and Its Treatments.* Springer International Publishing: USA, **2017**

Blaber, S. P., Webster, R. A., Hill, C. J., Breen, E. J., Kuah, D., Vesey, G. et al. Analysis of in-vitro secretion profiles from adipose-derived cell populations. *J Transl Med.* **2012,** 10: 172.

Boink, M. A., Roffel, S., Breetveld, M., Thon, M., Haasjes, M. S., Waaijman, T. et al. Comparison of advanced therapy medicinal product gingiva and skin substitutes and their *in vitro* wound healing potentials. *J Tissue Eng Regen Med.* **2018,** 12: 1088–1097.

Caló, E., Ballamy, L. and Khutoryanskiy, V. V. Hydrogels in wound management. *Hydrogels: Design, Synthesis and Application in Drug Delivery and Regenerative Medicine*, **2018**, 128.

Capanema, N. S. V., Mansur, A. A. P., De Jesus, A. C., Carvalho, S. M., De Oliveira, L. C. and Mansur, H. S. Superabsorbent cross-linked carboxymethyl cellulose-PEG hydrogels for potential wound dressing applications. *Int J Biol Macromol.* **2018**, 106: 1218–1234.

Caravaggi, C., De Giglio, R., Pritelli, C., Sommaria, M., Dalla Noce, S., Faglia, E. et al. HYAFF 11-based autologous dermal and epidermal grafts in the treatment of noninfected diabetic plantar and dorsal foot ulcers: a prospective, multicenter, controlled, randomized clinical trial. *Diabetes Care.* **2003**, 26: 2853–2859.

Carsin, H., Ainaud, P., Le Bever, H., Rives, J. M., Lakhel, A., Stephanazzi, J. et al. Cultured epithelial autografts in extensive burn coverage of severely traumatized patients: a five year single-center experience with 30 patients. *Burns.* **2000**, 26: 379–387.

Cerqueira, M. T., Pirraco, R. P. and Marques, A. P. Stem cells in skin wound healing: are we there yet? *Adv Wound Care.* **2016**, 5: 164–175.

Chakavala, S. R., Patel, N. G., Pate, N. V., Thakkar, V. T., Patel, K. V. and Gandhi, T. R. Development and *in vivo* evaluation of silver sulfadiazine loaded hydrogel consisting polyvinyl alcohol and chitosan for severe burns. *J Pharm Bioallied Sci.* **2012**, 4: S54–56.

Chen, S. H., Tsao, C. T., Chang, C. H., Lai, Y. T., Wu, M. F., Chuang, C. N. et al. Assessment of reinforced poly(ethylene glycol) chitosan hydrogels as dressings in a mouse skin wound defect model. *Mater Sci Eng C.* **2013**, 33: 2584–2594.

Cheng, L., Ji, K., Shih, T. Y., Haddad, A., Giatsidis, G., Mooney, D. J. et al. Injectable shape-memorizing three-dimensional hyaluronic acid cryogels for skin sculpting and soft tissue reconstruction. *Tissue Eng Part A.* **2017**, 23: 243–251.

Cho, Y. S., Lee, J. W., Lee, J. S., Lee, J. H., Yoon, T. R., Kuroyanagi, Y. et al. Hyaluronic acid and silver sulfadiazine-impregnated polyurethane foams for wound dressing application. *J Mater Sci Mater Med.* **2002**, 13: 861–865.

Choi, W. I., Hwang, Y., Sahu, A., Min, K., Sung, D., Tae, G. et al. H. An injectable and physical levan-based hydrogel as a dermal filler for soft tissue augmentation. *Biomater Sci.* **2018**, 6: 2627–2638.

Chouhan, D., Thatikonda, N., Nilebäck, L., Widhe, M., Hedhammar, M. and Mandal, B. B. Recombinant spider silk functionalized silkworm silk matrices as potential bioactive wound dressings and skin grafts. *ACS Appl Mater Interfaces.* **2018**, 10: 23560–23572.

Collins, M. N. and Birkinshaw, C. Hyaluronic acid-based scaffolds for tissue engineering—A review. *Carbohyd Polym.* 2013, 92: 1262–1279.

Cremar, L., Gutierrez, J., Martinez, J., Materon, L., Gilkerson, R., Xu, F. et al. Development of antimicrobial chitosan-based nanofiber dressings for wound healing applications. *Nanomed J.* **2018**, 5: 6–14.

Dabiri, G., Heiner, D. and Falanga, V. The emerging use of bone marrow-derived mesenchymal stem cells in the treatment of human chronic wounds. *Exp Opin Emerg Drugs.* **2013**, 18: 405–419.

Davison-Kotler, E., Sharma, V., Kang, N. V. and García-Gareta, E. A universal classification system of skin substitutes inspired by factorial design. *Tissue Eng Part B Rev.* **2018**, 24: 279–288.

Dhasmana, A., Singh, L., Roy, P., Dinda, A., Bhattacharyya, S. and Mishra, N. Extracellular matrix-based skin grafts from goat skin for wound healing and skin tissue engineering. *Madridge J Dermatol Res.* **2018a**, 3: 59–67.

Dhasmana, A., Singh, S., Kadian, S. and Singh, L. Skin tissue engineering: principles and advances. *J Dermatol Skin Care*. **2018b**, 1.

Dong, R., Liu, X., Liu, Y., Deng, Z., Nie, X., Wang, X. et al. Enrichment of epidermal stem cells by rapid adherence and analysis of the reciprocal interaction of epidermal stem cells with neighboring cells using an organotypic system. *Cell Biol Int*. **2007**, 31: 733–740.

Dubin-Thaler, B. J., Giannone, G., Döbereiner, H. G. and Sheetz, M. P. Nanometer analysis of cell spreading on matrix-coated surfaces reveals two distinct cell states and STEPs. *Biophys J*. **2004**, 86: 1794–1806.

El-Sherbiny, I. M. and Yacoub, M. H. Hydrogel scaffolds for tissue engineering: progress and challenges. *Glob Cardiol Sci Pract*. **2013**, 3: 316–342.

Erginer, M., Akcay, A., Coskunkan, B., Morova, T., Rende, D., Bucak, S. et al. Sulfated levan from Halomonas smyrnensis as a bioactive, heparin-mimetic glycan for cardiac tissue engineering applications. *Carbohyd Polym*. **2016**, 149: 289–296.

Farhadihosseinabadi, B., Farahani, M., Tayebi, T., Jafari, A., Biniazan, F., Modaresifar, K. et al. Amniotic membrane and its epithelial and mesenchymal stem cells as an appropriate source for skin tissue engineering and regenerative medicine. *Artif Cells Nanomed Biotechnol*. **2018**, 3: 1–10.

Farokhi, M., Mottaghitalab, F., Fatahi, Y., Khademhosseini, A. and Kaplan, D. L. Overview of silk fibroin use in wound dressings. *Trends Biotechnol*. **2018**, 36: 907–922.

Feng, J., Mineda, K., Wu, S. H., Mashiko, T., Doi, K., Kuno, S. et al. An injectable non-cross-linked hyaluronic-acid gel containing therapeutic spheroids of human adipose-derived stem cells. *Sci Rep*. **2017**, 7: 1548.

Fortunel, N. O., Vaigot, P., Cadio, E. and Martin, M. T. Functional investigations of keratinocyte stem cells and progenitors at a single-cell level using multiparallel clonal microcultures. *Epidermal Cells*. **2010**, 585: 13–23.

Frykberg, R. G. and Banks, J. Challenges in the treatment of chronic wounds. *Adv Wound Care*. **2015**, 4: 560–582.

Getachew, A., Berhanu, A. and Birhane, A. Production of sterilized medium chain length polyhydroxyalkanoates (Smcl-PHA) as a biofilm to tissue engineering application. *J Tissue Sci Eng*. **2016**, 7: 2.

Ghannam, S., Korayem, H., Farghaly, L. and Hosny, S. The effect of chitosan nanosilver dressing versus mesenchymal stem cells on wound healing. *J Afr Assoc Physiol Sci*. **2018**, 6: 23–31.

Gholipourmalekabadi, M., Samadikuchaksaraei, A., Seifalian, A. M., Urbanska, A. M., Ghanbarian, H., Hardy, J. G. et al. Silk fibroin/amniotic membrane 3D bilayered artificial skin. *Biomed Mater*.**2018**, 13.

Gordley, K., Cole, P., Hicks, J. and Hollier, L. A comparative, long term assessment of soft tissue substitutes: AlloDerm, Enduragen, and Dermamatrix. *J Plast Reconstr Aestet Surg*. **2009**, 62: 849–850.

Gravante, G., Di Fede, M., Araco, A., Grimaldi, M., De Angelis, B., Arpino, A. et al. A randomized trial comparing ReCell® system of epidermal cells delivery versus classic skin grafts for the treatment of deep partial thickness burns. *Burns*. **2007**, 33: 966–972.

Green, J. J. and Elisseeff, J. H. Mimicking biological functionality with polymers for biomedical applications. *Nature*. **2016**, 540: 386.

Groeber, F., Holeiter, M., Hampel, M., Hinderer, S. and Schenke-Layland, K. Skin tissue engineering—*in vivo* and *in vitro* applications. *Adv Drug Deliv Rev*. **2011**, 63: 352–366.

Gupta, S., Yadav, B. S., Kesharwani, R., Mishra, K. P. and Singh, N. K. The role of nanodrugs for targeted drug delivery in cancer treatment. *Arch Appl Sci Res.* **2010,** 2(1): 37–51.

Gurtner, G. C., Bhatt, K. and Rajadas, J. Pullulan regenerative matrix. US Patents. 9636362B2, March 3, **2011**.

Hamedi, H., Moradi, S., Hudson, S. M. and Tonelli, A. E. Chitosan based hydrogels and their applications for drug delivery in wound dressings: a review. *Carbohyd Polym.* **2018,** 199: 445–460.

He, P., Zhao, J., Zhang, J., Li, B., Gou, Z., Gou, M. and Li, X. Bioprinting of skin constructs for wound healing. *Burns Trauma.* **2018,** 6: 5.

Herman, A. R. The history of skin grafts. *J Drugs Dermatol.* **2002,** 1: 298–301.

Hixon, K. R., Lu, T. and Sell, S. A. A comprehensive review of cryogels and their roles in tissue engineering applications. *Acta Biomater.* **2017,** 62: 29–41.

Ho, J., Walsh, C., Yue, D., Dardik, A. and Cheema, U. Current advancements and strategies in tissue engineering for wound healing: a comprehensive review. *Adv Wound Care.* **2017,** 6: 191–209.

Horch, R. E., Kopp, J., Kneser, U., Beier, J. and Bach, A. D. Tissue engineering of cultured skin substitutes. *J Cell Mol Med.* **2005,** 9: 592–608.

Hu, L., Wang, J., Zhou, X., Xiong, Z., Zhao, J., Yu, R., Huang, F., Zhang, H. and Chen, L. Exosomes derived from human adipose mensenchymal stem cells accelerates cutaneous wound healing via optimizing the characteristics of fibroblasts. *Sci Rep.* **2016,** 6: 329–393.

Huang, X. W., Wei, J. J., Liu, T., Zhang, X. L., Bai, S. M. and Yang, H. H. Silk fibroin-assisted exfoliation and functionalization of transition metal dichalcogenide nanosheets for antibacterial wound dressings. *Nanoscale.* **2017,** 9: 17193–17198.

Hussain, Z., Thu, H. E., Katas, H. and Bukhari, S. N. A. Hyaluronic acid-based biomaterials: a versatile and smart approach to tissue regeneration and treating traumatic, surgical, and chronic wounds. *Polym Rev.* **2017,** 57: 594–630.

Hüsing, B., Bührlen, B. and Gaisser, S. *Human Tissue Engineered Products: Today's Markets and Future Prospects*, EUR 21838, Fraunhofer Institute for Systems and Innovation Research Karlsruhe, European Commision, Germany. **2003**.

Iqbal, N., Khan, A. S., Asif, A., Yar, M., Haycock, J. W. and Rehman, I. U. Recent concepts in biodegradable polymers for tissue engineering paradigms: a critical review. *Int Mater Rev.* **2018,** 64: 1–36.

Jackson, W. M., Nesti, L. J. and Tuan, R. S. Concise review: clinical translation of wound healing therapies based on mesenchymal stem cells. *Stem Cells Transl Med.* **2012,** 1: 44–50.

Janeway, C. A., Travers, P., Walport, M. and Shlomchik, M. J. *Immunobiology: The Immune System In Health and Disease*, 5th edition. Garland Science: New York, **2001**.

Jeong, K. H., Park, D. and Lee, Y. C. Polymer-based hydrogel scaffolds for skin tissue engineering applications: a mini-review. *J Polym Res.* **2017,** 24: 112.

Kamoun, E. A., Kenawy, E. R. S. and Chen, X. A review on polymeric hydrogel membranes for wound dressing applications: PVA-based hydrogel dressings. *J Adv Res.* **2017,** 8: 217–233.

Keservani, R. K. Kesharwani, R. K. and Sharma, A. K. "Nanobiomaterials involved in medical imaging technologies", In: *Applications of NanoBioMaterials*, Volume VIII: Nanobiomaterials in Medical Imaging, Edited by Alexandru Mihai Grumezescu, William Andrew, Elsevier. 10, 2016, 301–323.

King, A., Balaji, S., Keswani, S. G. and Crombleholme, T. M. The role of stem cells in wound angiogenesis. *Adv Wound Care*. **2014,** 3: 614–625.

Kirdponpattara, S., Phisalaphong, M. and Kongruang, S. Gelatin-bacterial cellulose composite sponges thermally cross-linked with glucose for tissue engineering applications. *Carbohyd Polym*. **2017,** 177: 361–368.

Kirsner, R. S., Marston, W. A., Snyder, R. J., Lee, T. D., Cargill, D. I. and Slade, H. B. Spray-applied cell therapy with human allogeneic fibroblasts and keratinocytes for the treatment of chronic venous leg ulcers: a phase 2, multicentre, double-blind, randomised, placebo-controlled trial. *Lancet*. **2012,** 380: 977–985.

Koehler, J., Wallmeyer, L., Hedtrich, S., Goepferich, A. M. and Brandl, F. P. pH-Modulating poly(ethylene glycol)/alginate hydrogel dressings for the treatment of chronic wounds. *Macromol Biosci*. **2017,** 17: 1600369.

Kumar, P., Lakshmanan, V. K., Biswas, R., Nair, S. V. and Jayakumar, R. Synthesis and biological evaluation of chitin hydrogel/nano ZnO composite bandage as antibacterial wound dressing. *J Biomed Nanotechnol*. **2012,** 8: 891–900.

Kumbar, S. G., Nukavarapu, S. P., James, R., Nair, L. S. and Laurencin, C. T. Electrospun poly(lactic acid-co-glycolic acid) scaffolds for skin tissue engineering. *Biomaterials*. **2008,** 29: 4100–4107.

Leigh, I. and Watt, F. The culture of human epidermal keratinocytes. *Keratinocyte Handb*. 1994, 45.

Li, A., Pouliot, N., Redvers, R. and Kaur, P. Extensive tissue-regenerative capacity of neonatal human keratinocyte stem cells and their progeny. *J Clin Invest*. **2004,** 113: 390–400.

Lim, F. and Sun, A. M. Microencapsulated islets as bioartificial endocrine pancreas. *Science*. **1980,** 210: 908–910.

Límová, M. Active wound coverings: bioengineered skin and dermal substitutes. *Surg Clin North Am*. **2010,** 90: 1237–1255.

Lin, Z., Gao, W., Ma, L., Xia, H., Xie, W., Zhang, Y. et al. Preparation and properties of poly(ε-caprolactone)/bioactive glass nanofibre membranes for skin tissue engineering. *J Bioact Compact Polym*. **2018,** 33: 195–209.

Logeart-Avramoglou, D. and Jozefonvicz, J. Carboxymethyl benzylamide sulfonate dextrans (CMDBS), a family of biospecific polymers endowed with numerous biological properties: A review. *J Biomed Mater Res*. **1999,** 48: 578–590.

Madaghiele, M., Demitri, C., Sannino, A. and Ambrosio, L. Polymeric hydrogels for burn wound care: Advanced skin wound dressings and regenerative templates. *Burns Trauma*. **2014,** 2: 153–161.

Madhumathi, K., Kumar, P. S., Abhilash, S., Sreeja, V., Tamura, H., Manzoor, K. et al. Development of novel chitin/nanosilver composite scaffolds for wound dressing applications. *J Mater Sci Mater Med*. **2010,** 21: 807–813.

Maver, T., Maver, U., Kleinschek, K. S., Raščan, I. M. and Smrke, D. M. Advanced therapies of skin injuries. *Wien Klin Wochenschr*. **2015,** 127: 187–198.

Mccarthy, M. E., Brown, T. A., Bukowska, J., Bunnell, B. A., Frazier, T., Wu, X. et al. Therapeutic applications for adipose-derived stem cells in wound healing and tissue engineering. *Curr Stem Cell Rep*. **2018,** 4: 127–137.

Mearian, L. 3D-printed skin holds promise for burn victims and others. **2015.**

Mehrabani, M. G., Karimian, R., Mehramouz, B., Rahimi, M. and Kafil, H. S. Preparation of biocompatible and biodegradable silk fibroin/chitin/silver nanoparticles 3D scaffolds as a bandage for antimicrobial wound dressing. *Int J Biol Macromol*. **2018,** 114: 961–971.

Mishra, S., Rani, P., Sen, G. and Dey, K. P. Preparation, properties and application of hydrogels: a review. *Hydrogels (Springer)*. **2018**, 3: 145–173.

Moghaddam, A. B., Shirvani, B., Aroon, M. A. and Nazari, T. Physicochemical properties of hybrid electrospun nanofibers containing polyvinylpyrrolidone (PVP), propolis and aloe vera. *Mater Res Express*. **2018, 5**.

Mogoşanu, G. D. and Grumezescu, A. M. Natural and synthetic polymers for wounds and burns dressing. *Int J Pharm*. **2014**, 463: 127–136.

Mohebichamkhorami, F. and Alizadeh, A. Skin substitutes: an updated review of products from the year 1980 to 2017. *Appl Biotechnol*. **2018**, 4: 615–623.

Monstrey, S., Hoeksema, H., Verbelen, J., Pirayesh, A. and Blondeel, P. Assessment of burn depth and burn wound healing potential. *Burns*. **2008**, 34: 761–769.

Murphy, S. V., Skardal, A., Song, L., Sutton, K., Haug, R., Mack, D. L. et al. Solubilized amnion membrane hyaluronic acid hydrogel accelerates full-thickness wound healing. *Stem Cells Transl Med*. **2017**, 6: 2020–2032.

Naahidi, S., Jafari, M., Logan, M., Wang, Y., Yuan, Y., Bae, H. et al. Biocompatibility of hydrogel-based scaffolds for tissue engineering applications. *Biotechnol Adv*. **2017**, 35: 530–544.

Nahain, A. A., Ignjatovic, V., Monagle, P., Tsanaktsidis, J. and Ferro, V. Heparin mimetics with anticoagulant activity. *Med Res Rev*. **2018, 38**.

Nikkhah, D., Gilbert, P., Booth, S. and Dheansa, B. Should we be using silver-based compounds for donor site dressing in thermal burns? *Burns*. **2013**, 39: 1324–1325.

Noordenbos, J., Doré, C. and Hansbrough, J. F. Safety and efficacy of TransCyte* for the treatment of partial-thickness burns. *J Burn Care Rehabil*. **1999**, 20: 275–281.

Olmos-Zuñiga, J. R., Silva-Martínez, M., Jasso-Victoria, R., Baltazares-Lipp, M., Hernández-Jiménez, C., Buendía-Roldan, I. et al. Effects of pirfenidone and collagen-polyvinylpyrrolidone on macroscopic and microscopic changes, TGF-β1 expression, and collagen deposition in an experimental model of tracheal wound healing. *Biomed Res Int*. **2017**.

Oner, E. T., Hernandez, L. and Combie, J. Review of levan polysaccharide: From a century of past experiences to future prospects. *Biotechnol Adv*. **2016**, 34: 827–844.

Osman, A., Oner, E. T. and Eroglu, M. S. Novel levan and pNIPA temperature-sensitive hydrogels for 5-ASA controlled release. *Carbohyd Polym*. **2017**, 165: 61–70.

Park, I. S., Chung, P. S. and Ahn, J. C. Enhanced angiogenic effect of adipose-derived stromal cell spheroid with low-level light therapy in hindlimb ischemia mice. *Biomaterials*. **2014**, 3: 9280–9289.

Pellevoisin, C., Bouez, C. and Cotovio, J. Cosmetic industry requirements regarding skin models for cosmetic testing. *Skin Tissue Models*. **2018**, 2: 33–37.

Petrie, R. J. and Yamada, K. M. At the leading edge of three-dimensional cell migration. *J Cell Sci*. **2012**, 125: 5917–5926.

Pezeshki-Modaress, M., Zandi, M. and Rajabi, S. Tailoring the gelatin/chitosan electrospun scaffold for application in skin tissue engineering: an *in vitro* study. *Prog Biomater*. **2018**, 3: 1–12.

Pittenger, M. F., Mackay, A. M., Beck, S. C., Jaiswal, R. K., Douglas, R., Mosca, J. D. et al. Multilineage potential of adult human mesenchymal stem cells. *Science*. **1999**, 284: 143–147.

Poranki, D., Whitener, W., Howse, S., Mesen, T., Howse, E., Burnell, J. et al. Evaluation of skin regeneration after burns *in vivo* and rescue of cells after thermal stress *in vitro* following treatment with a keratin biomaterial. *J Biomater Appl*. **2014**, 29: 26–35.

Pourchet, L. J., Thepot, A., Albouy, M., Courtial, E. J., Boher, A., Blum, L. J. et al. Human skin 3D bioprinting using scaffold-free approach. *Adv Healthc Mater*. **2017**, 6: 1601101.

Qian, L. W., Fourcaudot, A. B. and Leung, K. P. Silver sulfadiazine retards wound healing and increases hypertrophic scarring in a rabbit ear excisional wound model. *J Burn Care Res.* **2017**, 38: e418–e422.

Qiu, X., Wang, J., Wang, G. and Wen, H. Vascularization of Lando® dermal scaffold in an acute full-thickness skin-defect porcine model. *J Plast Surg Hand Surg.* **2018**, 3: 1–6.

Rahmani Del Bakhshayesh, A., Mostafavi, E., Alizadeh, E., Asadi, N., Akbarzadeh, A. and Davaran, S. Fabrication of three-dimensional scaffolds based on nano-biomimetic collagen hybrid constructs for skin tissue engineering. *ACS Omega*. **2018**, 3: 8605–8611.

Rashaan, Z., Krijnen, P., Allema, J., Vloemans, A., Schipper, I. and Breederveld, R. Usability and effectiveness of Suprathel® in partial-thickness burns in children. *Eur J Trauma Emerg Surg.* **2017**, 43: 549–556.

Rowan, M. P., Cancio, L. C., Elster, E. A., Burmeister, D. M., Rose, L. F., Natesan, S. et al. Burn wound healing and treatment: review and advancements. *Crit Care.* **2015**, 19: 243.

Scarritt, M., Murdock, M. and Badylak, S. F. Principles of *Regenerative Medicine: Biologic Scaffolds Composed of Extracellular Matrix for Regenerative Medicine*, 3rd edition, Academic Press: USA, **2019**.

Selden, C. and Fuller, B. Role of bioreactor technology in tissue engineering for clinical use and therapeutic target design. *Bioengineering.* **2018**, 5: 32.

Shevchenko, R. V., James, S. L. and James, S. E. A review of tissue-engineered skin bioconstructs available for skin reconstruction. *J R Soc Interface.* **2009**, 7: 229–258.

Silva-Correia, J., Zavan, B., Vindigni, V., Silva, T. H., Oliveira, J. M., Abatangelo, G. et al. Biocompatibility evaluation of ionic- and photo-cross-linked methacrylated gellan gum hydrogels: *in vitro* and *in vivo* study. *Adv Healthc Mater.* **2013**, 2: 568–575.

Sionkowska, A. Current research on the blends of natural and synthetic polymers as new biomaterials. *Prog Polym Sci.* **2011**, 36: 1254–1276.

Smith, A. M., Paxton, J. Z., Hung, Y. P., Hadley, M. J., Bowen, J., Williams, R. L. and Grover, L. M. Nanoscale crystallinity modulates cell proliferation on plasma-sprayed surfaces. *Mater Sci Eng C.* **2015**, 48: 5–10.

Song, H. J., Lim, H. Y., Chun, W., Choi, K. C., Lee, T. Y., Sung, J. H. and Sung, G. Y. Development of 3D skin-equivalent in a pump-less microfluidic chip. *J Ind Eng Chem.* **2018**, 60: 355–359.

Sorg, H., Tilkorn, D. J., Hager, S., Hauser, J. and Mirastschijski, U. Skin wound healing: an update on the current knowledge and concepts. *Eur Surg Res.* **2017**, 58: 81–94.

Strong, A. L., Bowles, A. C., Maccrimmon, C. P., Frazier, T. P., Lee, S. J., Wu, X. et al. Adipose stromal cells repair pressure ulcers in both young and elderly mice: potential role of adipogenesis in skin repair. *Stem Cells Transl Med.* **2015**, 4: 632–642.

Sturzoiu, C., Petrescu, M., Galateanu, B., Anton, M., Nica, C., Simionca, G. I. et al. Zymomonas mobilis Levan is involved in metalloproteinases activation in healing of wounded and burned tissues. *Scientif Papers Animal Sci Biotechnol.* **2011**, 44: 453–458.

Su, A. and Al'aref, S. J. 3D Printing Applications in Cardiovascular Medicine: History of 3D Printing, 1st edition, Academic Press: USA, **2018**.

Summa, M., Russo, D., Penna, I., Margaroli, N., Bayer, I. S., Bandiera, T. et al. A biocompatible sodium alginate/povidone iodine film enhances wound healing. *Eur J Pharm Biopharm.* **2018**, 122: 17–24.

Sun, G., Zhang, X., Shen, Y. I., Sebastian, R., Dickinson, L. E., Fox-Talbot, K. et al. Dextran hydrogel scaffolds enhance angiogenic responses and promote complete skin regeneration during burn wound healing. *Proc Natl Acad Sci India.* **2011,** 108: 20976–20981.

Supp, D. M. and Boyce, S. T. Engineered skin substitutes: practices and potentials. *Clin Dermatol.* **2005a,** 23: 403–412.

Supp, D. M. and Boyce, S. T. Engineered skin substitutes: practices and potentials. *Clin Dermatol.* **2005b,** 23: 403–412.

Ter Horst, B., Chouhan, G., Moiemen, N. S. and Grover, L. M. Advances in keratinocyte delivery in burn wound care. *Adv Drug Deliv Rev.* **2018,** 123: 18–32.

Thangapazham, R., Darling, T. and Meyerle, J. Alteration of skin properties with autologous dermal fibroblasts. *Int J Mol Sci.* **2014,** 15: 8407–8427.

Toyserkani, N. M., Christensen, M. L., Sheikh, S. P. and Sørensen, J. A. Adipose-derived stem cells: new treatment for wound healing? *Ann Plast Surg.* **2015,** 75: 117–123.

Ucuzian, A. A., Gassman, A. A., East, A. T. and Greisler, H. P. Molecular mediators of angiogenesis. *J Burn Care Res.* **2010,** 31: 158–175.

Van Den Broek, L. J., Kroeze, K. L., Waaijman, T., Breetveld, M., Sampat-Sardjoepersad, S. C., Niessen, F. B. et al. Differential response of human adipose tissue-derived mesenchymal stem cells, dermal fibroblasts, and keratinocytes to burn wound exudates: potential role of skin-specific chemokine CCL27. *Tissue Eng Part A.* **2013,** 20: 197–209.

Van Der Veen, V. C., Van Der Wal, M. B., Van Leeuwen, M. C., Ulrich, M. M. and Middelkoop, E. Biological background of dermal substitutes. *Burns.* **2010,** 36: 305–321.

Varkey, M., Ding, J. and Tredget, E. E. Advances in skin substitutes—potential of tissue engineered skin for facilitating anti-fibrotic healing. *J Funct Biomater.* **2015,** 6: 547–563.

Venkatesan, J., Bhatnagar, I., Manivasagan, P., Kang, K. H. and Kim, S. K. Alginate composites for bone tissue engineering: a review. *Int J Biol Macromol.* **2015,** 72: 269–281.

Vig, K., Chaudhari, A., Tripathi, S., Dixit, S., Sahu, R., Pillai, S., Dennis, V. A. and Singh, S. R. Advances in skin regeneration using tissue engineering. *Int J Mol Sci.* **2017,** 18: 789.

Vilela, M. D., Pedrosa, H. A., Sampaio, F. D. and Carneiro, J. L. Matriderm for management of scalp necrosis following surgical treatment of giant parietal encephalocele. *World Neurosurg.* **2018,** 110: 30–34.

Wang, X., Zhang, D., Wang, J., Tang, R., Wei, B. and Jiang, Q. Succinyl pullulan-crosslinked carboxymethyl chitosan sponges for potential wound dressing. *Int J Polym Mater Po.* **2017,** 66: 61–70.

Wang, Y., Beekman, J., Hew, J., Jackson, S., Issler-Fisher, A. C., Parungao, R. et al. Burn injury: Challenges and advances in burn wound healing, infection, pain and scarring. *Adv Drug Deliv Rev.* **2018,** 123: 3–17.

Wong, D. J. and Chang, H. Y. Skin tissue engineering. **2009.**

Woodley, D. T., Peterson, H. D., Herzog, S. R., Stricklin, G. P., Burgeson, R. E., Briggaman, R. A. et al. Burn wounds resurfaced by cultured epidermal autografts show abnormal reconstitution of anchoring fibrils. *JAMA.* **1988,** 259: 2566–2571.

Xu, W., Dong, S., Han, Y., Li, S. and Liu, Y. Hydrogels as Antibacterial Biomaterials. *Curr Pharm Des.* **2018,** 24: 843–854.

Yan, W. C., Davoodi, P., Vijayavenkataraman, S., Tian, Y., Ng, W. C., Fuh, J. Y. et al. 3D bioprinting of skin tissue: from preprocessing to final product evaluation. *Adv Drug Deliv Rev.* **2018a,** 132: 270–295.

Yan, W., Liu, H., Deng, X., Jin, Y., Wang, N. and Chu, J. Acellular dermal matrix scaffolds coated with connective tissue growth factor accelerate diabetic wound healing by increasing fibronectin through PKC signalling pathway, *Tissue Eng Regen Med.* **2018b,** 12: e1461–e1473.

Yang, X., Yang, K., Wu, S., Chen, X., Yu, F., Li, J. et al. Cytotoxicity and wound healing properties of PVA/ws-chitosan/glycerol hydrogels made by irradiation followed by freeze–thawing. *Radiant Phys Chem.* **2010,** 79: 606–611.

Yildirimer, L., Thanh, N. T. and Seifalian, A. M. Skin regeneration scaffolds: a multimodal bottom-up approach. *Trends Biotechnol Res.* **2012,** 30: 638–648.

Yoon, K. Ethical Issues of 3D Printing, **2014.**

Zhang, Y. S., Oklu, R., Dokmeci, M. R. and Khademhosseini, A. Three-dimensional bioprinting strategies for tissue engineering. *Cold Spring Harb Perspect Med.* **2017,** 8: a025718.

Zhao, S., Li, L., Wang, H., Zhang, Y., Cheng, X., Zhou, N. et al. Wound dressings composed of copper-doped borate bioactive glass microfibers stimulate angiogenesis and heal full-thickness skin defects in a rodent model. *Biomaterials.* **2015,** 53: 379–391.

Zhong, S., Zhang, Y. and Lim, C. T. Fabrication of large pores in electrospun nanofibrous scaffolds for cellular infiltration: a review. *Tissue Eng Part B Rev.* **2011,** 18: 77–87.

Zielins, E. R., Brett, E. A., Longaker, M. T. and Wan, D. C. Autologous fat grafting: the science behind the surgery. *Aesthet Surg J.* **2016,** 36: 488–496.

Zmejkoski, D., Spasojević, D., Orlovska, I., Kozyrovska, N., Soković, M., Glamočlija, J. et al. Bacterial cellulose-lignin composite hydrogel as a promising agent in chronic wound healing. *Int J Biol Macromol.* **2018,** 118: 494–503.

Zulkifli, F. H., Hussain, F. S. J., Zeyohannes, S. S., Rasad, M. S. B. A. and Yusuff, M. M. A facile synthesis method of hydroxyethyl cellulose-silver nanoparticle scaffolds for skin tissue engineering applications. *Mater Sci Eng C.* **2017,** 79: 151–160.

CHAPTER 6

Biomaterials in Bone and Muscle Regeneration

SHESAN JOHN OWONUBI[1*], ERIC G AYOM[1], BLESSING A. ADERIBIGBE,[2] and NEERISH REVAPRASADU[1]

[1]Department of Chemistry, University of Zululand, KwaDlangezwa, KwaZulu-Natal 3886, South Africa

[2]Department of Chemistry, Alice Campus, University of Fort Hare, Eastern Cape, South Africa, 5700

*Corresponding author. E-mail: oshesan@gmail.com

ABSTRACT

Biomaterials have been employed over the years in the regeneration of bones and muscles. The regeneration or repair of skeletal muscle tissue or muscles is necessary when innate muscle or bones cannot initiate their own repair. Complex damage to muscles or bones could result in irreparable cells and loss of related function, hence requiring assistance with regeneration. This chapter introduces biomaterial and the advancement of biomaterials, then it indicates exactly what both bone and muscle regeneration involves and with numerous research findings reported, it dwells on biomaterials in bone regeneration. Then similarly, biomaterials in tissue regeneration are highlighted shedding light on both scaffolds derived from biological or synthetic materials and relevant references made. But, it is important to mention that although synthetic materials used to design scaffolds are tunable, over the years they still are not able to fully and functionally replace biologic scaffolds, but progress is constantly made. Also, although numerable *in vitro* studies are reported, more confirmatory functional *in vivo* studies are encouraged.

6.1 INTRODUCTION

6.1.1 WHAT ARE BIOMATERIALS?

Over the years, there has been diverse understanding of biomaterials, but for the purpose of this chapter we will refer to a biomaterial simply as any natural or man-made material/surface comprising part or all of a living biological system or biomedical device. Being more descriptive, a biomaterial is any nondrug material, natural/synthetic used as a substitute to any part of a living system or to function in close contact with any living tissue or organ (Donglu, 2005; Heness and Ben-Nissan, 2004). The history involving the science of biomaterials has been explored for quite some time (Helmus et al., 2008). Early applications involved ancient Phoenicia binding their loose teeth with gold wires, utilizing shell materials in primeval Mesoamerican dentistry, the knowledge that bone plates could be used for stabilization of bone fractures and that they accelerated healings in the early 1900s and also the coating of silver, gold, or other metals in the tooth and in different parts of the body (Parida et al., 2012; Pramanik et al., 2005; Batista et al., 2004; Heness and Ben-Nissan, 2004). The science of biomaterials is interdisciplinary encompassing broadly: material science and engineering, biology, clinical sciences, and tissue engineering (Hench, 1991). The specific biomaterial and its design are of uttermost importance for their application. Research involving biomaterial for bone and muscle regeneration encompasses the investigation of materials, which are not only synthetic such as: composites, ceramics, polymers, and metals, but also materials of biological nature and biocompatible as tissues, cells, and proteins (Ruys, 2013). It is important to mention that biomaterials used in regeneration of muscles and bones over the years were advanced from being bioinert to bioactive and in recent times, researchers design them to be multifunctional biomaterials encompassing growth factors and genes or in some cases cells (Yu et al., 2015). These biomaterials are mainly used as systems to encourage the proliferation, migration, and differentiation of cells, which eventually aid to promote new bone formation.

6.2 BONE REGENERATION

Bones are dynamic, greatly vascularized living tissues constituting of nerves and blood vessels, constantly being remodeled through the lifetime of individuals. They possess important roles for locomotion, ensuring the human skeleton possesses necessary load-bearing capacity, for the protection of delicate internal organs, and also in the regulation of particular electrolytes in blood (Stevens, 2008). Another vital role of bones is that they provide a suitable environment for the production of blood cells (the marrow) constituting minerals, vitamins and proteins, growing and repairing themselves by their own blood vessels. Bones, unlike other tissues, possess an efficient self-healing capacity, thus in the event of injury or bone fracture, in cases without complications, by necessary reduction and fixation of bone fractures, the formation of new bone can be appreciated after a few weeks. Total/complete bone union and total recovery may be obtainable only within a month. Conversely, in severe cases with complications, pathological cases, spinal fusion, joint replacement, bone tumor extraction, or some form of birth defect, the normal regenerative capacity of the bone is absent and thus, the patient will require some form of surgery (Kanczler and Oreffo, 2008; Stevens, 2008). At younger ages, the capacity for bones to regenerate is quite high, but this gradually reduces as individuals' age.

Thus, the ability of fractures in young people to heal without major intervention is high when compared to their aged counterparts. As a result of this inability to heal, the early 20th century upheld "autografting" as the standard technique for patients with bone defects. It involved the harvesting of a "donor" bone from the patient's skeletal system, one which typically from a nonload-bearing location and it transplanted to the defective site (Bauer and Muschler, 2000) (Figure 6.1).

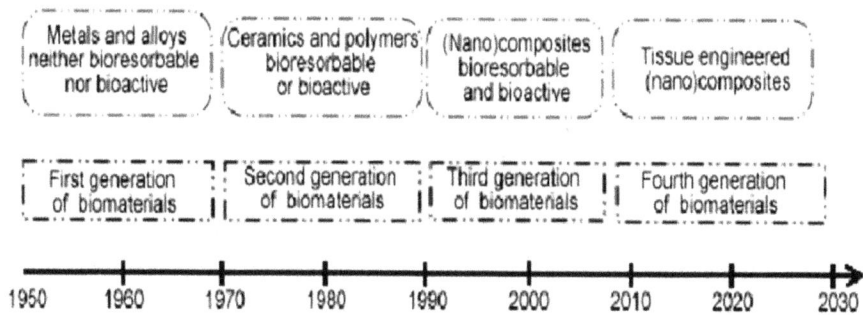

FIGURE 6.1   History of biomaterials used for different applications.

It was clinically successfully and effective as it involved bone transplanting from the patient, which integrated perfectly without autoimmune- or disease-related complications as opposed to bone transplants from human cadavers or animals, but it had the challenges of short supply of sites where the "donor" bones could be harvested, need for a secondary surgery, and also complications were reported in about one in five cases (Silber et al., 2003; Lord et al., 1988; Dimitriou et al., 2011; Zimmermann et al., 2001; Nakajima et al., 2007; Kretlow and Mikos, 2007). Unfortunately, no satisfactory solutions for cases of irreparable bone replacements were achieved due to the unmet complete regenerative potential of bones and this led to further research into new strategies such as use of allografts for bone regeneration which have been reportedly successful in lowering the complication rates to about one in 15, but these new strategies are still costly and rather invasive when compared to the previously accepted technique (Dimitriou et al., 2011; Nodzo et al., 2014).

The use of donor tissues from similar species have also been explored as a result of the challenges involved with quantity of required graft materials, but the risk of disease transmission and infection rates have led to the research into graft substitutes, which are effective, safe, and abundant (Control, 1988; Mankin et al., 2005; Laurencin et al., 1999; Buck et al., 1989; Lewandrowski et al., 2001; Moreau et al., 2000). This led to researchers exploring biomaterials such as calcium-based ceramics, hydroxyapatite (HA), tricalcium phosphate, bioactive ceramics, bioactive glasses, biphasic calcium phosphate, noncalcium-based ceramics, metals, polymers, and composite materials to investigate feasibility. It is of importance to highlight that biomaterials have roles in the regenerative engineering of bones. Biomaterials to be employed in regenerative bone engineering must possess the capability of osteoconduction, which refers to the capacity of the biomaterials to encourage formation of new bones on its surface (Albrektsson and Johansson, 2001; Urist et al., 1984); osteoinduction, which is that property of a biomaterial, which enables it to form bones at ectopic sites (Urist, 1965); vascularization, which is an important process for the formation of blood vessels, which is a requirement for tissues with size greater than 200 μm, the *in vivo* oxygen diffusion limit (Muschler et al., 2004); cell-surface interactions, which refer to cells adhesion and interactions between the biomaterial surface and the cell needed to impact the bone regeneration (Tirrell et al., 2002); and host tissue integration, the prerequisite confirmation of the integration of the bone tissue newly formed into its natural environment are the evidences of the functional bone regenerative capacity of the biomaterial. For example, a functional biomaterial for bone regeneration should not only serve as a scaffold for cell infiltration and tissue deposition, but should also perform roles of induction of signals facilitating connection of tissues with necessary host surfaces and nerve systems (Figure 6.2) (Wang et al., 2004).

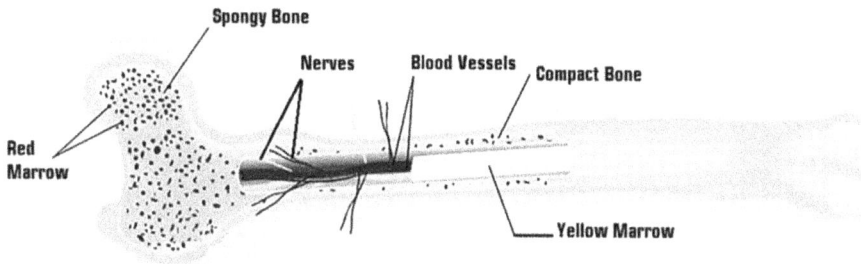

FIGURE 6.2 Process of bone regeneration.

6.3 MUSCLE REGENERATION

Skeletal muscle constitutes between 40% and 45% of an adults body mass and it aids bones in locomotion and facilitates voluntary movements (Liu et al., 2018). Figure 6.3 represents a skeletal muscle and being quite similar to bones, they possess the capability to regenerate inherently in response to minor injuries, but complex damage to muscles could result in irreparable muscles and loss of related function (Kwee and Mooney, 2017). Such compound damages are quite common during sporting activities, strains from rapid movement, crush trauma from accidents, laceration, aggressive tumor ablation, myopathies, etc., and the resultant inability of the muscle to regenerate tends to result in possible fatty degeneration of the muscles and scar formation (Kwee and Mooney, 2017; Järvinen and Lehto, 1993). The ability for muscles to regenerate has been traced to the activation of "satellite cells", which are multipotent stem cells with a capacity to self-renew themselves by maintaining an undifferentiated population in the tissue (Relaix and Zammit, 2012; Brack and Rando, 2012; Kuang et al., 2008; Shi and Garry, 2006). Akin to bones, in cases where regeneration is nonexistent, the required treatments to replace the injured muscle are the goal. These treatments could be in the forms of muscle transplantation from alternate sites of the injured patients' muscles or in some cases ex vivo muscle cells implantation. But, limited successes have been recorded by these techniques (Chuang, 2008); as a result of donor site morbidity and in some cases immune system rejection, these have led to research into techniques to aid in successful muscle regeneration in cases of irreparable injuries (Palmieri et al., 2010). The research into the adoption and use of biomaterials for muscle regeneration has been the focus of academics for sometime with some levels of successes reported. By developing techniques, which combine the peculiar biomaterial with cells, some researchers have been able to report regeneration and these strategies could enable the creation of artificially engineered muscle constructs *in vitro* for the replacement of these irreparable muscles.

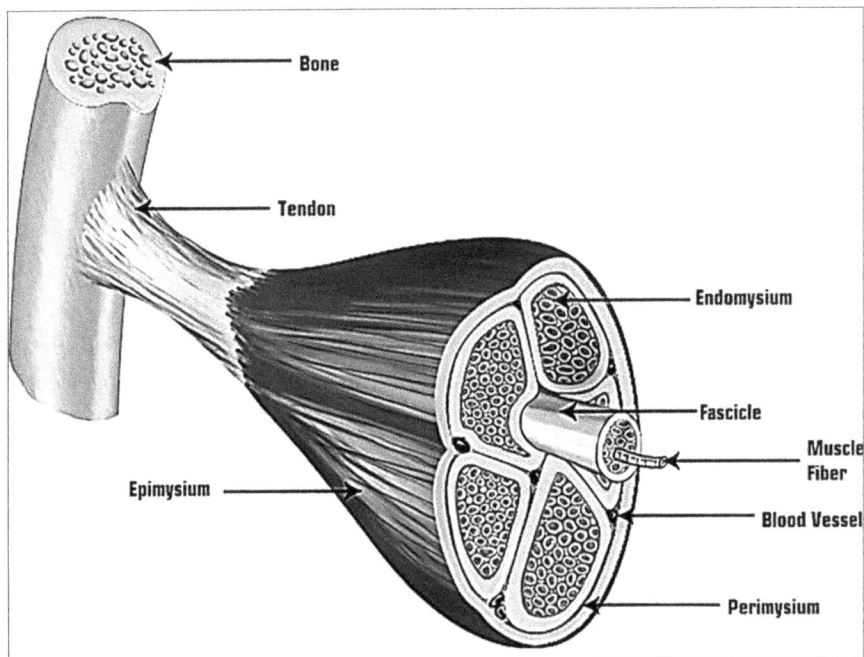

FIGURE 6.3   Diagrammatic representation of muscle regeneration.

6.4   BIOMATERIALS IN BONE REGENERATION

Researchers over the years have reported employing biomaterials of various classes and sources in bone regeneration, confirming their feasibility by substituting biomaterials with irreparable bones. In the past, biomaterials were designed to be bioinert, but over the years scientists desired that biomaterials are bioactive with a capacity to regenerate tissues and integrate with the body by biomimicking biological molecules (Langer and Vacanti, 1993; Hench and Polak, 2002). Biomaterial-related substitutes in the forms of bioactive ceramics, bioactive glasses, biphasic calcium phosphate, noncalcium-based ceramics, polymers, and composite materials have been employed with some levels of successes recorded. The general notion of researchers using biomaterials for bone regeneration is that the substitute materials will be resorbed and overtime replaced by the body's own newly regenerated biological tissue (Langer and Vacanti, 1993).

Calcium-based ceramics have been adopted by scientists as substitutes for bone regeneration; as a result of the similarity in mineral composition with bones, they are generally classified into calcium phosphates (CPs) and glass ceramics. They are of interest to researchers because they are excellent synthetic material, which can be beneficial in filling up bone cavities, discontinuities, or defects (Koutsoukos et al., 1980; Dorozhkin, 2007). Calcium phosphate cements (CPCs) are usually obtained by sintering at high temperature; for example, HA is obtained by sintering at temperatures above 1,000°C, while other phases as tetracalcium phosphate (TTCP) and α- and β-tricalcium phosphate (α-, β-TCP) can be obtained by other sintering methods, all employing the granular forms of the byproducts obtained. CPCs are generally biocompatible and injectable cement pastes that possess the capability to self-set in a bone cavity (Brown, 1983), hence avoiding the need to be precast or needing to fit required bone surgical sites using any means that can eventually lead to possible bone loss (Laurencin et al., 1999). Quite a lot of researchers have investigated CPs as implants and there have been reports employing 3D printing of CPCs for fabrication of specific implants (Klammert et al., 2010; Butscher et al., 2012; Inzana et al., 2015; Komlev et al., 2015; Bergmann et al., 2014; Inzana et al., 2014; Habibovic et al., 2008). Yuan and his colleagues implanted calcium phosphate biomaterials (CPBs) in dogs to study the osteoinduction of the implanted biomaterials (Yuan et al., 1998). The experiment involved the comparison of different composite of CPCs and they reported that the CPBs with micropores (HA ceramic, HA/TCP ceramic, CP cement, and β-TCP ceramic) encouraged bone formation in comparison to the other CP composites. They concluded that the CPBs exhibited osteoinductive capacity when certain chemical and structural characteristics were observed by the CPB mixes. Similarly, Tsukanaka and coworkers implanted highly purified porous β-TCP materials into FVB mice to investigate its osteoinductive potential (Tsukanaka et al., 2015). It has been reported by Kondo and colleagues (2006) that highly purified porous β-TCP materials are 100% osteoinductive by 16 weeks in dogs. In this experiment, they compared the oseteoinductive capacity of 60% and 75% porous β-TCP materials. They classified the pore sizes by the mercury intrusion porosimeter with 60% porous materials having between ≥0.2 and <2 μm, while 75% porous materials with pore sizes between ≥100 and <200 μm. After the mice were anesthetized, the materials were implanted and the investigation of their osteoinductive capacity, number of vessels, and newly formed bone areas were reported, although other parameters were also investigated and reported.

Newly formed bones were observed only in the materials with 60% porosity and the identification was gotten by histological evaluation using the Hematoxylin and Eosin (H&E) staining protocol. They concluded that the osteoinductive capacity of highly purified porous β-TCP materials was evident, but not as compared to that in dogs. Davison and coworkers investigated the relationship between surface architecture of TCP, osteoinduction, and biological resorption (Davison et al., 2014). To achieve this, they prepared two TCP ceramics with varying levels of surface architecture (one at a submicron scale and the other at a micron scale) and evaluated the effect of the surface architecture on the formation of osteoclast and activity of some osteogenic signals *in vitro*; also the resorbability of the material and inductive capacity of the bone were evaluated by *in vivo* experiments.

Similarly, Zhang and colleagues revealed that the size of the surface microstructures of CPCs is an osteogenic factor (Zhang et al., 2014). They showed this by having two classes of TCP ceramics: TCP-S (0.99 ± 0.20 μm grain size and 0.65 ± 0.25 μm micropore size) and TCP-B (3.08 ± 0.52 μm grain size and 1.58 ± 0.65 μm micropore size). After *in vitro*, they observed that TCP-S provided suitable surface for enhanced cell proliferation and differentiation of cultured human bone marrow without bone marrow stromal cells when compared to TCP-B ceramic granules. They went further to implant these ceramic granules *in vivo* for 12 weeks in paraspinal muscles of dogs and bone formation was recorded in TCP-S ($21 \pm 10\%$ bone in the available space) and no bone formed in TCP-B. Over the years, scientists have become more focused on improving the properties of CPs and CPCs properties such as: mechanical strength, resorbability, and injectability. Although, CPs generally are quite close in mineral composition to bones, HA [$Ca_5(PO_4)_3(OH)$] is the CP which is closest to bone when taking into consideration its mineral phase (Kasir et al., 2017). It is characterized by very slow biodegradation rates and it is biocompatible (Draenert et al., 2013), but although it is challenged with properties such as brittleness, low tensile strength, and impact resistance, it has been successfully studied as a substitute for bone as an osteoconductive material for implant since the early 1980s (Jarcho, 1981). Researchers have been investigating and designing HA with or without pores and over numerous reports with varying animals, the necessity of pores (macro or micro) has been testified for osteoinduction (Yuan et al., 1998, 1999; Wang et al., 2013; Akiyama et al., 2011; Ripamonti, 1996). Table 6.1 summarizes some studies and the reported osteoinductive capacity of the calcium-based ceramics was investigated. Although the issue of CPs being hardened material lacking interconnected network for possible vascularization still lingers, scientists are constantly investigating the possibility of encapsulation of cells and drugs within CPCs creating an avenue for possible encapsulation of scaffolds or polymers to improve biological properties of the injectable cement paste (Zhao et al., 2010).

TABLE 6.1 Summary of Osteoinductive Capacity of Some Calcium-Based Ceramics

Materials	Pore Sizes Investigated	*In vivo* Test Animal	Induced Osteogenic Signals	References
Hydroxyapatite	Macro- + Micropore sizes	Rats	Yes	(Lee et al., 2013)
		Dogs	Yes	(Yuan et al., 1999; Ripamonti, 1996; Wang et al., 2013)
		Goats	No	(Habibovic et al., 2008)
	Macroporous	Dogs	No	(Yuan et al., 1999)
	Microporous	Dogs	Yes	(Yuan et al., 1998)
	Nonporous	Dogs	No	(Yuan et al., 1998)
Biphasic calcium phosphate	Macro- + Micropore sizes	Dogs	Yes	(Duan et al., 2003)
		Rats	Yes	(Miron et al., 2016; Duan et al., 2003)
		Rabbits	Yes	(Duan et al., 2003)
		Goats	No	(Fellah et al., 2008)
		Mice	Yes	(Cheng et al., 2010; Yang et al., 2011; Wang et al., 2014)
	Microporous	Rats	No	(Cheng et al., 2013)
		Rabbits	No	(Cheng et al., 2013)
		Dogs	Yes	(Davison et al., 2015; Yuan et al., 1998)
	Nonporous	Dogs	No	(Davison et al., 2015)
Beta-tricalcium phosphate	Macro- + Micropore sizes	Dogs	Yes	(Kondo et al., 2006)
	60% porosity macro- + micropores	Mice	Yes	(Tsukanaka et al., 2015)
	75% porosity macro- + micropores	Mice	No	(Tsukanaka et al., 2015)

TABLE 6.1   *(Continued)*

Materials	Pore Sizes Investigated	*In vivo* Test Animal	Induced Osteogenic Signals	References
	Microporous	Dogs	Yes	(Yuan et al., 1998)
	Microporous— small pores	Dogs	Yes	(Davison et al., 2015)
	Microporous— large pores	Dogs	No	(Davison et al., 2015)
	Nonporous	Dogs	No	(Davison et al., 2015)
Alpha-tricalcium phosphate	Microporous	Dogs	No	(Yuan et al., 1998)
Calcium phosphate cements	Macro- + Micropore sizes	Goat	No	(Bodde et al., 2007)
Brushite	Macro- + Micropore sizes	Goat	Yes	(Habibovic et al., 2008)
Monetite	Macro- + Micropore sizes	Goat	Yes	(Habibovic et al., 2008)
Calcium metaphosphate	Macro- + Micropore sizes	Rats	Yes	(Lee et al., 2013)

Polymers have been employed in the regeneration of bones since the early 1960s; its use to support shaft to prosthesis for the anchor of femoral head was reported by Charnley using self-polymerizing synthetic polymethyl methacrylate (PMMA) as a bone cement (Charnley, 1960). He observed that the inertness and properties of PMMA allowed for excellent fixation of the prosthesis to the femur shaft and hence allow for secondary biological fixation. He also reported challenges with exothermic polymerization reaction, which he indicated could allow for unreacted monomers to reside within the bloodstream, which during polymerization could lead to shrinkage of the cement as a result of possibly fat embolism. More recently, other polymers have been employed; a modified form of ultra-high-molecular-weight polyethylene (UHMWPE) was used by Italian researchers as inserts in joint replacements (Del Prever et al., 2009). Failures in joint replacements based on UHMWPE were previously reported, but Brach and his coworkers investigated cross-linked and noncross-linked UHMWPE identifying that the challenges were observed with UHMWPE. UHMWPE had benefits of having low friction, biocompatibility, unparalleled toughness, ease of fabrication, and high abrasion resistance, but a challenge of oxidative degradation, which eventually leads to low mechanical properties and wear resistance.

By employing cross-linked polyethylene, Brach and his colleagues prevented oxidation and by other modification, other beneficial properties were achieved (Del Prever et al., 2009). Researchers have employed polyetheretherketone (PEEK), a thermoplastic polymer in medical devices as an alternative to titanium. Sagomonyants and his colleagues reported on the response of human osteoblasts *in vitro* to substrates made of PEEK in comparison to pure titanium (Sagomonyants et al., 2008). Synthetic polymer-based scaffolds have been designed to include: polyglycolic acid (PGA), polylactic acid (PLA), poly(ε-caprolactone) (PCL), polyhydroxyalkanoates (PHAs), poly(propylene fumarate), and poly(lactide-*co*-glycolide) (PLGA), with an intention of controlling the mechanical properties by varying the cross-linking densities, concentrations, and copolymerization ratios. Investigations involving controlling of the synthesis conditions to ensure reproducible properties, which negate factors of immunogenicity and infections have been reported. For example, PLGA is mostly blended with PLA, PGA, and poly(α-hydroxyl) esters for improved mechanical stability, resorbability, and cytocompatibility (Gunatillake and Adhikari, 2003).

Researchers overtime are knowledgeable about the compressive strength and low osteoconductivity properties of PGA and PLA, which make them not suitable for use as scaffolds for bone regeneration, but blending PLGA with varying ratios of PGA and PLA gives rise to a mechanically more stable material, which is also more soluble, with enhanced osteoconductivity and enhanced controllable degradation rate (Gentile et al., 2014; Remya et al., 2013). PCL, although its appreciable flexibility and controllable degradation rates, approval by the Food and Drug Administration (FDA) for use in tissue engineering, its byproducts after degradation tend to be acidic. Its acidic byproducts often lead to undesirable changes in the pH condition of its existing locale and its absence of functional group tends to result in osteoinduction and its hydrophobic nature tends to be unsuitable for cell attachment. But, by blending with other polymers and natural materials such as collagen, chitosan, and hybrid scaffolds for use in bone regenerations have been designed with properties of mechanical stability, superior osteogenic capacity, stimulatory, and the biomimicry effect of the natural polymers (Baylan et al., 2013; Fu et al., 2012; Yang et al., 2009). Natural polymers such as silk, chitosan, gelatin, and collagen have been used in bone regeneration, as they mimic the biochemical properties, chemical composition, and the biological structure of bones organic matrix. They also tend to stimulate positive cell responses, possess low immunogenic properties, and can be functional while supporting bone and tissue regeneration (Stoppel et al., 2015; Tsai et al., 2010; Themistocleous et al., 2007; Shih et al., 2006; O'brien, 2011; Yoshioka and Goissis, 2008; Yunoki and Matsuda, 2008). Although some of these natural polymers have drawbacks of poor mechanical properties and the potential risk of allergic reactions or infections in some cases (Lynn et al., 2004; Adachi et al., 2006), these challenges can be evaded by blends of polymers.

Natural polymeric scaffolds such as alginate and chitosan have the capacity for surface interactions with anionic biological molecules such as lipids, cell membranes, proteins, and deoxyribonucleic acid as a result of their cationic surfaces. Their cationic amino surfaces enable the possibility for them to stimulate growth factors and cytokines, which aid in bone and tissue generation (Costa-Pinto et al., 2011, 2012; Wang and Stegemann, 2010) and this has been reported by quite a number of researchers studying chitosan-based models promoting new bone formation *in vivo*. It has been reported that silk fibroin, although possesses low compressive strength, encourages cell proliferation, *in vitro* osteogenesis, and *in vivo* bone formation in calvarial defect models (Meechaisue et al., 2007; Uebersax et al., 2013; Zhang et al., 2010; Mata et al., 2010; Holmes, 2002; Hartgerink et al., 2001; Kantlehner et al., 2000; Gandavarapu et al., 2013). Thus, they have been reportedly biocompatible, possess osteoconductive properties, but only applied to bone tissue sites where load bearing is not required (Stoppel et al., 2015). Overtime, the fabrication of biomaterials to possess blend of nanofibrous polymer matrices has been via techniques such as chemical etching, phase separation, electrospinning, and 3D printing worldwide.

6.5 BIOMATERIALS IN TISSUE REGENERATION

Biomaterials have been successful in aiding researchers to overcome the limitations of contemporary therapies involving skeletal muscle repair and regeneration. By providing physical and chemical conditions for muscle cells growth from the host, in the case of minor repair or transplantation from a foreign host, biomaterials have allowed for promotion of functional maturation, enhancement of survival rates, provided protection from foreign bodies, and enhancement of vascularization of repair sites. To achieve these, biomaterials have been employed as carriers of isolated muscle cells and supporting cells for eventual *in vivo* implantation at muscle injury sites or to encourage functional development of cells *in vitro* prior to implantation. In some other situations, biomaterials are used in combination with cytokines or paracrine signaling to encourage endogenous regeneration by inducing changes in nearby cells, altering the behavior of those cells. Normally, the repair response to an injury to muscle occurs in five stages:

1. Degradation
2. Inflammation
3. Regeneration
4. Remodeling
5. Maturation

These responses are defined by the expression of different cytokines, growth factors released, and various cells recruitment and activities. Depending on the level of muscle injury, replacement can be achieved by the satellite cells within the muscles themselves, but with over 20% volumetric muscle loss, the muscle will need to be assisted to be repaired (Grogan et al., 2011; Sicari et al., 2012; Wu et al., 2012). Scaffolds used in the regeneration of muscles and/or tissues could be designed in the form of synthetic or biological forms.

6.5.1 BIOLOGIC SCAFFOLDS

Synthetic biologic scaffolds have been designed to encourage the proliferation of cells and production of contractile tissues under *in vitro* and *in vivo* conditions. Hydrogels, collagens, scaffolds having acellular extracellular matrix (ECM), and materials made of polymers have been designed to have cells ranging from human stem cells to differentiated myoblasts seeded within to allow for tissue repairs (Wolf et al., 2015). These scaffolds have been designed with varying materials and therapeutically delivered as hydrogels, tissue constructs, sheets, etc. (Wolf et al., 2015). These FDA-approved scaffolds with acellular ECM do not only encourage attachment of cells, but also immune degradation of the ECM and a conducive environment for regeneration (Badylak et al., 2016; Dziki et al., 2016a, 2016b). The investigation into the use of scaffolds based on ECM to repair skeletal muscles in animal models has been reported since the mid-90s by researchers (Badylak et al., 1995). The urinary bladder or small intestinal submucosa (SIS) of pigs provided the ECM therapeutic scaffold for repairs and various tissues.

The first study revealed the biocompatibility potential of employing SIS as vascular grafts in canines (Lantz et al., 1990; Badylak et al., 1989). It was reportedly found that stripping the cells reduced the host systems immune response, which is one of the major challenge faced in transplantation studies. They also revealed that porcine SIS, which was decellularized, was effective scaffolds, encouraging infiltration of host cells while still maintaining the tissues structural integrity with the host tissue (Lantz et al., 1990). The host cells and ECM eventually replaced the vascular grafts when total recovery had taken place (Sandusky Jr et al., 1992). These observations led Dr Stephen Badylak and his coworkers to investigate using decullularized porcine SIS and the urinary bladder's submucosa for the repair of tissues. In subsequent years, they reported findings on esophageal, dural tissue, and bladder wall repair using porcine SIS (Kropp et al., 1995, 1996; Cobb et al., 1999; Badylak et al., 2000). Porcine SIS has also been employed as a patch for wound healing in a rodent model (Prevel et al., 1995a, 1995b). SIS bioscaffolds regenerative capacities of muscles, bones, and tendons were investigated by researchers. The study of tendon repair revealed that using decellularized porcine SIS, there is a possibility of defects of the Achilles tendon in canines (Badylak et al., 1995).

Badylak and his colleagues determined that the repaired portion of the tendon had a better strength than the distal or proximal ends of the tendon 12 weeks after recovery and achieving this by measuring the uniaxial longitudinal tensile strength. 8 weeks postimplantation, the SIS bioscaffold had degraded and had been replaced by host tissue and revealed by immunohistological analysis. SIS was firstly reported to encourage regeneration in muscle defects by Prevel and his colleagues in the mid-90s (Prevel et al., 1995a) using a rodent model. The defect in the abdominal wall of the rodent was developed by a 2 cm by 2 cm abdominal wall skeletal muscle defect and to confirm regeneration of skeletal muscle, they subjected thin muscle sections to qualitative histological analysis by determining that the SIS was incorporated in the abdominal wall after 2 months after with minimal inflammation and no evidence of host rejection of the donor tissue (Prevel et al., 1995a). Employing porcine SIS to repair volumetric muscle loss in animal models was reported by Tuner and his colleagues. They initiated a defect in the proximal half of associated Achilles tendon of canines and the distal third of the gastrocnemius muscle (Turner et al., 2010). Similarly, Sicari and his colleagues made defects in murine quadriceps (Sicari et al.,

2012). They both employed similar techniques to determine the capacity to which SIS assists in the repair of the defects in skeletal muscles. They both probed the vascularization of the wound site, infiltration of the myoblasts, and nascent myofiber formation. They observed degradation of the SIS scaffold in the site of the wound. They reported that the repair occurred similarly to researchers previously reported models with abdominal wall defects, which showed rapid degradation of the scaffold, neovascularization, and myoblasts formation of isolation myofibers within the defects (Turner et al., 2010; Sicari et al., 2012). It is of importance to mention that Badylak and his colleagues confirmed wound repair and formation or regeneration of muscles by histological studies and not *in vivo* functional studies, although they have employed ex vivo functional studies to support findings (Turner et al., 2010).

The comparison of regeneration potential of SIS to ECM derived from skeletal muscle as a bioscaffold to encourage repair was investigated (Wolf et al., 2012). They revealed that differences existed in the structural protein of basement membrane, structural proteins, glycosaminoglycans, and growth factors of ECM scaffolds. But, employing the same conditions as previous studies, the two scaffold kinds revealed little differences in the capacity to regenerate defect in the abdominal walls (Wolf et al., 2012). They came to a conclusion that "superior tissue remodeling outcomes are not universally dependent upon homologous tissue-derived ECM scaffold materials." Sicari and his colleagues again reported the repair of muscles in rat models and five human patients using ECM derived from porcine urinary bladder.

It was indicated that the porcine urinary bladder matrix derived from ECM was biochemically and structurally similar to that obtained from porcine SIS, but that in three of the five human patients, there were functional improvements observed (Sicari et al., 2014). Sicari and his colleagues did not tag this response "regeneration", but "constructive remodeling" and although "complete clarity" were not made; recent review by Badylak highlighted the distinction between both responses (Badylak et al., 2016). *Nature Medicine* in 2008 featured the decellularization of a mammalian heart by Ott and his colleagues and it was one of the highlight of decellularized tissues (Ott et al., 2008). Ott and his colleagues attempted to make a scaffold heart by decullularizing a mammalian heart and harvest the cells in a scaffold for return to the host. They were successful in the repopulation of the scaffold with smooth muscle cells, endothelial cells, fibrocytes, and neonatal cardiomyocytes. But though after 8 days, the scaffold heart responded to chemical and electrical stimuli, only 2% contractile force of adult rat heart function was possible. They recorded contractions and rhythmic depolarizations up to 5 minutes after the heart was taken off the electric pacer. Ott and his colleagues indicated that only 34% of tissues in the scaffold were recellularized by injected cells, but the study confirmed the regenerative capacity of scaffolds. Injectable skeletal muscle matrix hydrogel was designed by DeQuach and his colleagues for the repair of peripheral artery disease in hindlimb ischemia rat model (DeQuach et al., 2012). The femoral artery was resected in the model rat to imitate ischemia, "inadequate blood supply to an organ or part of the body". A week after confirmation of hindlimb ischemia, either collagen or decellularized skeletal muscle (DSM) hydrogel was intramuscularly injected below the defected site. There was reportedly a significant increase in desmin-positive cells coexpressing Ki67, which indicates proliferation of satellite cells observed at the injection sites of DSM hydrogels. It is of important to mention that cell-based therapies have their drawbacks when compared to therapies involving ECMs derived from DSM (DeQuach et al., 2012). Drawbacks in the form of transdifferentiation of the implanted cells, which could lead to cancerous growths, difficulty in cell delivery, and short supply of fresh donor cells (Dumont et al., 2011) encourage researchers to rather employ later. The supply of donor cells is a drawback relating to organ transplantation or donation and host rejection response.

6.5.2   SYNTHETIC SCAFFOLDS

Scaffolds have been designed with synthetic materials for the regeneration of muscle and tissue. The uses of synthetic materials for scaffold designs possess benefits from the engineerable standpoint. Synthetic scaffolds can be crafted with specifics in relation to architecture, composition, materials used, etc. (Wolf et al., 2015). Considering the robust possibility available in designing synthetic scaffolds and customizing them for specific applications, they have not been more successful than the bioscaffolds for regeneration in animal models. Quite a number of polymers have been evaluated for their capacity as substitutes in muscle trauma and they include, but are not limited to, PLA, PGA, PCL, PLGA, and polyurethanes (Wolf et al., 2015). Cronin and his colleagues reported the viability and proliferation of both mouse skeletal and human skeletal muscle cell lines on PLA. They utilized PLA as both a film and as a fiber coating it with gelatin, laminin, fibronectin, or ECM gel and then seeded it with cells. The PLA-ECM-coated scaffolds outperformed the rest of the prepared scaffolds in respect to attachment of cells and related genes expression (Cronin et al., 2004).

Although the study was limited to *in vitro* studies, which limited any potential evidence of further therapeutic advantage of PLA for skeletal muscle tissue engineering. Due to the nontoxic byproducts of PLGA, glycolic acid, and lactic acid, PLGA has gained popularity as a scaffold of choice for fabrication purposes by researchers. Fabrication of biomimetic constructs using PLGA has been investigated by a number of researchers *in vitro* for skeletal muscle repair and other applications. Shandalov and his colleagues implanted a PLA-PLGA scaffold for the treatment of an abdominal wall defect in a mouse (Shandalov et al., 2014). This stem cell seeded PLA-PLGA scaffold was initially implanted around the femoral artery and vein and isolated from the surrounding tissue. This form of *in vivo* preparation allowed for initial vessel formation within the scaffold before subsequent transplantation into the abdominal wall. 2 weeks postimplantation, they reported anastomosis with the host's vasculature and robust perfusion of the scaffolds. Similar to this study, although PLGA scaffolds have been successful *in vivo* with other animal models, yet the evidence of functional recovery from extreme volumetric muscle loss repair (Levenberg et al., 2005; Laschke et al., 2008). For close to two decades, scaffolds of PGA have been employed in the repair of skeletal muscle tissue. Saxena and his colleagues, as far back as the late 1990s, revealed that regeneration of tissue resembling skeletal muscle tissue could occur by implantation of seeded myoblast primary cell lines within PGA absorbable meshes into Fisher 344 rat (Saxena et al., 1999).

Further immunohistochemistry (IHC) studies 45 days postimplantation displayed cells of the degraded synthetic grafts which stained positive for desmin and α-sarcomeric actin, which are proteins depicting possible skeletal tissue growth/presence. It is important to mention that the locale of implantation was the omentum and the graft was evidently vascularized. Biocompatibility of the PGA grafts was evident, but they could not conclude that a direct extrapolation with myoblast-PGA construct could be effective for regeneration of muscles in defected skeletal muscle. Compatibility is one of the major challenges of synthetic scaffolds and due to the apparent compatibility of PCL proffers; researchers have employed it in fabrication of scaffolds using techniques such as electrospinning. It is a method by which synthetic constructs can be arranged by extruding a polymer onto a plate which is charged the variation of the deposition rate and charge encourages the variation in alignment of scaffold microstructure, which can encourage cell proliferation, adhesion, or division (Choi et al., 2008). PCL electrospun scaffolds have been designed by numerous researchers; Choi and his colleagues designed PCL electrospun scaffolds with aligned fibers and revealed their capacity to encourage *in vitro* myotube formation (Choi et al., 2008). Scaffolds of polyurethane have also been designed using the electrospinning technique by researchers reporting proliferation and differentiation of multiple cell lines such as human satellite cells, L6, and C2C12 cell lines (Riboldi et al., 2005). Encouraging mechanical properties have been identified for polyesterurethane scaffolds, but the high tensile modulus of PLGA, PGA, and PLA fibers observed will definitely influence their application in skeletal muscle tissue engineering (Riboldi et al., 2005). Fibers of polyesterurethane have been reported to show elastomeric properties and also shown to provide a conducive substrate for attachment, proliferation, and differentiation of skeletal muscle progenitor cells (Riboldi et al., 2005, 2008; Sirivisoot and Harrison, 2011).

Generally, synthetic scaffold materials morphology—fiber alignment and sizes of pores are tunable and they are usually tuned to mimic ECM (Klumpp et al., 2010). The fiber organization has been directed by researchers since these synthetic materials do not possess similar biochemical composition to ECM (Choi et al., 2008; Aviss et al., 2010). For example, pristine hydrogels do not possess organization for cell attachment, but by modification of their surfaces, researchers have been employed in skeletal muscle tissue engineering. Similarly, using soft photolithography, micropatterning has been employed to encourage cell adherence and proliferation by researchers (Huang et al., 2010). In addition to developing scaffolds, some researchers have sought to engineer skeletal muscle tissue from cells. Tissue-engineered skeletal muscle can function as a model for pharmacological research, a tool for understanding embryological development and/or myogenesis or a therapeutic intervention for repairing skeletal muscle trauma. Two separate groups have been using tissue-engineered skeletal muscle under *in vivo* conditions and, more importantly, within skeletal muscle tissue. Dr Juhas and Dr Bursac from Duke University and Dr Larkin from the University of Michigan have developed constructs that produce contractile force and, in the case of Dr Larkin's research, have successfully integrated into damaged host muscle. Juhas et al. fabricated engineered skeletal muscle by first molding a Matrigel hydrogel with primary rat myoblasts in a polydimethylsiloxane mold (Juhas et al., 2016).

The authors noted the first objective was to create an *in vitro* environment that more accurately reproduces the *in vivo* environment of the myogenic tissue niche. Satellite cell was proliferated and differentiated under *in vitro* conditions and the researchers were directed the development of cells into an engineering skeletal muscle tissue. The engineered construct was capable of contractile force generation before it was implanted into a dorsal window on a rat. At 2 weeks postimplantation, the construct was producing 3.5× more contractile force than the preimplanted engineered muscle. The engineered muscle also showed robust vascular ingrowth from the host vasculature and a 40.7% increase in myofiber diameter. The authors reported that engineered muscle appeared to have a myogenic response to implantation even though it was not within a skeletal muscle niche. In addition, the authors reported vigorous recovery from an *in vitro* cardiotoxin injury. Juhas et al. concluded that the results from their research support using *in vitro* engineered muscle as a tool for drug and toxicology studies. Dr. Larkin's group has also developed tissue-engineered muscle tissue and has used their construct to specifically repair volumetric muscle loss in an animal model. In a paper authored by VanDusen et al., they reported that a rat tibialis anterior (TA) muscle with a volumetric muscle loss injury receiving therapeutic intervention with their construct produced significantly more *in vivo* tetanic contractile force than an unrepaired TA (VanDusen et al., 2014). The fabrication of their engineered muscle used techniques similar to those by Dr Bursac's group. Muscle progenitor cells, along with isolated bone marrow cells, were harvested from the soleus muscle of 120–150 g female Fisher 344 rats. Bone marrow cells were cultured in appropriate media to produce engineered bone-tendon anchors used to implant the engineered muscle tissue. The muscle progenitor cells were grown to confluence until elongating myotubes began to form and the monolayer was delaminated and rolled into a cylindrical muscle construct. In addition to determining *in vivo* peak tetanic force, the researchers also evaluated the regenerative potential of the engineered muscle through histological data. Fluorescent imaging revealed aligned myofibers that had developed advanced sarcomeric structure. At 28 days postimplantation, there was evidence of innervation of the engineered construct through IHC staining for panaxonal filaments and the presence of acetylcholine receptors through α-bungarotoxin staining. Immunostaining with CD31 also showed the presence of a well-developed capillary network throughout the engineered muscle tissue. The capillary network was morphologically similar to those found in native muscle, with vessels running parallel to the muscle fibers. The results from this study and others performed by Dr Larkin's group have motivated further investigations using engineered muscle tissue to repair volumetric muscle loss in larger volume models and to explore entire muscle replacement. As previously discussed, skeletal muscle tissue is highly aligned and the force production of a muscle is heavily influenced by the muscle's architecture.

Muscle architecture, the arrangement of muscle fibers in relation to the axis of force generation, is constrained by the length of the muscle, the length of myofibers, the pennation angle, and the physiological cross-sectional area (Lieber and Fridén, 2000). Even in pennate muscles, adjacent myofibers have parallel alignment and the surrounding ECM is highly uniform in direction. When designing bioreactors for tissue-engineered skeletal muscle, researchers are deliberate in developing alignment within their constructs (Aubin et al., 2010; Aviss et al., 2010; Vandenburgh and Karlisch, 1989). Parallel alignment of myofibers has been shown to be important for developing phenotypically normal muscle tissue under *in vitro* conditions (Aubin et al., 2010; Lam et al., 2009; Vandenburgh and Karlisch, 1989; Wang et al., 2015). Researchers obtain parallel alignment through micropatterning (Cimetta et al., 2009; Flaibani et al., 2009; Huang et al., 2010; Shimizu et al., 2009), aligned deposition of fibers (Aviss et al., 2010; Choi et al., 2008; Wang et al., 2015), or by selecting a scaffold that has native parallel alignment. Myofiber alignment indicative of a mature muscle phenotype has also been induced *in vitro* using bioreactors that deliver mechanical or electrical stimulation to cells and/or tissue constructs (Flaibani et al., 2009; Ahadian et al., 2013; Boonen et al., 2010; Donnelly et al., 2010; Grossi et al., 2007; Langelaan et al., 2011; Powell et al., 2002; Vandenburgh and Karlisch, 1989).

6.6 CONCLUSION

Biomaterials have had marked successes *in vitro* in the regeneration of bones and skeletal muscle tissues, although research involving *in vivo* studies is not reported widely. In bone regeneration, blending of polymers has encouraged successes recorded and although numerous synthetic scaffolds have been employed in regeneration and repair of skeletal muscle tissues, mainly only *in vitro* studies have also been reported. Though cell viability and proliferation are of importance to encourage implantation, *in vivo* testing must be investigated for confirmation of functional applications. The vast knowledge of bone and skeletal muscle tissue morphology and physiology reveals the complicated nature of muscular injury with numerous spatiotemporal concerns to consider. Most researchers have investigated and reported successful *in vitro* findings regarding skeletal muscle tissues, but are lacking with advancement with *in vivo* results, beyond reports on abdominal wall defects models and host infiltration analysis. It is important from an engineering perspective to identify thoroughly the varied ramification of the engineered material for possible contractile force production possibly *in vivo* or within cases of skeletal muscle repair.

ACKNOWLEDGMENTS

The authors thank the University of Zululand, Medical Research Council (MRC) and the National Research Foundation, South Africa through the South African Research Chair Initiative (SARChI) for their financial assistance toward this research. SJO specially thanks the National Research Foundation (NRF) for SARChI Postdoctoral Research Fellowship.

KEYWORDS

- **biomaterials**
- **bone**
- **muscle**
- **tissue**
- **regeneration**
- **repair**

REFERENCES

Adachi, T., Tomita, M., Shimizu, K., Ogawa, S. and Yoshizato, K. Generation of hybrid transgenic silkworms that express Bombyx mori prolyl-hydroxylase α-subunits and human collagens in posterior silk glands: production of cocoons that contained collagens with hydroxylated proline residues. *J Biotechnol.* **2006,** 126(2): 205–219.

Ahadian, S., Ramón-Azcón, J., Ostrovidov, S., Camci-Unal, G., Kaji, H., Ino, K., Shiku, H., Khademhosseini, A. and Matsue, T. A contactless electrical stimulator: application to fabricate functional skeletal muscle tissue. *Biomed Microdevices.* **2013,** 15(1): 109–115.

Akiyama, N., Takemoto, M., Fujibayashi, S., Neo, M., Hirano, M. and Nakamura, T. Difference between dogs and rats with regard to osteoclast-like cells in calcium-deficient hydroxyapatite-induced osteoinduction. *J Biomed Mater Res A.* **2011,** 96(2): 402–412.

Albrektsson, T. and Johansson, C. Osteoinduction, osteoconduction and osseointegration. *Eur Spine J.* **2001,** 10(2): S96–S101.

Aubin, H., Nichol, J. W., Hutson, C. B., Bae, H., Sieminski, A. L., Cropek, D. M. et al. Directed 3D cell alignment and elongation in microengineered hydrogels. *Biomaterials.* **2010,** 31(27): 6941–6951.

Aviss, K., Gough, J. and Downes, S. Aligned electrospun polymer fibres for skeletal muscle regeneration. *Eur Cell Mater.* **2010,** 19(1): 193–204.

Badylak, S., Meurling, S., Chen, M., Spievack, A. and Simmons-Byrd, A. Resorbable bioscaffold for esophageal repair in a dog model. *J Pediatr Surg.* **2000,** 35(7): 1097–1103.

Badylak, S. F., Dziki, J. L., Sicari, B. M., Ambrosio, F. and Boninger, M. L. Mechanisms by which acellular biologic scaffolds promote functional skeletal muscle restoration. *Biomaterials.* **2016,** 103: 128–136.

Badylak, S. F., Lantz, G. C., Coffey, A. and Geddes, L. A. Small intestinal submucosa as a large diameter vascular graft in the dog. *J Surg Res.* **1989,** 47(1): 74–80.

Badylak, S. F., Tullius, R., Kokini, K., Shelbourne, K. D., Klootwyk, T., Voytik, S. L., Kraine, M. R. and Simmons, C. The use of xenogenic small intestinal submucosa as a biomaterial for Achilles tendon repair in a dog model. *J Biomed Mater Res.* **1995,** 29(8): 977–985.

Batista, G., Ibarra, M., Ortiz, J. and Villegas, M. Engineering biomechanics of knee replacement. *Appl Eng Mech Med.* **2004;** 2: 1–12.

Bauer, T. W. and Muschler, G. F. Bone graft materials: an overview of the basic science. *Clin Orthop Relat Res.* **2000,** 371: 10–27.

Baylan, N., Bhat, S., Ditto, M., Lawrence, J. G., Lecka-Czernik, B. and Yildirim-Ayan, E. Polycaprolactone nanofiber interspersed collagen type-I scaffold for bone regeneration: a unique injectable osteogenic scaffold. *Biomed Mater.* **2013,** 8(4): 045011.

Bergmann, C. J., Odekerken, J. C., Welting, T. J., Jungwirth, F., Devine, D., Bouré, L. et al. Calcium phosphate based three-dimensional cold plotted bone scaffolds for critical size bone defects. *Biomed Res Int.* **2014,** 2014: 852610.

Bodde, E. W., Cammaert, C. T., Wolke, J. G., Spauwen, P. H. and Jansen, J. A. Investigation as to the osteoinductivity of macroporous calcium phosphate cement in goats. *J Biomed Mater Res B Appl Biomater.* **2007,** 83(1): 161–168.

Boonen, K. J., Langelaan, M. L., Polak, R. B., van der Schaft, D. W., Baaijens, F. P. and Post, M. J. Effects of a combined mechanical stimulation protocol: value for skeletal muscle tissue engineering. *J Biomech.* **2010,** 43(8): 1514–1521.

Brack, A. S. and Rando, T. A. Tissue-specific stem cells: lessons from the skeletal muscle satellite cell. *Cell Stem Cell.* **2012,** 10(5): 504–514.

Brown, W. A new calcium phosphate setting cement. *J Dent Res.* **1983,** 63: 672.

Buck, B., Malinin, T. I. and Brown, M. D. Bone transplantation and human immunodeficiency virus. An estimate of risk of acquired immunodeficiency syndrome (AIDS). *Clin Orthop Relat Res.* **1989,** 240: 129–136.

Butscher, A., Bohner, M., Roth, C., Ernstberger, A., Heuberger, R., Doebelin, N. et al. Printability of calcium phosphate powders for three-dimensional printing of tissue engineering scaffolds. *Acta Biomater.* **2012,** 8(1): 373–385.

Charnley, J. Anchorage of the femoral head prosthesis to the shaft of the femur. *J Bone Joint Surg Br.* **1960,** 42(1): 28–30.

Cheng, L., Shi, Y., Ye, F. and Bu, H. Osteoinduction of calcium phosphate biomaterials in small animals. *Mater Sci Eng C.* **2013,** 33(3): 1254–1260.

Cheng, L., Ye, F., Yang, R., Lu, X., Shi, Y., Li, L. et al. Osteoinduction of hydroxyapatite/β-tricalcium phosphate bioceramics in mice with a fractured fibula. *Acta Biomater.* **2010,** 6(4): 1569–1574.

Choi, J. S., Lee, S. J., Christ, G. J., Atala, A. and Yoo, J. J. The influence of electrospun aligned poly(epsilon-caprolactone)/collagen nanofiber meshes on the formation of self-aligned skeletal muscle myotubes. *Biomaterials.* **2008,** 29(19): 2899–2906.

Chuang, D. C. C. Free tissue transfer for the treatment of facial paralysis. *Facial Plast Surg.* **2008,** 24(2): 194–203.

Cimetta, E., Pizzato, S., Bollini, S., Serena, E., De Coppi, P. and Elvassore, N. Production of arrays of cardiac and skeletal muscle myofibers by micropatterning techniques on a soft substrate. *Biomed Microdevices.* **2009,** 11(2): 389–400.

Cobb, M. A., Badylak, S. F., Janas, W., Simmons-Byrd, A. and Boop, F. A. Porcine small intestinal submucosa as a dural substitute. *Surg Neurol.* **1999,** 51(1): 99–104.

Control, C. F. D. Transmission of HIV through bone transplantation: case report and public health recommendations. *Morb Mortal Wkly Rep.* **1988,** 37(39): 597.

Costa-Pinto, A. R., Reis, R. L. and Neves, N. M. Scaffolds-based bone tissue engineering: the role of chitosan. *Tissue Eng Part B Rev.* **2011,** 17(5): 331–347.

Costa-Pinto, A., Correlo, V., Sol, P., Bhattacharya, M., Srouji, S., Livne, E. et al. Chitosan–poly(butylene succinate) scaffolds and human bone marrow stromal cells induce bone repair in a mouse calvaria model. *J Tissue Eng Regen Med.* **2012,** 6(1): 21–28.

Cronin, E. M., Thurmond, F. A., Bassel-Duby, R., Williams, R. S., Wright, W. E., Nelson, K. D. et al. Protein-coated poly(L-lactic acid) fibers provide a substrate for differentiation of human skeletal muscle cells. *J Biomed Mater Res A.* **2004,** 69(3): 373–381.

Davison, N., Luo, X., Schoenmaker, T., Everts, V., Yuan, H., Barrere-de Groot, F. et al. Submicron-scale surface architecture of tricalcium phosphate directs osteogenesis *in vitro* and *in vivo*. *Eur Cell Mater.* **2014,** 27(2): 281–297.

Davison, N., Su, J., Yuan, H., van den Beucken, J. and de Bruijn, J. D. Influence of surface microstructure and chemistry on osteoinduction and osteoclastogenesis by biphasic calcium phosphate discs. *Eur Cell Mater.* **2015,** 29: 314–329.

Del Prever, E. M. B., Bistolfi, A., Bracco, P. and Costa, L. UHMWPE for arthroplasty: past or future? *J Orthop Traumatol.* **2009,** 10(1): 1–8.

DeQuach, J. A., Lin, J. E., Cam, C., Hu, D., Salvatore, M. A., Sheikh, F. et al. Injectable skeletal muscle matrix hydrogel promotes neovascularization and muscle cell infiltration in a hindlimb ischemia model. *Eur Cell Mater.* **2012,** 23: 400.

Dimitriou, R., Mataliotakis, G. I., Angoules, A. G., Kanakaris, N. K. and Giannoudis, P. V. Complications following autologous bone graft harvesting from the iliac crest and using the RIA: a systematic review. *Injury.* **2011,** 42: S3–S15.

Donglu, S. (**2005**). *Introduction to Biomaterials.* World Scientific.

Donnelly, K., Khodabukus, A., Philp, A., Deldicque, L., Dennis, R. G. and Baar, K. A novel bioreactor for stimulating skeletal muscle *in vitro*. *Tissue Eng Part C Methods.* **2010,** 16(4): 711–718.

Dorozhkin, S. V. Calcium orthophosphates. *J Mater Sci.* **2007,** 42(4): 1061–1095.

Draenert, M., Draenert, A. and Draenert, K. Osseointegration of hydroxyapatite and remodeling-resorption of tricalcium phosphate ceramics. *Microsc Res Tech.* **2013,** 76(4): 370–380.

Duan, Y., Wu, Y., Wang, C., Chen, J. and Zhang, X. A study of bone-like apatite formation on calcium phosphate ceramics in different kinds of animals *in vivo*. *J Biomed Eng.* **2003,** 20(1): 22–25.

Dumont, N. A., Bentzinger, C. F., Sincennes, M. C. and Rudnicki, M. A. Satellite cells and skeletal muscle regeneration. *Compr Physiol.* **2011,** 5(3): 1027–1059.

Dziki, J., Badylak, S., Yabroudi, M., Sicari, B., Ambrosio, F., Stearns, K. et al. An acellular biologic scaffold treatment for volumetric muscle loss: results of a 13-patient cohort study. *NPJ Reg Med.* **2016a,** 1: 16008.

Dziki, J. L., Sicari, B. M., Wolf, M. T., Cramer, M. C. and Badylak, S. F. Immunomodulation and mobilization of progenitor cells by extracellular matrix bioscaffolds for volumetric muscle loss treatment. *Tissue Eng Part A.* **2016b,** 22(19–20): 1129–1139.

Fellah, B. H., Gauthier, O., Weiss, P., Chappard, D. and Layrolle, P. Osteogenicity of biphasic calcium phosphate ceramics and bone autograft in a goat model. *Biomaterials.* **2008,** 29(9): 1177–1188.

Flaibani, M., Boldrin, L., Cimetta, E., Piccoli, M., Coppi, P. D. and Elvassore, N. Muscle differentiation and myotubes alignment is influenced by micropatterned surfaces and exogenous electrical stimulation. *Tissue Eng Part A.* **2009,** 15(9): 2447–2457.

Fu, S., Ni, P., Wang, B., Chu, B., Zheng, L., Luo, F. et al. Injectable and thermosensitive PEG-PCL-PEG copolymer/collagen/n-HA hydrogel composite for guided bone regeneration. *Biomaterials.* **2012,** 33(19): 4801–4809.

Gandavarapu, N. R., Mariner, P. D., Schwartz, M. P. and Anseth, K. S. Extracellular matrix protein adsorption to phosphate-functionalized gels from serum promotes osteogenic differentiation of human mesenchymal stem cells. *Acta Biomater.* **2013,** 9(1): 4525–4534.

Gentile, P., Chiono, V., Carmagnola, I. and Hatton, P. An overview of poly(lactic-co-glycolic) acid (PLGA)-based biomaterials for bone tissue engineering. *Int J Mol Sci.* **2014,** 15(3): 3640–3659.

Grogan, B. F., Hsu, J. R. and Consortium, S. T. R. Volumetric muscle loss. *J Am Acad Orthop Surg.* **2011,** 19: S35–S37.

Grossi, A., Yadav, K. and Lawson, M. A. Mechanical stimulation increases proliferation, differentiation, and protein expression in culture: stimulation effects are substrate dependent. *J Biomech.* **2007,** 40(15): 3354–3362.

Gunatillake, P. A. and Adhikari, R. Biodegradable synthetic polymers for tissue engineering. *Eur Cell Mater.* **2003,** 5(1): 1–16.

Habibovic, P., Gbureck, U., Doillon, C. J., Bassett, D. C., van Blitterswijk, C. A. and Barralet, J. E. Osteoconduction and osteoinduction of low-temperature 3D-printed bioceramic implants. *Biomaterials.* **2008,** 29(7): 944–953.

Hartgerink, J. D., Beniash, E. and Stupp, S. I. Self-assembly and mineralization of peptide-amphiphile nanofibers. *Science.* **2001,** 294(5547): 1684–1688.

Helmus, M. N., Gibbons, D. F. and Cebon, D. Biocompatibility: meeting a key functional requirement of next-generation medical devices. *Toxicol Pathol.* **2008,** 36(1): 70–80.

Hench, L. Molecular design of bioactive glasses and ceramics for implants. *Ceram Soc Japan.* **1991;** 3: 519–534.

Hench, L. L. and Polak, J. M. Third-generation biomedical materials. *Science.* **2002,** 295(5557): 1014–1017.

Heness, G. and Ben-Nissan, B. (**2004**). Innovative bioceramics. In *Mater Forum*: Institute of Materials Engineering Australia Ltd.

Holmes, T. C. Novel peptide-based biomaterial scaffolds for tissue engineering. *Trends Biotechnol.* **2002,** 20(1): 16–21.

Huang, N. F., Lee, R. J. and Li, S. Engineering of aligned skeletal muscle by micropatterning. *Am J Transl Res.* **2010,** 2(1): 43.

Inzana, J. A., Olvera, D., Fuller, S. M., Kelly, J. P., Graeve, O. A., Schwarz, E. M. et al. 3D printing of composite calcium phosphate and collagen scaffolds for bone regeneration. *Biomaterials.* **2014,** 35(13): 4026–4034.

Inzana, J. A., Trombetta, R. P., Schwarz, E. M., Kates, S. L. and Awad, H. A. 3D-printed bioceramics for dual antibiotic delivery to treat implant-associated bone infection. *Eur Cell Mater.* **2015,** 30: 232.

Jarcho, M. Calcium phosphate ceramics as hard tissue prosthetics. *Clin Orthop Relat Res.* **1981,** 157: 259–278.

Järvinen, M. J. and Lehto, M. U. The effects of early mobilisation and immobilisation on the healing process following muscle injuries. *Sports Med.* **1993,** 15(2): 78–89.

Juhas, M., Ye, J. and Bursac, N. Design, evaluation, and application of engineered skeletal muscle. *Methods.* **2016,** 99: 81–90.

Kanczler, J. and Oreffo, R. Osteogenesis and angiogenesis: the potential for engineering bone. *Eur Cell Mater.* **2008,** 15(2): 100–114.

Kantlehner, M., Schaffner, P., Finsinger, D., Meyer, J., Jonczyk, A., Diefenbach, B. et al. Surface coating with cyclic RGD peptides stimulates osteoblast adhesion and proliferation as well as bone formation. *ChemBioChem.* **2000,** 1(2): 107–114.

Kasir, R., Vernekar, V. N. and Laurencin, C. T. Inductive biomaterials for bone regeneration. *J Mater Res.* **2017,** 32(6): 1047–1060.

Klammert, U., Gbureck, U., Vorndran, E., Rödiger, J., Meyer-Marcotty, P. and Kübler, A. C. 3D powder printed calcium phosphate implants for reconstruction of cranial and maxillofacial defects. *J Craniomaxillofac Surg.* **2010,** 38(8): 565–570.

Klumpp, D., Horch, R. E., Kneser, U. and Beier, J. P. Engineering skeletal muscle tissue—new perspectives *in vitro* and *in vivo. J Cell Mol Med.* **2010,** 14(11): 2622–2629.

Komlev, V. S., Popov, V. K., Mironov, A. V., Fedotov, A. Y., Teterina, A. Y., Smirnov, I. V., Bozo, I. Y., Rybko, V. A. and Deev, R. V. 3D printing of octacalcium phosphate bone substitutes. *Front Bioeng Biotech.* **2015,** 3: 81.

Kondo, N., Ogose, A., Tokunaga, K., Umezu, H., Arai, K., Kudo, N. et al. Osteoinduction with highly purified β-tricalcium phosphate in dog dorsal muscles and the proliferation of osteoclasts before heterotopic bone formation. *Biomaterials.* **2006,** 27(25): 4419–4427.

Koutsoukos, P., Amjad, Z., Tomson, M. and Nancollas, G. Crystallization of calcium phosphates. A constant composition study. *J Am Chem Soc.* **1980,** 102(5): 1553–1557.

Kretlow, J. D. and Mikos, A. G. Mineralization of synthetic polymer scaffolds for bone tissue engineering. *Tissue Eng.* **2007,** 13(5): 927–938.

Kropp, B. P., Eppley, B. L., Prevel, C., Rippy, M., Harruff, R., Badylak, S. et al. Experimental assessment of small intestinal submucosa as a bladder wall substitute. *Urology.* **1995,** 46(3): 396–400.

Kropp, B. P., Rippy, M. K., Badylak, S. F., Adams, M. C., Keating, M. A., Rink, R. C. et al. Regenerative urinary bladder augmentation using small intestinal submucosa: urodynamic and histopathologic assessment in long-term canine bladder augmentations. *J Urol.* **1996,** 155(6): 2098–2104.

Kuang, S., Gillespie, M. A. and Rudnicki, M. A. Niche regulation of muscle satellite cell self-renewal and differentiation. *Cell Stem Cell.* **2008,** 2(1): 22–31.

Kwee, B. J. and Mooney, D. J. Biomaterials for skeletal muscle tissue engineering. *Curr Opin Biotechnol.* **2017,** 47: 16–22.

Lam, M. T., Huang, Y. C., Birla, R. K. and Takayama, S. Microfeature-guided skeletal muscle tissue engineering for highly organized three-dimensional free-standing constructs. *Biomaterials.* **2009,** 30(6): 1150–1155.

Langelaan, M. L., Boonen, K. J., Rosaria-Chak, K. Y., van der Schaft, D. W., Post, M. J. and Baaijens, F. P. Advanced maturation by electrical stimulation: Differences in response between C2C12 and primary muscle progenitor cells. *J Tissue Eng Regen Med.* **2011,** 5(7): 529–539.

Langer, R. and Vacanti, J. P. Tissue engineering. *Science.* **1993,** 260(5110): 920–926.

Lantz, G. C., Badylak, S. F., Coffey, A. C., Geddes, L. A. and Blevins, W. E. Small intestinal submucosa as a small-diameter arterial graft in the dog. *J Invest Surg.* **1990,** 3(3): 217–227.

Laschke, M., Rücker, M., Jensen, G., Carvalho, C., Mülhaupt, R., Gellrich, N. C. et al. Incorporation of growth factor containing Matrigel promotes vascularization of porous PLGA scaffolds. *J Biomed Mater Res A.* **2008,** 85(2): 397–407.

Laurencin, C. T., Ambrosio, A., Borden, M. and Cooper Jr, J. Tissue engineering: orthopedic applications. *Ann Rev Biomed Eng.* **1999,** 1(1): 19–46.

Lee, H. R., Kim, H. J., Ko, J. S., Choi, Y. S., Ahn, M. W., Kim, S. et al. Comparative characteristics of porous bioceramics for an osteogenic response *in vitro* and *in vivo*. *PLoS One.* **2013,** 8(12): e84272.

Levenberg, S., Rouwkema, J., Macdonald, M., Garfein, E. S., Kohane, D. S., Darland, D. C. et al. Engineering vascularized skeletal muscle tissue. *Nat Biotechnol.* **2005,** 23(7): 879.

Lewandrowski, K. U., Rebmann, V., Päßler, M., Schollmeier, G., Ekkernkamp, A., Grosse-Wilde, H. et al. Immune response to perforated and partially demineralized bone allografts. *J Orthop Sci.* **2001,** 6(6): 545–555.

Lieber, R. L. and Fridén, J. Functional and clinical significance of skeletal muscle architecture. *Muscle Nerve.* **2000,** 23(11): 1647–1666.

Liu, J., Saul, D., Böker, K. O., Ernst, J., Lehman, W. and Schilling, A. F. Current methods for skeletal muscle tissue repair and regeneration. *Biomed Res Int.* **2018,** 2018: 1984879.

Lord, C., Gebhardt, M., Tomford, W. and Mankin, H. Infection in bone allografts. Incidence, nature, and treatment. *J Bone Joint Surg Am.* **1988,** 70(3): 369–376.

Lynn, A., Yannas, I. and Bonfield, W. Antigenicity and immunogenicity of collagen. *J Biomed Mater Res B.* **2004,** 71(2): 343–354.

Mankin, H. J., Hornicek, F. J. and Raskin, K. A. Infection in massive bone allografts. *Clin Orthop Relat Res.* **2005,** 432: 210–216.

Mata, A., Geng, Y., Henrikson, K. J., Aparicio, C., Stock, S. R., Satcher, R. L. et al. Bone regeneration mediated by biomimetic mineralization of a nanofiber matrix. *Biomaterials.* **2010,** 31(23): 6004–6012.

Meechaisue, C., Wutticharoenmongkol, P., Waraput, R., Huangjing, T., Ketbumrung, N., Pavasant, P. et al. Preparation of electrospun silk fibroin fiber mats as bone scaffolds: a preliminary study. *Biomed Mater.* **2007,** 2(3): 181.

Miron, R. J., Sculean, A., Shuang, Y., Bosshardt, D. D., Gruber, R., Buser, D. et al. Osteoinductive potential of a novel biphasic calcium phosphate bone graft in comparison with autographs, xenografts, and DFDBA. *Clin Oral Implants Res.* **2016,** 27(6): 668–675.

Moreau, M. F., Gallois, Y., Baslé, M. F. and Chappard, D. Gamma irradiation of human bone allografts alters medullary lipids and releases toxic compounds for osteoblast-like cells. *Biomaterials.* **2000,** 21(4): 369–376.

Muschler, G. F., Nakamoto, C. and Griffith, L. G. Engineering principles of clinical cell-based tissue engineering. *J Bone Joint Surg.* **2004,** 86(7): 1541–1558.

Nakajima, T., Iizuka, H., Tsutsumi, S., Kayakabe, M. and Takagishi, K. Evaluation of posterolateral spinal fusion using mesenchymal stem cells: differences with or without osteogenic differentiation. *Spine (Phila Pa 1976).* **2007,** 32(22): 2432–2436.

Nodzo, S. R., Kaplan, N. B., Hohman, D. W. and Ritter, C. A. A radiographic and clinical comparison of reamer–irrigator–aspirator versus iliac crest bone graft in ankle arthrodesis. *Int Orthop.* **2014,** 38(6): 1199–1203.

O'brien, F. J. Biomaterials and scaffolds for tissue engineering. *Mater Today.* **2011,** 14(3): 88–95.

Ott, H. C., Matthiesen, T. S., Goh, S. K., Black, L. D., Kren, S. M., Netoff, T. I. et al. Perfusion-decellularized matrix: using nature's platform to engineer a bioartificial heart. *Nat Med.* **2008,** 14(2): 213.

Palmieri, B., Tremblay, J. P. and Daniele, L. Past, present and future of myoblast transplantation in the treatment of Duchenne muscular dystrophy. *Pediatr Transplant.* **2010,** 14(7): 813–819.

Parida, P., Behera, A. and Mishra, S. C. Classification of biomaterials used in medicine. *Int J Adv App Sci.* **2012,** 1(3): 125–129.

Powell, C. A., Smiley, B. L., Mills, J. and Vandenburgh, H. H. Mechanical stimulation improves tissue-engineered human skeletal muscle. *Am J Physiol Cell Physiol.* **2002,** 283(5): C1557–C1565.

Pramanik, S., Agarwal, A. K. and Rai, K. Chronology of total hip joint replacement and materials development. *Trends Biomater Artif Organs.* **2005,** 19(1): 15–26.

Prevel, C. D., Eppley, B. L., Summerlin, D. J., Jackson, J. R., McCarty, M. and Badylak, S. F. Small intestinal submucosa: utilization for repair of rodent abdominal wall defects. *Ann Plast Surg.* **1995a,** 35(4): 374–380.

Prevel, C. D., Eppley, B. L., Summerlin, D. J., Sidner, R., Jackson, J. R., McCarty, M. and Badylak, S. F. Small intestinal submucosa: utilization as a wound dressing in full-thickness rodent wounds. *Ann Plast Surg.* **1995b,** 35(4): 381–388.

Relaix, F. and Zammit, P. S. Satellite cells are essential for skeletal muscle regeneration: the cell on the edge returns centre stage. *Development.* **2012,** 139(16): 2845–2856.

Remya, K., Joseph, J., Mani, S., John, A., Varma, H. and Ramesh, P. Nanohydroxyapatite incorporated electrospun polycaprolactone/polycaprolactone–polyethyleneglycol–polycaprolactone blend scaffold for bone tissue engineering applications. *J Biomed Nano.* **2013,** 9(9): 1483–1494.

Riboldi, S. A., Sadr, N., Pigini, L., Neuenschwander, P., Simonet, M., Mognol, P. et al. Skeletal myogenesis on highly orientated microfibrous polyesterurethane scaffolds. *J Biomed Mater Res A.* **2008,** 84(4): 1094–1101.

Riboldi, S. A., Sampaolesi, M., Neuenschwander, P., Cossu, G. and Mantero, S. Electrospun degradable polyesterurethane membranes: potential scaffolds for skeletal muscle tissue engineering. *Biomaterials.* **2005,** 26(22): 4606–4615.

Ripamonti, U. Osteoinduction in porous hydroxyapatite implanted in heterotopic sites of different animal models. *Biomaterials.* **1996,** 17(1): 31–35.

Ruys, A. J. (**2013**). *Biomimetic biomaterials: structure and applications.* Elsevier.

Sagomonyants, K. B., Jarman-Smith, M. L., Devine, J. N., Aronow, M. S. and Gronowicz, G. A. The *in vitro* response of human osteoblasts to polyetheretherketone (PEEK) substrates compared to commercially pure titanium. *Biomaterials.* **2008,** 29(11): 1563–1572.

Sandusky Jr, G., Badylak, S., Morff, R., Johnson, W. and Lantz, G. Histologic findings after *in vivo* placement of small intestine submucosal vascular grafts and saphenous vein grafts in the carotid artery in dogs. *Am J Path.* **1992,** 140(2): 317.

Saxena, A. K., Marler, J., Benvenuto, M., Willital, G. H. and Vacanti, J. P. Skeletal muscle tissue engineering using isolated myoblasts on synthetic biodegradable polymers: preliminary studies. *Tissue Eng.* **1999**, 5(6): 525–531.

Shandalov, Y., Egozi, D., Koffler, J., Dado-Rosenfeld, D., Ben-Shimol, D., Freiman, A. et al. An engineered muscle flap for reconstruction of large soft tissue defects. *Proc Natl Acad Sci.* **2014**, 111(16): 6010–6015.

Shi, X. and Garry, D. J. Muscle stem cells in development, regeneration, and disease. *Genes Dev.* **2006**, 20(13): 1692–1708.

Shih, Y. R. V., Chen, C. N., Tsai, S. W., Wang, Y. J. and Lee, O. K. Growth of mesenchymal stem cells on electrospun type I collagen nanofibers. *Stem Cells.* **2006**, 24(11): 2391–2397.

Shimizu, K., Fujita, H. and Nagamori, E. Alignment of skeletal muscle myoblasts and myotubes using linear micropatterned surfaces ground with abrasives. *Biotechnol Bioeng.* **2009**, 103(3): 631–638.

Sicari, B. M., Agrawal, V., Siu, B. F., Medberry, C. J., Dearth, C. L., Turner, N. J. et al. A murine model of volumetric muscle loss and a regenerative medicine approach for tissue replacement. *Tissue Eng Part A.* **2012**, 18(19–20): 1941–1948.

Sicari, B. M., Dearth, C. L. and Badylak, S. F. Tissue engineering and regenerative medicine approaches to enhance the functional response to skeletal muscle injury. *Anat Rec.* **2014**, 297(1): 51–64.

Silber, J. S., Anderson, D. G., Daffner, S. D., Brislin, B. T., Leland, J. M., Hilibrand, A. S., Vaccaro, A. R. and Albert, T. J. Donor site morbidity after anterior iliac crest bone harvest for single-level anterior cervical discectomy and fusion. *Spine (Phila Pa 1976).* **2003**, 28(2): 134–139.

Sirivisoot, S. and Harrison, B. S. Skeletal myotube formation enhanced by electrospun polyurethane carbon nanotube scaffolds. *Int J Nanomedicine.* **2011**, 6: 2483.

Stevens, M. M. Biomaterials for bone tissue engineering. *Mater Today.* **2008**, 11(5): 18–25.

Stoppel, W. L., Ghezzi, C. E., McNamara, S. L., Black III, L. D. and Kaplan, D. L. Clinical applications of naturally derived biopolymer-based scaffolds for regenerative medicine. *Ann Biomed Eng.* **2015**, 43(3): 657–680.

Themistocleous, G. S., Katopodis, H. A., Khaldi, L., Papalois, A., Doillon, C., Sourla, A. et al. Implants of type I collagen gel containing MG-63 osteoblast-like cells can act as stable scaffolds stimulating the bone healing process at the sites of the surgically-produced segmental diaphyseal defects in male rabbits. *In Vivo.* **2007**, 21(1): 69–76.

Tirrell, M., Kokkoli, E. and Biesalski, M. The role of surface science in bioengineered materials. *Surf Sci.* **2002**, 500(1–3): 61–83.

Tsai, K. S., Kao, S. Y., Wang, C. Y., Wang, Y. J., Wang, J. P. and Hung, S. C. Type I collagen promotes proliferation and osteogenesis of human mesenchymal stem cells via activation of ERK and Akt pathways. *J Biomed Mater Res A.* **2010**, 94(3): 673–682.

Tsukanaka, M., Fujibayashi, S., Otsuki, B., Takemoto, M. and Matsuda, S. Osteoinductive potential of highly purified porous β-TCP in mice. *J Mater Sci Mater Med.* **2015**, 26(3): 132.

Turner, N. J., Yates Jr, A. J., Weber, D. J., Qureshi, I. R., Stolz, D. B., Gilbert, T. W. et al. Xenogeneic extracellular matrix as an inductive scaffold for regeneration of a functioning musculotendinous junction. *Tissue Eng Part A.* **2010**, 16(11): 3309–3317.

Uebersax, L., Apfel, T., Nuss, K. M., Vogt, R., Kim, H. Y., Meinel, L. et al. Biocompatibility and osteoconduction of macroporous silk fibroin implants in cortical defects in sheep. *Eur J Pharm Biopharm.* **2013**, 85(1): 107–118.

Urist, M. R. Bone: formation by autoinduction. *Science.* **1965,** 150(3698): 893–899.

Urist, M. R., Lietze, A. and Dawson, E. Beta-tricalcium phosphate delivery system for bone morphogenetic protein. *Clin Orthop Relat Res.* **1984,** 187: 277–280.

Vandenburgh, H. H. and Karlisch, P. Longitudinal growth of skeletal myotubes *in vitro* in a new horizontal mechanical cell stimulator. *In Vitro Cell Dev Biol.* **1989,** 25(7): 607–616.

VanDusen, K. W., Syverud, B. C., Williams, M. L., Lee, J. D. and Larkin, L. M. Engineered skeletal muscle units for repair of volumetric muscle loss in the tibialis anterior muscle of a rat. *Tissue Eng Part A.* **2014,** 20(21–22): 2920–2930.

Wang, D. A., Williams, C. G., Yang, F. and Elisseeff, J. H. Enhancing the tissue-biomaterial interface: tissue-initiated integration of biomaterials. *Adv Funct Mater.* **2004,** 14(12): 1152–1159.

Wang, H., Zhi, W., Lu, X., Li, X., Duan, K., Duan, R. et al. Comparative studies on ectopic bone formation in porous hydroxyapatite scaffolds with complementary pore structures. *Acta Biomater.* **2013,** 9(9): 8413–8421.

Wang, J., Chen, Y., Zhu, X., Yuan, T., Tan, Y., Fan, Y. et al. Effect of phase composition on protein adsorption and osteoinduction of porous calcium phosphate ceramics in mice. *J. Biomed Mater Res A.* **2014,** 102(12): 4234–4243.

Wang, L. and Stegemann, J. P. Thermogelling chitosan and collagen composite hydrogels initiated with β-glycerophosphate for bone tissue engineering. *Biomaterials.* **2010,** 31(14): 3976–3985.

Wang, L., Wu, Y., Guo, B. and Ma, P. X. Nanofiber yarn/hydrogel coreshell scaffolds mimicking native skeletal muscle tissue for guiding 3D myoblast alignment, elongation, and differentiation. *ACS Nano.* **2015,** 9(9): 9167–9179.

Wolf, M. T., Daly, K. A., Reing, J. E. and Badylak, S. F. Biologic scaffold composed of skeletal muscle extracellular matrix. *Biomaterials.* **2012,** 33(10): 2916–2925.

Wolf, M. T., Dearth, C. L., Sonnenberg, S. B., Loboa, E. G. and Badylak, S. F. Naturally derived and synthetic scaffolds for skeletal muscle reconstruction. *Adv Drug Del Rev.* **2015,** 84: 208–221.

Wu, X., Corona, B. T., Chen, X. and Walters, T. J. A standardized rat model of volumetric muscle loss injury for the development of tissue engineering therapies. *Bioresearch.* **2012,** 1(6): 280–290.

Yang, R. N., Ye, F., Cheng, L. J., Wang, J. J., Lu, X. F., Shi, Y. J. et al. Osteoinduction by CaP biomaterials implanted into the muscles of mice. *J Zhejiang Uni Sci B.* **2011,** 12(7): 582–590.

Yang, X., Chen, X. and Wang, H. Acceleration of osteogenic differentiation of preosteoblastic cells by chitosan containing nanofibrous scaffolds. *Biomacromolecules.* **2009,** 10(10): 2772–2778.

Yoshioka, S. A. and Goissis, G. Thermal and spectrophotometric studies of new crosslinking method for collagen matrix with glutaraldehyde acetals. *J Mater Sci Mater Med.* **2008,** 19(3): 1215–1223.

Yu, X., Tang, X., Gohil, S. V. and Laurencin, C. T. Biomaterials for bone regenerative engineering. *Adv Healthc Mater.* **2015,** 4(9): 1268–1285.

Yuan, H., Kurashina, K., de Bruijn, J. D., Li, Y., De Groot, K. and Zhang, X. A preliminary study on osteoinduction of two kinds of calcium phosphate ceramics. *Biomaterials.* **1999,** 20(19): 1799–1806.

Yuan, H., Yang, Z., Li, Y., Zhang, X., De Bruijn, J. and De Groot, K. Osteoinduction by calcium phosphate biomaterials. *J Mater Sci Mater Med.* **1998,** 9(12): 723–726.

Yunoki, S. and Matsuda, T. Simultaneous processing of fibril formation and cross-linking improves mechanical properties of collagen. *Biomacromolecules.* **2008,** 9(3): 879–885.

Zhang, J., Luo, X., Barbieri, D., Barradas, A. M., de Bruijn, J. D., Van Blitterswijk, C. A. et al. The size of surface microstructures as an osteogenic factor in calcium phosphate ceramics. *Acta Biomater.* **2014,** 10(7): 3254–3263.

Zhang, Y., Wu, C., Friis, T. and Xiao, Y. The osteogenic properties of CaP/silk composite scaffolds. *Biomaterials.* **2010,** 31(10): 2848–2856.

Zhao, L., Weir, M. D. and Xu, H. H. Human umbilical cord stem cell encapsulation in calcium phosphate scaffolds for bone engineering. *Biomaterials.* **2010,** 31(14): 3848–3857.

Zimmermann, C., Börner, B. I., Hasse, A. and Sieg, P. Donor site morbidity after microvascular fibula transfer. *Clin Oral Investig.* **2001,** 5(4): 214–219.

CHAPTER 7

Tissue Engineering in Reconstruction and Regeneration of Visceral Organs

SOMA MONDAL GHORAI[1*] and SUDHANSHU MISHRA[2]

[1]*Department of Zoology, Hindu College, University of Delhi, Delhi-110007, India*

[2]*Department of Advanced Science & Technology, Nims University Rajasthan, Jaipur-303121, India*

Corresponding author. E-mail: somamghorai@hindu.du.ac.in

ABSTRACT

The last half of the century witnessed great strides in the field of transplantation medicine. However, there are limitations due to impeding shortage of donor tissues/organs and low rate of successful surgeries mainly in the pediatric patients. Tissue engineering is an innovative field, which combines engineering with biology and is the answer to the abovementioned limitation. This strategy helps to reconstruct and regenerate damaged and diseased tissues/organs. This chapter discusses the bioengineering of visceral organs and the various challenges that are faced in the field of tissue engineering and reconstructive surgery.

7.1 INTRODUCTION

Tissue engineering (TE) is a knowledge base field, which has principles of engineering and bioscience and it results in development of biological substitutes that restore, maintain, or improve damaged tissues or organs (Langer and Vacanti, 1993). TE uses advances in cell science, surgery, and engineering wherein engineered tissues and organs may be transplanted into patients to assist restore or improve their function. The construct of TE was projected by several researchers for treatment of tissue defect and organ failure, which is now being revolutionized. It will be distinguished from antecedently developed techniques by its use of advanced technologies (incorporating regenerative medication and advanced materials engineering, together with nanotechnology) and by the actual fact that its products contain living tissue. Tissues built through TE contain three basic components: cells, scaffolds, and signals. The flexibility to create tissues within the body upon transplantation depends upon the ability to fill the tissue void by scaffold matrices, so as to provide structural support and deliver the growth factors to the desired cells (Howard et al., 2008).

In the last half century, tremendous breakthrough is made in the field of transplantation of damaged organs. High technological medical advances coupled with innovative drugs and medical devices have helped in availability of many organs for transplantation. Although, even after such great strides, there are still huge challenges in terms of high costs, procedural faults, intensive postoperative care, and most importantly shortage of donor organs (Vacanti, 1988; Mohand-Said et al., 2000). In such a scenario, TE has made a great progress to reconstruct organs without the need of donor organs. Apart from skin and bone tissue reconstruction, TE is widely being considered for development of 3D in-vitro models for many visceral organs (Caddeo et al., 2017). Visceral organs, by definition, mean those organs and tissues that are present in body cavity, especially those within chest cavity (heart and lungs) or peritoneal cavity (liver, pancreas, and intestines). This chapter mainly focuses on the advancement of TE with the reconstruction and regeneration of diseased and damaged visceral organs.

For reconstruction of visceral organs, specific cell types are usually preferred. Autologous cells are garnered via two procedures. In the first method, specific cells are aspirated through biopsy. This technique is well known for most organ structures such as liver, heart, and blood vessels whereas cells for heart valves cannot be retrieved through direct autopsy and peripheral vein segments are the suitable cell source (Ikada, 2006). Fibroblast stem cells are also used for TE of cardiac myoblasts (Ramkisoensing et al., 2014). The basic architecture for reconstruction of tissues and organs in TE is provided by the scaffolds, which provide the cells, growth factors, and extracellular matrix (ECM) needed to organize and develop the desired organ. Within the scaffold, cells reorganize, develop, or replace the damaged tissue in the ECM, finally leading to the degradation of the scaffold. The newly formed cells or organs reassemble, restore, and preserve the tissue function. TE differs from guided tissue regeneration such as in the former, cells are seeded within matrices *in vitro* and in the later, acellular matrices are repopulated by the host after implantation (Abou Neel and Young, 2013). Scaffolds in TE employ a two-way approach; first the cells are seeded onto the matrix and then the cells itself lay the foundations by developing new matrices. The second approach encompasses combination of growth factors with the scaffolds in the in-vivo system, where the cells from the body repopulate the scaffold and the matrices. Both these approaches are mutually exclusive and care should be taken to prudently select the composition, topography, and the architecture of the scaffold (Ripamonti and Duneas, 1996).

Nano- to microscale topography has been incontestable to have an effect on cell behavior by modification of anatomical structure arrangements (Meredith et al., 2007). Moreover, totally different cell varieties react to different materials; as an example, different scaffolds material produce diverse levels of glycosaminoglycans in the regenerated tissue (Freed et al., 1993). Also, the selection and source of seed cells are vital for scaffolds (Francioli et al., 2007). A scaffold for TE must be biocompatible and is able to provide adequate nutrition and other biological needs to the growing tissue. Mostly, decellularized matrices are used, which are derived after enzymatic or detergent digestion from the allogeneic or xenogeneic tissues. Theoretically, these decellularized matrices are degraded by metalloproteinases and are bioreabsorbed for appropriate cell seeding (Lee and Shin, 2007). The use of xenogeneic tissues for TE has both advantages and disadvantages. The advantage is clearly noted in TE of heart valves, where ample supply is obtained from pigs with good stress-resistant capacity; but, at the same time, there are certain subtle anatomical differences too. For instance, the normal human aortic valve-root system has an asymmetric sinus dimension that diverges significantly from pigs (Cooper, 2012). There are some other materials considered as matrices for scaffolds. Collagen-based structures such as meniscus and blood vessels are used in TE (Yao et al., 2008). Small intestinal mucosa and inverted small intestine are other potential matrices considered for the purpose of TE (Le Visage et al., 2006).

Synthetic materials such as lactic-glycolic acid or polyacrylonitrile-polyvinyl chlorides are most commonly used to encapsulate mammalian cells (Makadia and Siegel, 2011). Poly-4-hydroxybutyrate is nowadays considered for its high elasticity and a controllable degradation profile (Crow, 2004). Apart from these polymers, alginate hydrogels are in high demand due to its high porosity, ability to change physical states from liquid to gel, and easy deliverability through catheters or by endoscopic techniques (Sun and Tan, 2013). The material processing techniques, such as 3D printing along with polymer chemistry, enable manufacture of highly complex matrices and help in achieving a multidisciplinary tactic in the field of TE. TE matrices can be tailor-made for the ideal properties of scaffold materials by prudent mix of specific side chains and cross-linkages and molecular weights. Furthermore, in-vivo usage of biodegradable surgical sutures such as polyhydroxyl acid materials can be used as drug delivery devices (Grund et al., 2011).

Scaffolds are considered not only for support in TE, but also as drug delivery vehicle. They are deliberated for delivery of growth factors/drugs to the sites of repair, thus hastening the retrieval development. The release of growth factors is one of the most important challenges as it should match the kinetics of physiological processes. Growth factors such as vascular endothelial growth factor (VEGF), a peptide growth factor when incorporated into polylactic acid (PLA) scaffolds, encouraged the vascularization of the scaffold and retained the angiogenic properties (Kanczler et al., 2007). Similarly, basic fibroblast growth factors added to the alginate gel surface via an NH functional group, provided a microenvironment for the growth and differentiation of neuronal tissues (Narine et al., 2006). Further the function of growth factors can be enhanced by zoning, where PLA/polyethylene glycol microparticles are laden with proteins such as bone morphogenetic protein-2, trypsin, and horseradish peroxidase and are zonally or locally released for a longer period of time (Suciati et al., 2006). Gene therapy is also being explored to deliver the growth factors by incorporating the gene of interest for specific proteins and delivering them to the site of tissue regeneration (Heyde et al., 2007). TE absolutely avoids the risk of immune rejections (hyperacute and delayed), as well as viral infections, by the use of autologous cells (Vaquette et al., 2018). Appropriate incorporation of acceptable physical and cellular signals are the main underlying factors that help in integration and interaction among cells and tissues involved in TE/regenerative medicine. Therefore, inclusion of modifying factors such as biologically active proteins and DNA are crucial to success. Currently, less complicated procedures are being followed to replace injured cartilage by primary chondrocytes (Brittberg and Lindahl, 2008; Richardson et al., 2010) as well as skin cell sheets for ruined skin (MacNeil, 2008). However, some larger and additional complicated tissue, notably the bladder, is reconstructed with considerable success (Eberli and Atala, 2006), giving hope for many other complicated tissue to be reconstructed in the near future. Though basic useful TE strategies are the key, there is still extended scope for future developments in terms of cell sources, discrete tailored cell supports, immune modulation, vascularization, and also the prognostic skills of computational and mathematical modeling for additional complicated materials. Though TE faces an impressive information gap within the challenge to totally recapitulate complicated organ-specific topographies, but still it is the only novel and translational approach to restore injured or damaged whole tissues/organs.

7.2   VISCERAL ORGAN REGENERATION AND MODELING VIA TISSUE ENGINEERING

Worldwide, there is great demand for organ donation with a long waiting list for specific organs such as kidney, liver, heart, and lungs (Kellar, 2015; Magee et al., 2007). There are many challenges, which are encountered in organ transplantation. Firstly, in traditional transplantation, getting the histocompatible donor is in itself a great task, which may further get complicated with immunological incompetency. Secondly, procuring a xenologous organ graft has animal ethics concerns. Use of animals in biomedical research is a topic of huge debate and animal welfare in science is currently being incorporated in national and international legislation (Festing, 2004; Pound and Bracken, 2014). Though animal's usage has contributed tremendously to the understanding of human biology and physiology, the transplanted animal organs has its own limitations in human-specific conditions (Dixit and Boelsterli, 2007). Apart from the subtle anatomical differences, the molecular mechanisms propelling their inception and progress are often significantly dissimilar (Dixit and Boelsterli, 2007; Pound and Bracken, 2014). The inefficacies of some drugs in human system; which have been successfully tested in animal models, are proof of inability to recapitulate human physiology. Another potent challenge in organ transplantation is the excessive costs that are incurred for transforming a drug candidate from a new molecular entity to a clinical product (DiMasi et al., 2016). It has been noted that 2D monocultures for tissues and organs usually lack the requisite characters needed for successful assays (Grainger, 2014). These 2D monocultures encounter cell death and loss of function due to the buildup of waste products, restricted nutrient resource, and absence of cell-specific mechanostimulation (Mosig, 2016).

Based on the abovementioned challenges, TE has adapted procedures to encompass successful, ethical, and cost-effective methods to grow in-vivo tissues and organs in 3D environment, which allows active interactions with the surrounding extracellular matrices and the soluble factors for a successful gene expression and organ development (Mikos et al., 2006; Atala et al., 2012). Each visceral organ has precise physiognomies to sustain its function, for instance, the types of cells and the matrices, architecture and the biophysical ambience (pressure and force), and biochemical stimuli (reactive oxygen species, cytokines, and growth factors) (Figure 7.1). In this chapter, we highlight mainly on the visceral organ-specific cells, source of matrices, in-vivo architectures, as well as focus on the bottlenecks and prospective for organ-specific TE.

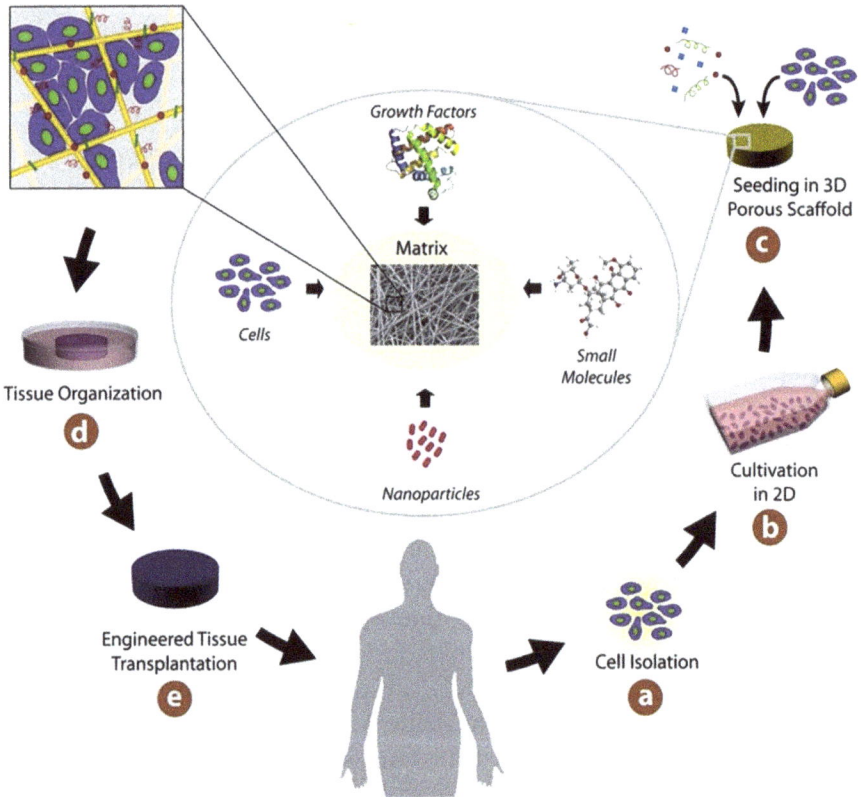

FIGURE 7.1 Steps in tissue engineering for visceral organs are: (a) autologous tissues sample from the patient's body; (b) retrieval of organ-specific cells from the cell bank; (c) cells are seeded in an engineered scaffold to help grow, connect, and communicate; (d) transferred from the scaffolds, organs are grown in 3D tissues; and (e) implanted in the body and recreate the cell structure and function.

Source: Reprinted from https://tissueengineeringproject.weebly.com/

7.3 OUTLINING TOPOGRAPHIES OF THE KIDNEY, LIVER, HEART, PANCREAS, INTESTINE, AND LUNG

Human body is a complex and sophisticated organization where each organ is built on specific tissues and performs specific functions. All the visceral organs namely the kidney, heart, lungs, liver, intestine, and pancreas achieve functional uniqueness by repeating their structural units or the mass in each organ. Kidneys filter toxins and produce urine, heart pumps blood to the entire body, lungs exchange gases, intestine digests the food, and pancreas acts both as an endocrine and an exocrine gland. Thus, it is important to understand the topographies of each organ.

7.3.1   VISCERAL ORGANS OF THE CHEST CAVITY: HEART AND LUNGS

7.3.1.1   HEART

Heart is a delicate and powerful muscular pump and with each contraction cycle drives unidirectional blood flow into the systemic and pulmonary circulation (Buckberg et al., 2008). To generate an efficient and rhythmical contractile force and to provide sufficient nutrient support, a highly organized vasculature is required (Young and Cowan, 2012). From the outermost to the innermost, heart is basically comprised of three main layers: epicardium, myocardium, and endocardium (Figure 7.2). The epicardium comprises the nerves and coronary blood vessels for the sustenance of heart's metabolic demand and provision of rhythmic electrical propagation in the myocardium. Two coronary arteries arise from the epicardial surface, which further penetrate deep into the myocardium as smaller arterioles and capillaries. The dynamic coronary vascular resistance enables the coronary blood to adapt to fluctuating mechanical and metabolic conditions. The myocardium is a thick muscular helical structure designed in a manner such that each contraction is propagated in an asynchronous way leading to maximum efficiency (Kocica et al., 2006; Poveda et al., 2013). The cellular components of the myocardium comprise cardiomyocytes, large number of cardiac fibroblasts, and supporting vasculature. Within a space of 20 mm, each and every myocardial cell is perfused by a capillary to facilitate not only to provide oxygen and nutrients but also to eliminate the toxic wastes (Korecky, 1982). Endometrium is the innermost layer, which lies in direct vicinity of the blood and the circulatory system. It has a specialized endothelial layer, a thick connective tissue and muscle layer, and a deep layer of connective fibers to initiate the rhythmic pumping of blood. The most complex and delicate structures of the heart are the heart valves that control the flow between the chambers of ventricles and auricles. As the valves are thin, they are likely subjected to damage and injury. Therefore, in most of the cardiological medical problems, the affected or the damaged valves need to get replaced (Schoen and Levy, 1999; Cheung et al., 2015).

Tissue engineering for cardiac tissues is focused onto: (1) remuscularize the heart via myocardial transplant or cell injection; (2) recreate live mechanically strong heart valves. Although much progress has been attained, still medical and engineering progress has to go a long way to make an efficient myocardium as seen in in-vivo environment. The critical challenges that are faced to recreate 3D state-of-the-art engineered cardiac constructs are the exquisite hierarchical organization of the cardiomyocytes, vascularization, and the interactions between vasculature and perfusion with cardiomyocytes (Schoen and Levy, 1999; Cheung et al., 2015).

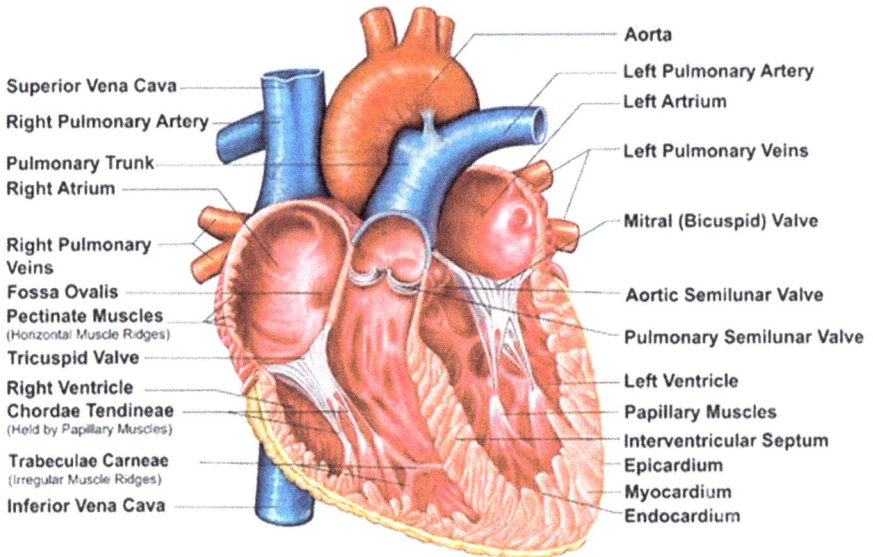

FIGURE 7.2   The internal anatomy of human heart.

Source: Image by OpenStax College. https://commons.wikimedia.org/wiki/File:2008_Internal_Anatomy_of_the_HeartN.jpg (https://creativecommons.org/licenses/by/3.0/deed.en)

7.3.1.2   *LUNGS*

The lungs are highly specialized airways that branch into innumerable narrow, short tubes that ends in alveolar sacs, each with diameter about 0.2 mm (Mercer et al., 1994; Hsia et al., 2016). The alveoli of the lungs are the most important structure for gas-blood exchange in the respiratory zone and they increase along the bronchioles. The alveolar septum comprising of collagen and elastin fibers separate the neighboring alveoli; thus, the alveolar space, septum, and the adjoining capillaries form an air-blood double membrane barrier system (Figure 7.3) (Itoh et al., 2004). The thin portion of the barrier is the surfactant layer made up of type I pneumocyte and the capillary endothelial cells with its basal lamina. The thick portion of the barrier is made up of connective tissue and fibers juxtaposed in between the two layers of basal laminae. This is the site where accretion of fluid occurs that finally drains into the lymphatic system (Weibel and Knight, 1964; West, 2009). The 3D hierarchical structure coupled with biochemical intricate functions that permits exchange of gases presents enough challenges to replicate lung tissues using modern engineering approaches. Moreover, the entire vascular and alveolar compartments of lungs are organized within a dynamic and flexible matrix. Thus, to overcome these challenges, limited structural and functional recapitulation of lung tissue is attempted.

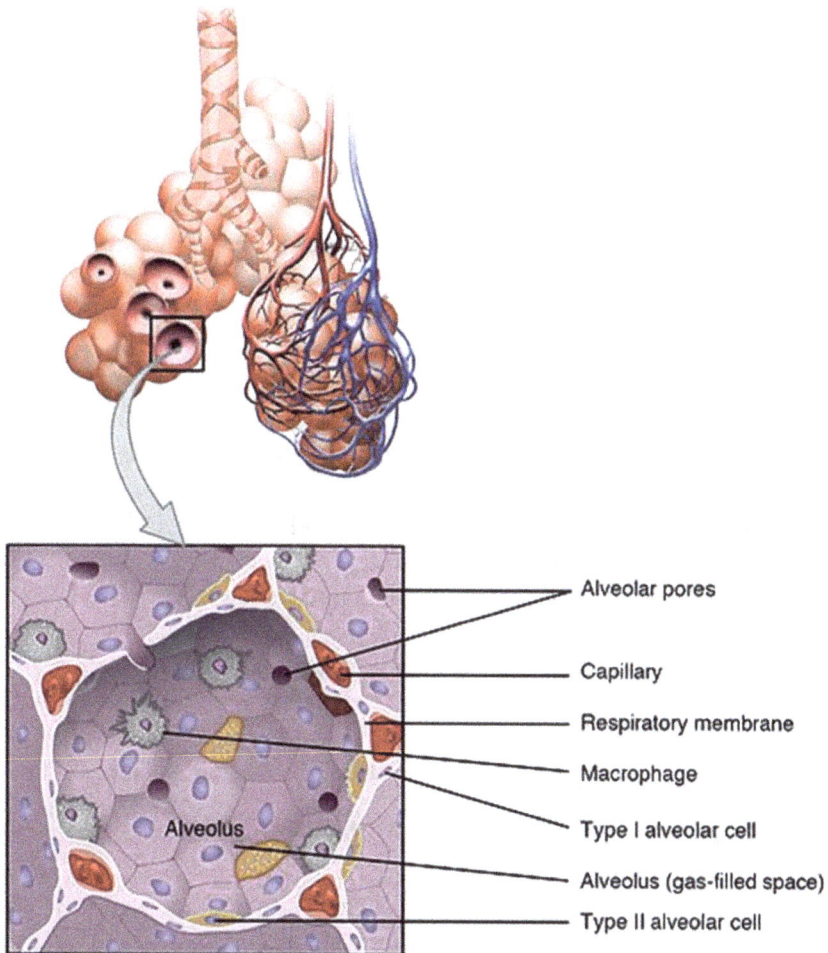

FIGURE 7.3   Internal anatomy of the lungs.

Source: Image by OpenStax College. https://commons.wikimedia.org/wiki/File:2309_The_Respiratory_Zone.jpg (https://creativecommons.org/licenses/by/4.0/)

7.3.2 VISCERAL ORGANS OF THE PERITONEAL CAVITY: KIDNEY, LIVER, PANCREAS, AND INTESTINE

7.3.2.1 KIDNEY

Kidney is a highly vascular organ whose main components are the nephrons encircled within dense meshwork of kidney capillaries. Each kidney usually contains 6×10^5 and 1.4×10^6 nephrons, which filter, reabsorb solutes, secrete, regulate the volume and composition of the extracellular fluid, and uphold blood pressure (Pocock et al., 2013). The capillaries participate in dual function of receiving about 25% of cardiac output and provide nourishment to the nephrons (Jen et al., 2011). Both the nephrons and the capillaries are susceptible to injury and have limited regeneration capacity, leading to fibrosis, inflammation, tissue ischemia, tubular dysfunction, and chronic kidney failure (Basile, 2004, 2007, and 2011).

Engineering kidney tissues are challenging as it is difficult to recapitulate the kidney exchange interface, which are a specialized network of vessels and tubules at close proximity with suitable cell phenotypes and matrices. The kidney exchange interface mainly comprises of three compartments: the tubular lumen, a thin layer of basement membrane, and the capillary lumen and each lumen is lined with unique cells (Figure 7.4) (Bulger and Dobyan, 1983). The capillary lumen is lined with endothelial cells rich in glycocalyx. The tubular lumen has epithelial cells with microvilli on the apical surface; the lateral surface has Na^+/K^+-ATPase transporters and transmembrane water channels (aquaporin-1) to control absorption and fluid transport and fenestrated by narrow tight junctions. The visceral layer of Bowman's capsule is lined by specialized cells called podocytes that interdigitate extensively leaving small gaps in between (~25 nm wide). The basement membrane matrix is rich in collagen IV and laminin and is ~1 μm in thickness (Salmon et al., 2009; Shirato et al., 1991). Other cells such as mesangial cells and perivascular cells provide nourishment and structural support as well as secrete signals during tissue injury (Cortes et al., 2000).

7.3.2.2 LIVER

Liver is a specialized structure supported by four major compartments: the hepatocytes that carry metabolic functions, the sinusoidal capillaries to maintain vascular flow within hepatocytes, the perisinusoidal space between the hepatocytes and the capillaries, and the stroma comprising of connective

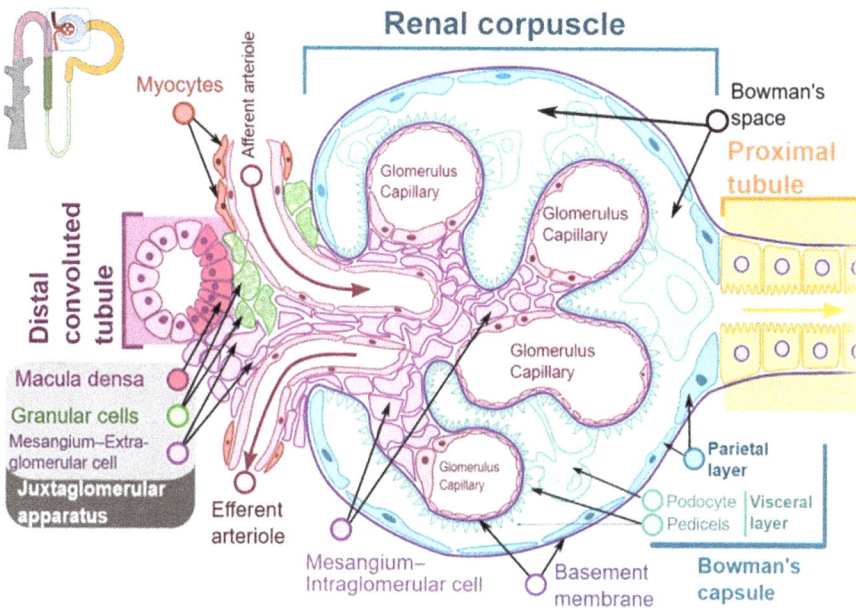

FIGURE 7.4   Diagram of renal corpuscle structure and nephron histology.

Source: Image by Shypoetess. https://commons.wikimedia.org/wiki/File:Renal_corpuscle-en.svg (https://creativecommons.org/licenses/by-sa/4.0/)

tissue (Figures 7.5) (Krishna, 2013). Each lobule of the hepatocytes is hexagonal in shape surrounding a central vein and each corner has the triad of hepatic artery, hepatic portal vein, and the bile duct (Rappaport et al., 1954). The portal vein and the artery carry deoxygenated and oxygenated blood that travels through the sinusoid to drain into the central vein, thus maintaining efficient transport within the hepatocytes. Hepatic sinusoids are the unique structure that imparts special function to the liver. They are composed of intermittent endothelium, with large gaps between adjacent cells and house the Kupffer cells; the interstellate sinusoidal macrophages are meant to provide innate immunity to the liver (Bilzer et al., 2006). The perisinusoidal space allows substantial exchange among blood plasma and the hepatocytes. Additionally, the lack of continuous basal lamina, presence of microvilli on the basal side of the hepatocytes, and gaps within the sinusoids increase the exchange efficiency. These perisinusoidal spaces also contain hepatic stellate cells, which are involved in vitamin A storage (Puche et al., 2013). In response to any tissue injury, these cells are involved in vascular resistance and help in restructuring the extracellular matrices of the liver. Thus, engineering the liver is a daunting task as it highly organized biomimetic architecture with specialized cells that involves a hierarchical vasculature and perfusion support to maintain adequate mass for physiological function.

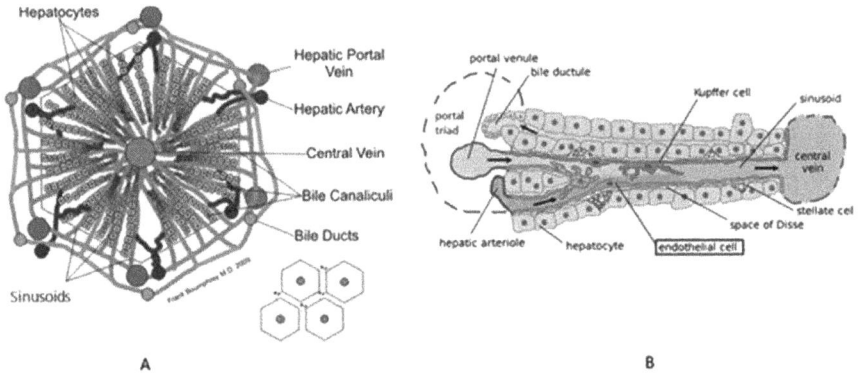

FIGURES 7.5   Structural details of liver.

Source: Source: Image by Shypoetess. https://commons.wikimedia.org/wiki/File:Renal_corpuscle-en.svg (https://creativecommons.org/licenses/by-sa/4.0/)

7.3.2.3   PANCREAS

Pancreas lies in the upper abdomen and is a part of gastrointestinal system and acts both as an exocrine and an endocrine organ. It secretes digestive juices into the intestine as well as hormones into the blood for metabolism and storage. Basically, it is made up of clusters of cells known as the pancreatic acini that produce digestive enzymes and some other structures called pancreatic islets or the islets of Langerhans are involved in endocrine function (Figure 7.6). The exocrine part of the pancreas is a complex tubular network of acini and the cells are situated along with a small ductile at the intersection of acinar tubule or acinus. The complex duct system is a key to prevent the entry of exocrine enzymes into the interstitial space, which, if disrupted, may cause tissue damage that manifest as pancreatitis. The central and interlobular ducts have thick compact collagenous walls. The connective tissue becomes narrow and progressively becomes thin as the ducts branch out, arising incidence of leakage of the duct system. To prevent this, intercellular tight junctions (zonula occludens) are found between duct cells, the acinar cells, and the centroacinar cells (Longnecker, 2014). The endocrine part of the pancreas constitutes islets of Langerhans that substantially differ in size. In humans, the average size ranges between 100 and

150 m wherein about 70% are in the size range of 50–250 m in diameter (Hellman, 1959a). Most islets are spherical or ellipsoid, wherein the smaller islets are dispersed throughout the acinar lobules and larger islets underline the main and interlobular ducts of the pancreas. Glucagon secreted from α-cells, insulin secreted from β-cells, and somatostatin secreted from δ-cells are the main pancreatic islet cell types that produce the peptide hormones. Also, cells secreting pancreatic polypeptide are regarded as the fourth most predominant endocrine cell type in the islets (Hellman, 1959b). Thus, designing a tissue-engineered pancreatic substitute (TEPS), which consists of insulin-producing cells appropriately encapsulated to support cellular function, poses major challenge.

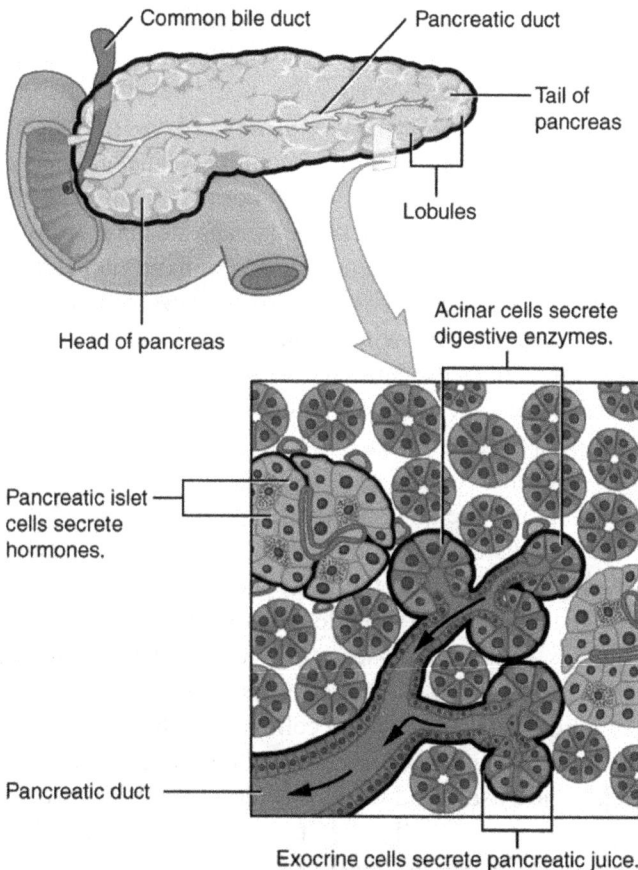

FIGURE 7.6   The exocrine and endocrine cells of pancreas.

Source: Image by OpenStax College. https://commons.wikimedia.org/wiki/File:2424_Exocrine_and_Endocrine_Pancreas.jpg (https://creativecommons.org/licenses/by/3.0/deed.en)

Moreover, it should be able to interact with the host tissues in regulating blood glucose for the treatment of insulin-dependent diabetes (IDD). Though improvements are made in the expression level of GLUTag-INS cells and/ or the number of viable cells confined within the TEPS, there is still much deliberation needed for successful treatment of IDD in humans. Incorporating implantable 3D TEPS is also plausible method for promoting proper cellular function of recombinant L-cells.

7.3.2.4   INTESTINE

The small intestine is segmented into three regions: these are the duodenum, jejunum, and ileum (Spoerri, 1949). Duodenum is the shortest of 25.4 cm and begins after the pyloric sphincter followed by jejunum of 0.9 m and ileum is the longest of about 1.8 m in length. Ileum is also the thickest and most vascular with well-developed folds than the other two. The entire intestine is innervated by parasympathetic nerve fibers from the vagus nerve and sympathetic nerve fibers from the thoracic splanchnic nerve. Intestine is also accompanied by a well-circulated portal system with the superior mesenteric artery and superior mesenteric vein as the main artery and vein to collect the nutrient-rich blood and carry it to the liver via the hepatic portal vein. Anatomically, intestine is composed of mucosa and submucosa and a highly absorptive surface area with numerous villi and microvilli and more than 600-fold, circular folds. Special lymphoid organ Peyer's patches are seen within the submucosa of the intestine, which impart immunity from the invading pathogens (Figure 7.7A).

The large intestine comprises of four main regions: the cecum, the colon, the rectum, and the anus. Draining of chyme from the small intestine to the large intestine is controlled by the ileocecal valve, which is located between the ileum and the large intestine. Large intestine differs from small intestine in some notable ways such as the wall of the large intestine contains few enzyme-secreting cells and there are no circular folds or villi. The mucosa of the colon is simple columnar epithelium composed of enterocytes (absorptive cells) and goblet cells (Figure 7.7B). Mucus secreted by the goblet cells prevents the intestine from the harmful effects of acids and gases produced by enteric bacteria as well as helps in easy movement of the feces (Lopez et al., 2019). Intestinal bacteria also synthesize vitamins, which are absorbed by enterocytes along with water and salts. Both the small and the large intestines display many diverse patterns and are controlled by chemical and electrical interactions within smooth muscle, interstitial cells, mucosal epithelial layers, and intramural innervation. Such intricate complexity requires a multidisciplinary approach to regenerate functional intestine.

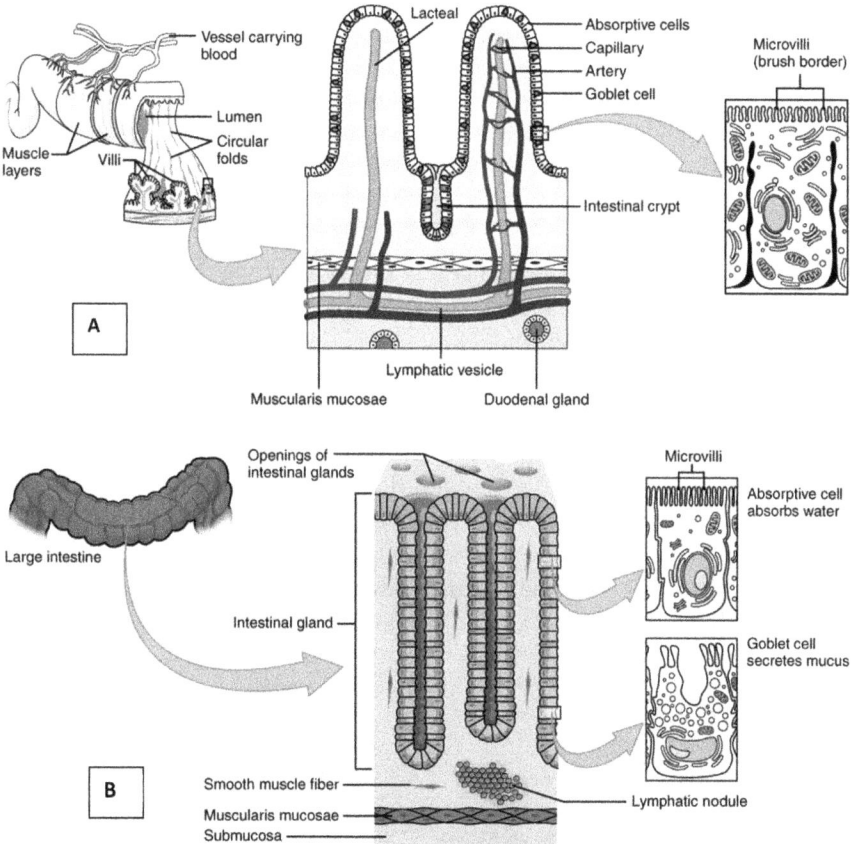

FIGURES 7.7   (A) Anatomy of small intestine and (B) anatomy of large intestine.

Source: Reprinted from https://opentextbc.ca/anatomyandphysiology/chapter/23-5-the-small-and-large-intestines/

7.4   FUNDAMENTAL PRINCIPLES UNDERLYING VISCERAL ORGAN REGENERATION

Translational medicine integrates engineering with varied fields of biology such as embryology, anatomy, physiology, cell and molecular biology, and immunology and enables technology such as 3D bioprinting using biocompatible biomaterials and biofabrication platforms. Organ recreation is, thus, an art, which merges many sciences with technical rigor. Restructuring whole organs involve maturation of varied cell types and complex tissues and their coordinated differentiation and morphogenesis (Kaushik et al., 2017). This is controlled by an intricate balance between the physicochemical and spatio-temporal cues of the various growth factors mainly fibroblast growth factors, wingless-type MMTV integration site family members (Wnts), and bone morphogenetic proteins (Ren et al., 2012; Martino et al., 2011). The prospects of TE have expanded our horizon in better understanding the developmental processes and empowering translational and precision medicine. The model organs developed have increased the possibility of next-generation drug testing platforms. Definitely, this has led to increased drug affordability and high yield efficiency due to precise accuracy with fewer false positives and low development costs (Paul et al., 2010; Aronson, 2015). It can be explained as follows: the new Food and Drug Administration (FDA) has steadily declined the number approved drugs while increasing the drug development cost by $2.6 billion (Helen, 2016). Thus, the FDA approves only 10.4% of all drugs that are allowed to enter a phase I clinical trial and gain market approval (Hay et al., 2014). Although the technique of organ engineering poses immense benefits, achieving such intricate complexity of developing a whole organ has proven to be a substantial engineering challenge. Neverthe-less, many advances are made to understand and recreate complex organs using biological designs and technological rigor (Figure 7.8).

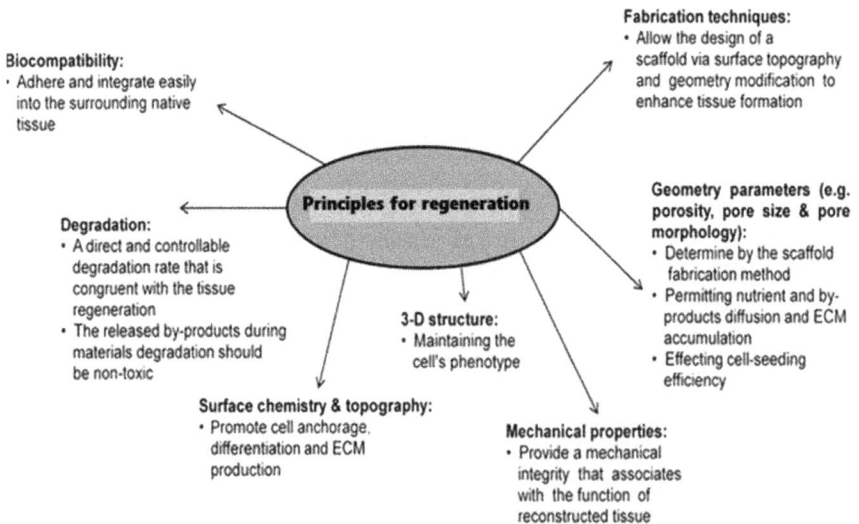

Fabrication techniques:
• Allow the design of a scaffold via surface topography and geometry modification to enhance tissue formation

Biocompatibility:
• Adhere and integrate easily into the surrounding native tissue

Principles for regeneration

Degradation:
• A direct and controllable degradation rate that is congruent with the tissue regeneration
• The released by-products during materials degradation should be non-toxic

Geometry parameters (e.g. porosity, pore size & pore morphology):
• Determine by the scaffold fabrication method
• Permitting nutrient and by-products diffusion and ECM accumulation
• Effecting cell-seeding efficiency

3-D structure:
• Maintaining the cell's phenotype

Surface chemistry & topography:
• Promote cell anchorage, differentiation and ECM production

Mechanical properties:
• Provide a mechanical integrity that associates with the function of reconstructed tissue

FIGURE 7.8   The factors that define successful bioengineering of organs and tissues.

Source: Reprinted with permission from Nayyer et al. (2012). © Wolters Kluwer Health, Inc.

7.4.1 STRUCTURE-FUNCTION BIOMIMICRY OF ORGANS

The organ's structural complexity underlies its functional capacity. For instance, the intricate internal structure of kidney enables it to filter and reabsorb body fluids; the dense vasculature of pancreas helps it to perform efficiently both exocrine and endocrine function. Thus, changing the organ's structural milieu will bring in pathophysiological conditions (Yamanaka and Yokoo, 2015; Bara and Sambanis, 2009). Similarly, any alterations in the structural complexity within the cell morphology or misalignment of chondrocytes will cause impaired heart function (Arnal-Pastor et al., 2013; Radisic, 2015). Thus, it is still impossible to restructure fully anatomically correct complex tissue structures *in vitro* (Takasato and Wymeersch, 2020). The first step toward TE is, thus, to have a thorough knowledge about the structural, mechanical, and biochemical cues of the organs. In terms of engineering intricacy, tissues and organs can be prearranged into three elementary groups in ascending order: 2D, hollow, and 3D/solid tissues (Loh and Choong, 2013). Sputter coating or simple printing of cells and materials are the simplest 2D deposition techniques, adapted first to replace damaged tissues (Bianchi et al., 2006; Lalwani et al., 2013). Structuring hollow organs such as large vessels and intestines are still a far-fetched method but if successfully attempted may help a large section of patients. Recently, bladder-shaped scaffold laden with autologous cells and composed of omentum-wrapped collagen polyglycolic acid were inserted into patients with cystoplasty (Atala et al., 2006). But above all, restructuring the solid organs poses the most difficult hurdle as restructuring them requires a delicate integration of previous iterations and approaches to emulate the native tissue's structures/functions.

7.4.2 MULTISCALE DIGITAL IMAGING DATA

Knowledge of the anatomy and the structure-function details helped the bioengineers to accurately recreate the organs in detail multiscale imaging data. Techniques such as computed tomography (CT) images and magnetic resonance imaging (MRI) have provided good amount of macroscale digital printing data to study historical histology. Although, the images by CT and MRI have low resolution of about few 100 μm and can only provide single histological section, especially the planar structural information about an organ. Therefore, these days, multi-image modality dataset is represented to print whole, functional organs by integrating imaging modalities across length scales. This is done by combining the immunohistochemical with histological data paired with MRI as well as clinical data, respectively (Kaushik et al., 2017). Thus, recreating the blueprints with high-resolution print designs is obtained through a collection of data via recent advances in bioimaging.

Another techniques known as CLARITY transforms tissues into transparent, porous hydrogels–tissue hybrids by removing the lipid content while maintaining intact tissue structures (Yue et al., 2015; Vashist and Ahmad, 2015). In this, a polymer that can increase in size within the matrices is achieved by removing the lipids using charged ionic sodium dodecyl sulfate (SDS) micelles via electrophoretic tissue clearing and then covalently linking the tissues nucleic acids and proteins. A resolution as high as 70 nm showing the tissue's structure and molecular composition can be pictured, thus enabling to map various proteins within a single tissue volume (Chen et al., 2015). Thus, CLARITY helps in generation of native-like tissues and organs by providing inclusive understandings into the spatial composition of a wide range of tissues as precise, repeatable immunolabeled molecules can be visualized (Yue et al., 2015; Vashist and Ahmad, 2015). Molecular imaging has enabled us to understand the distribution of various proteins within the cells, tissues, or organs, while techniques such as contrast-enhanced nano-computed tomography (nano-CT) (Kerckhofs et al., 2013), MRI (Xu et al., 2008), or histological data (Opitz et al., 2004) have provided structural information of a wide range of tissues. All the information on both structural and biochemical heterogeneity could be used to design multiphasic structures.

7.4.3   ACTIVE AND PASSIVE MECHANICAL FORCES REGULATE CELL FATE AND FUNCTION

A deep understanding of how cells grow, regulate, and function is necessary to bioengineer the organs (Clark, 2014). Among other factors, the concept that mechanical forces (mechanotransduction) increased our understanding of how cells regulate cell fate and function through the entire lifespan of an organ (Korossis et al., 2006; Parker and Ingber, 2007). Stem cells sense mechanical forces via protein-mediated signaling, cellular deformations, and membrane tension (Vining and Mooney, 2017), hence differentiates behave and age as they sense and respond to the various cellular cues (Inanç et al., 2008; Fehrer and Lepperdinger, 2005). Cells can also sense mechanotransduction via integrin-mediated and focal adhesions, thus remodel themselves based on external stimuli that trigger signaling cascades and change biological consequences of the cell behavior (Spanjaard and de Rooij, 2013).

Passive mechanical stimuli can affect how cells emulate and retort to their milieu. The stiffness of the surrounding microenvironment also partially determines the stem cell lineage commitment (Keung et al., 2010). A study by Berry et al. (2006) showed that mesenchymal stem cells (MSCs) seeded on hydrogels with a stiffness of ~0.5 kPa developed a neurogenic phenotype, while ~10 or ~30 kPa induced a myogenic or osteogenic phenotype, respectively. Another report by Guvendiren and Burdick (2012) showed a shift of stem cell differentiation from adipogenic to osteogenic when the culture containing MSCs with a 1:1 mix of osteogenic and adipogenic medium was stiffened from 1 to 10 kPa for a period of 2 weeks. Thus, the maintenance of the stiffness throughout the differentiation process is an important factor in how organs and tissues function (Weisbrod et al., 2013). MSCs via integrin alpha-5 respond to different levels of stiffness in 2D than in 3D, respectively (Huebsch et al., 2010). Also, actomyosin contractibility is essential to mechanosensing as it was noted that blockers such as cytochalasin D, Y27632, or blebbistatin prevents mechanosensing (Inoue et al., 2011). Moreover, a balance should be attained between biochemistry and mechanosensing as the focal adhesion-based signaling is as important as the stiffness in the ECM (Taylor-Weiner et al., 2015; Wen et al., 2014). Various mechanical cues can be sensed by cells through focal adhesions and integrin-mediated signal transduction that is able to distort its environment, animatedly alter in response to external stimuli, and trigger signaling cascades with a widespread range of biological consequences (Spanjaard and de Rooij, 2013).

Active forces come to foreright during embryogenesis when cells get affected by the active forces from their neighboring cells which decide the expression of the cell adhesion molecules and subsequently the morphogenetic movements (Duband and Thiery, 1990). For instance, uniaxial lateral deformation along the entire dorsal-ventral axis was triggered by mechanically-induced nuclear translocation of *Armadillo* gene (homolog for *Drosophila* *β*-catenin) resulting in distorted anterior gut formation (Farge, 2003). The polarity of the various molecules eventually decided the fate of the organs. It has also been seen that excessive shear forces on vascular endothelial cells cause vascular deformations and hypertension (Malek et al., 1999). Thus, active or informed mechanical force directly influences cell physiology from internal cell signaling to cell morphology (Rangamani et al., 2013).

The proper functioning of the organ in *in vivo* system is based on the continuous balanced mechanical feedback, neither too high nor too low. That is the reason, the organs degenerate when removed from the body or during the aging process which sees more stiffening of the tissues (Humphrey et al., 2016). An apt example is witnessed in case of hypertension, which happens due to increased ECM production, vascular thickness, and arterial stiffness. Bioengineering any organ or tissue should be presented with a balanced mechanical environment for sustaining proper tissue and organ function and avoiding improper remodeling.

7.4.4   *SPATIAL COMPONENT IN ORGAN REMODELING*

The most important component in TE is the removal of the target organ, decellularizing it completely by removing all soluble matters, and just leaving behind the "ghost-white" scaffold (Ott et al., 2008). This scaffold is then seeded with the desired cells, but such decellularized organs often face enforced spatial constraint. Mostly, a modest amount or organ structure-function is achieved but still enormous work is needed to overcome the spatial constraints (Bao et al., 2011; Badylak et al., 2011). Cells remodel according to the environment in which they exist and factors such as cell seeding density can affect the migration, proliferation, differentiation, and finally the cell metabolism (Erickson et al., 2012). 2D printing and micropatterning allow the cells to conform and deposit cell-adhesive molecules (Parker et al., 2008). Channels and pits are provided for cell alignment in soft photolithography techniques, so that roughness and curvature can be imparted (Pfeiffer et al., 2014). Nowadays, bioprinting has revolutionized 3D organ design where cell alignment can be controlled.

7.5   BIOENGINEERING VISCERAL ORGAN-SPECIFIC TISSUES AND FUNCTIONS

All the visceral organs show a great degree of complex architecture and function in terms of type of cells and cellular matrix at both the molecular and cellular level. Thus, reconstructing these organs is attempted by two competing principles, top-down, and bottom-up engineering. The top-down engineering is compelled by the cells and the scaffolds, wherein whole-organ scaffolds or the macroscopic scaffolds are seeded with cells of interest and the cells are allowed to repopulate by cellular modeling and self-assembly (Hasan et al., 2014). In the bottom-up engineering, the smallest component of the tissue is directly assembled onto a large construct and is built by brick-by-brick to explicitly specify fundamental units and organizations of cell–cell and cell–matrix interactions. In this, stem cells such as the human pluripotent stem cells are used to generate organoids and organ-specific parenchyma from a single-cell source (Fatehullah et al., 2016).

7.5.1   WHOLE-ORGAN SCAFFOLDS USING TOP-DOWN ENGINEERING

Success has been achieved on reconstruction of all the four organs namely liver, lungs, kidney, and heart by the progressive top-down method that uses whole organs as the scaffold (Ott et al., 2008, 2010; Petersen et al., 2010; Song et al., 2013; Crapo et al., 2011; Wu et al., 2015). Whole organs can be achieved from either the donor or from the cadavers that are decellularized using SDS and Triton X-100 (Keane et al., 2015). This method had the benefit of innate matrix configuration and multifaceted architecture to restore functional whole organs that may be used in therapeutics for organ transplantation. Scaffolds are obtained with both native structure and a complex matrix that maintains the spatial dispersal of ECM proteins (Nakayama et al., 2010). Cell seeding of these scaffolds has seen tremendous popularity with the advances in stem cell technology. Most notably, induced pluripotent stem cells (iPSCs) that are created by using reprogramming factors on adult somatic cells have the ability to differentiate into all cell types in the body (Malik and Rao, 2013; Shi et al., 2016). Thus, the regenerative property of the stem cells into multiple cell lineage differentiation may progress to higher level recellularization and organ-specific function (Ren et al., 2015; Huang et al., 2013; Lu et al., 2013).

7.5.2   ORGAN-SPECIFIC RECONSTRUCTION USING BOTTOM-UP ENGINEERING

Engineered organ-specific tissue has drawn substantial attention as a method to recapitulate organ functional units, which has enriched our understanding on organ microphysiological system (MPS), the disease progression, drug toxicity as well as mechanisms of injury, and the regeneration response. MPS encompasses minimal requirement of cells and reagents and has made a probable transference in the drug development process from animal models toward high-throughput screening in human (Sutherland et al., 2013; Stokes et al., 2015; Marx et al., 2016). This method also minutely controls the biophysical (i.e., pressure, flow, oxygen tension) and biochemical stimuli (organ-specific growth factors and cytokines), as well as the spatially controlled cell-to-cell and cell-to-matrix interactions. MPS monitors the diverse interactions among tissues and can be achieved on simple microfluidic flow chambers (Mathur et al., 2015) engineering platforms to complex 3D tissues with controlled interactions among various tissues (Vernetti et al., 2017; Miller and Shuler, 2016).

7.6 BIOENGINEERING OF HEART

Cardiovascular disease is the leading cause of death around the world. Heart is a complex organ, meticulously arranged in layers, and made up of smooth muscle cells, blood vessels, fibroblasts, cardiac myocytes, nerves, and ECM components such as cardiac interstitium and collagen (Di Donato et al., 2004). In the past, many therapeutic strategies have been employed to rectify the damaged ischemic tissue or ventricular dilation and also to develop new myocardial tissue. With the help of cellular therapy (so-called cellular cardiomyoplasty), cells of different origin are implanted onto the infarcted ventricle with the expectation that cells will electrically couple with the host myocardium and contribute to the generation of new contractile tissue to replace the damaged tissue (Chachques, 2011). Attempts, so far, have failed to successfully implanted cells, which die soon after transplantation, as they are unable to withstand the mechanical forces they experience in the host tissue (Wu et al., 2009). The underlying mechanisms that govern the cardiac structure-function relationship are not yet known completely. The roles of paracrine factors, which play an important role, are some critical issues that are still to be clarified. Many factors should be taken into account like, for example, from delivery of maximum cells to minimal death, the optimal time of cell administration, the minimum immune rejection owing to inflammation, and avoidance of fibroid scar formation (Zhou et al., 2006).

To overcome the abovementioned challenges, autologous cells or cells derived from allogeneic sources are entrapped in a cell-friendly gelling biomaterial. Gels have bioactive molecules that are injected onto the infarcted myocardium, thus avoid any invasive surgery (Vunjak-Novakovic et al., 2011). Cardiac cells combined with biogel increase, to some extent, the cells residence time at the site of interest and enhance cells adhesion and survival by providing them a better microenvironment (Shen et al., 2009). Conversely, these materials lose their mechanical properties and lead to nonsynchronous spreading of cells leading to dilated ventricle and postinfarct ventricular dysfunction.

The therapeutic efficiency of a material when compared showed that prefabricated scaffold or patch gave better results than the injectable gel. Use of 3D myocardial patches or scaffolds in recapitulating the heart are another alternative TE strategy helps cardiac cells to improve their survival, induces the formation of new blood vessels and ECM, and at the same time supports the native tissue mechanically within the host body (Nerem, 1997; Jawad et al., 2008). Nowadays, many fabrication techniques for the preparation of scaffolds are employed with the computer-assisted techniques providing wide versatility in terms of chemistry and morphology. Scaffolds laden with growth factors provided the right mechanical and electrical stimulation that help the cardiomyocytes to mature within the scaffolds and develop the characteristics and structures typical of cardiac tissue. Still, this method has the disadvantage of being invasive and needs to be vascularized in comparison to injectable gels to ensure the success of the graft. Figure 7.9 shows the various strategies for engineering the heart tissue.

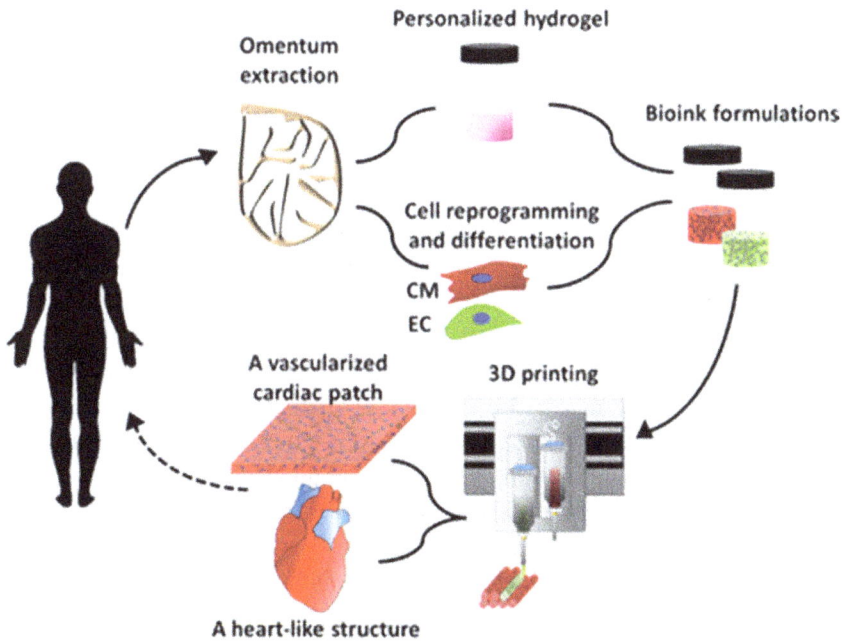

FIGURE 7.9 Schematic representation of bioengineering of heart. An autologous omentum tissue is processed into a personalized thermoresponsive hydrogel after being extracted and decellularized from the matrix. The cells are reprogrammed into pluripotent stem cells, so that they can differentiate into cardiomyocytes and endothelial cells. This is followed by encapsulation within the hydrogel to generate the bioinks used for printing. The bioinks are then printed to engineer vascularized patches and complex cellularized structures. The resulting autologous engineered tissues then repair or replace injured/diseased organs with low risk of rejection and finally transplanted back into the patient.
Source: Reprinted from Noor et al. (2019). https://creativecommons.org/licenses/by/4.0/)

7.7   BIOENGINEERING OF LUNGS

Developing a tissue-engineered lung has been in great demand among a substantial pediatric population and also in adults with lung damage. Scaffold for a tissue-engineered lung must be designed in manner that it can efficiently transfer the oxygen and the nutrients from the vascular chamber to the paren-chymal chamber, thus should have a robust vascular network (Figure 7.10). A thin porous membrane separates the vascular network from the contiguous alveolar chamber to maintain continuous oxygen flow. This membrane is engaged in exchange of oxygen and carbon dioxide between the blood and the alveolar chamber. The lung scaffold can be significantly scaled up to gain the maximum surface area for gas exchange. It was noted that a single planar scaffold with a surface area of 0.0018 m^2 can achieve oxygen transfer of 0.17 mL/min and carbon dioxide transfer of 0.16 mL/min. Efforts are being made to increase the surface area that is seen in a resting adolescent or young adult with 2.8 m^2 of surface area and oxygen transfer of 250 mL/min and carbon dioxide transfer of 265 mL/min. Mostly, silicone or traditional resorbable biomaterials are used to develop lung scaffolds. Nevertheless, these scaffolds lose their efficiency when implanted *in vivo* and efforts are underway to construct scaffolds using naturally occurring ECM proteins, possibly combined with resorbable polymer. A thin collagen membrane is established for the lung scaffold, which is seeded with pneumocytes and endothelial cells and is functionally similar to the alveolar membrane or air–blood interface in the lung. This setup worked well in in-vitro condition and was able to utilize flowing fresh blood over it by transferring oxygen and carbon dioxide across the membrane (Hoganson et al., 2008). Still, it requires a lot of optimization process to gain the combination of strength and the thickness of thin collagen membranes that can transfer the gases proficiently. Porous scaffolds for lungs are also developed using polyglycolic acid or Pluronic F-127 (PF-127) (Cortiella et al., 2006) seeded with ovine somatic lung progenitor cells. These are first grown *in vitro* and then implanted on the back of a nude mouse or into an ovine lung wedge resection site. It was seen that these worked well *in vitro* but generated inflammatory response to the polymer when implanted *in vivo*, though they developed morphologically similar tissues like that of lung alveoli. Andrade et al. also attained "alveolar-like structures" in an in-vivo lung TE model by engaging a simple porous scaffold (Andrade et al., 2007). Gelfoam sponges were seeded with fetal rat pneumocytes and implanted into a healthy lung of a rat, which later developed into structure resembling the native vascular alveoli. Similarly, fetal rat lung cells on a collagen glycosaminoglycan tissue-engineered scaffold were able to develop into achieved alveolar-like structures giving much prominence to the future of restructured lungs (Chen et al., 2005).

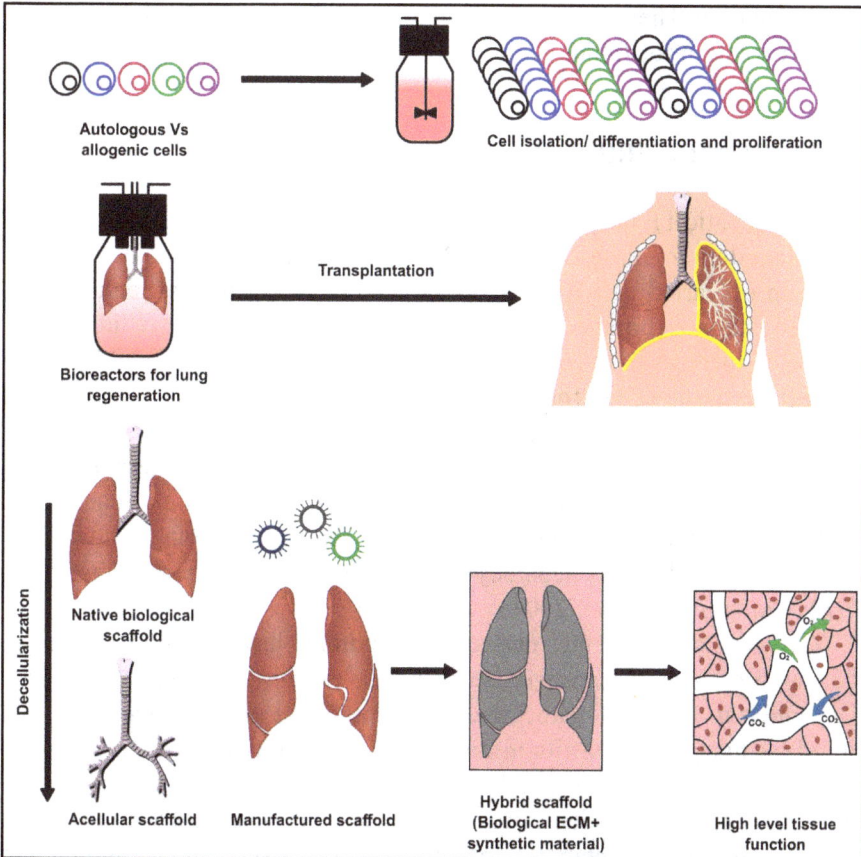

FIGURE 7.10   Schematic representation of bio-engineering of lung. A lung scaffold is seeded with autologous or allogeneic cells and is expanded to appropriate numbers in bioreactors for cell expansion. Either decellularised scaffolds or hybrid synthetic scaffolds (combined with biological extracellular matrix (ECM) are popularly used.

Source: Adapted from De Santis et al. (2018).

Though the literature for lung TE is scarce, the possibility to use autologous or allogeneic lung cells expanded *in vitro* can be considered for future endeavors. Human embryonic stem cells (hESCs) or other stem cell-based approaches hold much promise in the creation of a respiratory device for preterm infants (Samadikuchaksaraei et al., 2006). This process follows immediate retrieval of the umbilical vein and umbilical artery of a preterm infant and instantly cannulated, so that these vessels can supply blood to the tissue-engineered scaffold of the lung. The scaffold is developed into an endothelialized vascular network, so blood could flow through it avoiding anticoagulation. Therefore, the field of TE of lung has the potential to provide a potent solution for future clinical applications.

7.8   BIOENGINEERING OF LIVER

Liver or hepatic TE has a lot of potential to treat patients with inborn metabolic disorders to chronic liver failure. Liver is a compact solid structure made up of varied cell types such as hepatocytes, sinusoid, endothelial, Kupffer, stellate, biliary, epithelial, and pit cells and all are intricately connected through tight junctions and type I and IV collagen and laminins connective tissue (Crawford, 1999). The greatest challenge that is faced is the availability of functional hepatocytes, which maintain metabolic homeostasis, protein synthesis, and detoxification (Jungermann and Katz, 1982, 1989). Several animal hepatocytes, hepatocellular carcinoma (HepG2) cell lines, and human primary hepatocytes from normal liver have been considered as hepatocytes source for liver regeneration (Seglen, 1972; Kulig and Vacanti, 2004).

Xenogeneic hepatocytes derived from porcine have been considered in the past for TE of human liver because they exhibit metabolic characteristics similar to human hepatocytes, can be procured in large quantities, and stored for many months with minimal loss of viability (Krebs et al., 2007). Although, there are many disadvantages such as the zoonotic transmission of diseases such as porcine endogenous retrovirus (Demetriou et al., 2004) as well as the subtle metabolic differences exist between animal and human hepatocytes, which limit the performance of a tissue-engineered construct based on animal cells (Xu et al., 2004). Therefore, the ideal cell source for hepatic TE should clearly come from a human-derived source of hepatocytes.

Till date, the best source of human hepatocytes is derived from metastatic hepatic tumors because they exhibit immortality and unlimited growth *in vitro*. Cell line such as C3A subclone of the HepG2 is currently being explored for the same as they demonstrate high tolerance and good proliferation (Krebs et al., 2007; Kelly and Sussman, 1994). They also exhibit some normal hepatic metabolic function including albumin synthesis, p450 activity, and urea synthesis. Regrettably, these cells produce abnormal metabolic byproduct as alpha-fetoprotein, which also pose the risk of metastases development in any clinical application, thus relegating these cells to only in-vitro setup (Ichai and Samuel, 2004; Allen and Bhatia, 2002).

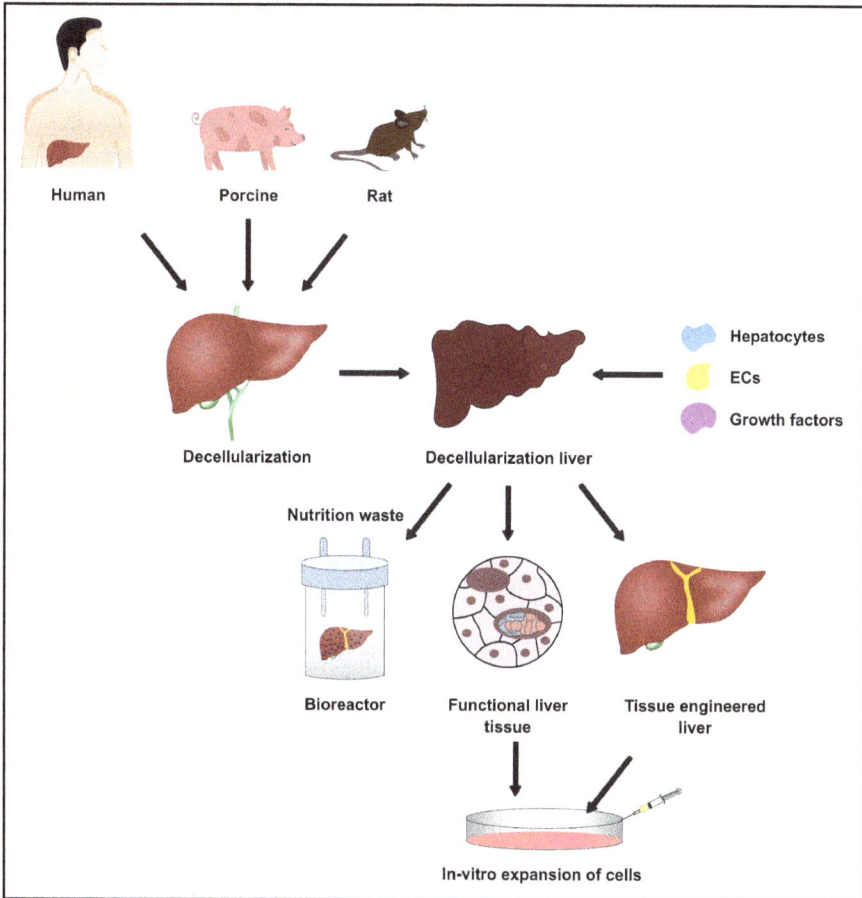

FIGURE 7.11 Autologous or allogenic liver tissues are decellularized for procuring the biological scaffold. Whole liver is recellularized by reseeding the scaffold by various cell types such as induced pluripotent stem cells (iPSCs), mesenchymal stem cells (MSCs) or liver progenitor cells (LPCs).

In such a scenario, primary hepatocytes isolated from the ECM of human liver are the best choice and can be either isolated from other humans (allogeneic) or from the patient's itself (autologous). The most limiting factor for deriving the primary hepatocytes of either variety is to obtain them in large numbers (Hengstler et al., 2005). Both the derived cells have their share of advantages and disadvantages. Tissue-engineered construct containing allogeneic hepatocytes would present all the immune risks of transplantation and could complicate the patient's future rejection risk (Pryor and Vacanti, 2008) whereas autologous cells exhibit the same immunomarkers as the patient thus, eliminating the possibility of an immune rejection (Krebs et al., 2007). However, it poses two main threats; firstly, patients with liver dysfunction may not have enough reservoirs of healthy hepatocytes to be considered for TE and secondly, once removed from in-vivo environment, these cells may completely lose their functional capacity (Pryor and Vacanti, 2008). These days, the primary hepatocytes are expanded and preserved through the use of immortalization techniques involving temperature-sensitive SV40Tag, suicide genes, and Cre-LoxP-mediated oncogene excision and have shown promise in in-vitro cultures (Krebs et al., 2007).

Embryonic stem cells have shown potential to differentiate into hepatocytes when treated with cytokines such as activin A and hepatocyte growth factor (Martin, 1981, Martin et al., 2006; Chen et al., 2006). Study by Soto-Gutierrez et al. demonstrated murine embryonic stem cells differentiated into mature hepatocytes by regulating through interactions with their environment along with developing the characteristics of broad plasticity of embryonic stem cells (Soto-Gutierrez et al., 2007). Unfortunately, use of human stem cells to generate hepatocytes is yet not successful. Adult MSCs were originally identified in the connective tissue matrices that can be used in tissue bioengineering. Human bone marrow-derived MSCs (BMSCs) have been mostly extensively research for this purpose (Fuchs and Segre, 2000). Lee at al. established that umbilical cord blood-derived BMSCs and MSCs readily differentiated into hepatocytes with functional capability (Lee et al., 2004). Other studies too demonstrated hematopoietic stem cells from bone marrow to transdifferentiate from the mesenchymal lineage to an endothelial lineage and expressing markers for hepatic cell type (Fuchs and Segre, 2000; Petersen et al., 1999; Oh et al., 2007). Also, there are reports where adipose-derived MSCs were shown to differentiate into osteogenic, adipogenic, and chondrogenic lineages with equal or greater efficiency than BMSCs (De Ugarte et al., 2003; Talens-Visconti et al., 2006; Song et al., 2007; Kern et al., 2006). However, there is still no definite breakthrough in bioengineering of liver from stem cells. Figure 7.11 gives an overview of TE of liver.

7.9 BIOENGINEERING OF KIDNEY

Regeneration of even 10% kidney function in terminally ill patients with end-stage kidney disease can greatly improve the quality of life in such patients. Though the regeneration of functional kidney still remains a huge challenge, but some advances are being made in kidney regeneration using iPSC (Evan and Kaufman, 1981; Takahashi and Yamanaka, 2006; Takahashi et al., 2007). The kidney is embryologically developed from a ureteric bud, which then follows precisely timed interactions between multiple signals to derive the intermediate mesoderm (IM) and metanephric mesenchyme (MM) (Blake and Rosenblum, 2014). Both IM and MM kidney-specific cells have been generated using nephron progenitor cells with growth factor such as the Wnt agonist CHIR99021 to promote mesoderm differentiation (Taguchi et al., 2014; Takasato et al., 2014; Xia et al., 2013; Mae et al., 2013; Gadue et al., 2006; Lam et al., 2014). Another protocol is developed to induce differentiation of IM cells from human iPSCs (hiPSCs)/hESCs using a combination of activin A and CHIR99021 to generate mesoderm followed by combined treatment with bone morphogenetic protein-7 and CHIR99021 (Mae et al., 2013; Gadue et al., 2006). It should be noted that developing the renal progenitor cells is important as only then it can allow a 3D construct from PSCs with a functional vascular system. Even, with many progresses in this field, a complete functional restructured kidney in in-vivo system has not been achieved.

For the development of complete whole kidney, native kidney ECM is crucial to provide a scaffold for cell seeding and a niche for stem cells to differentiate into whole organs (Song and Ott, 2011). Organogenesis and repair of the kidney tissues are controlled by the ECM molecules and their receptors. Additionally, ECM provides a scaffold for the spatial organization of the renal cells as well as secretes and stores growth factors and cytokines, thus regulates signal transduction for regeneration process (Song and Ott, 2011; Lelongt and Ronco, 2003; Salvatori et al., 2014; Haagsma and Pound, 1980; Cuppage and Tate, 1967; Oliver, 2011). The decellularization–recellularization technology has also been used in renal reconstruction in many animal studies (Sullivan et al., 2012; Nakayama et al., 2010; Ross et al., 2009). These studies failed to produce functional kidney. Only one study by Song et al. was able to successfully regenerate a whole kidney that produced urine after transplantation (Song et al., 2013). The work encompassed formation of 3D acellular renal scaffolds via perfusion decellularization of cadaveric rat, pig, and human kidneys. These scaffolds were then perfused with endothelial and epithelial cells leading to the formation of viable tissues for renal construction. However, this strategy too faced some challenges regarding the production of urine and later with the development of massive thrombi, despite robust anticoagulation prophylaxis. Nonetheless, it holds promise for future of regenerative medicine on organ transplantation and hopes to solve the acute shortage of donor organs.

7.10   BIOENGINEERING OF THE GUT

The bioengineered construct should mimic the native gut both anatomically and physiologically. Though, TE of gut is quite a daunting task, as it involves the restructuring of many layers of smooth muscles, specialized mucosa, epithelial, and the interstitial cells. Moreover, the constructs which are composed of both synthetic- and naturally-derived components should not elicit any adverse immune response in the host after implantation. Thus, as mentioned in all other visceral organs, the quest for autologous cells such as embryonic and adult stem cells, bone marrow-derived cells, neural crest-derived cells, and muscle-derived stem cells in TE of gut is of prime importance. Further, the scaffolding biomaterial should be biocompatible and biodegradable.

The most prominent cells used in TE of the gut are the bone marrow-derived cells that can be manipulated using soluble factors in the growth medium for regeneration of specifically the vascular and bladder smooth muscle (Tian et al., 2009; Kumar et al., 2009; Metharom et al., 2009). Muscle derived-stem cells have also been identified to differentiate into myotubes as well as smooth muscle phenotypes (Hwang et al., 2004). Similarly, neural crest-derived stem cells, which persist through adult development (Kruger et al., 2002), are too a potential source of autologous neuronal cells required to reengineer the gut neuromusculature (Schafer et al., 2009). These prospective autologous neuronal and glial progenitor cells express Ret and p75 markers (Young, 2005) that help in differentiating into enteric phenotype.

The biomaterials commonly preferred for TE of gut are the naturally-derived materials (collagen scaffolds, small intestinal submucosa-derived scaffolds) or synthetic polymer-based scaffolds [PLA, polyglycolic acid (PGA), poly(ε-caprolactone), etc.] (Hubbell, 1995; Kim and Mooney, 1998). These scaffolds are then combined with endothelial cells that form prevascular structures that aid in vascular ingrowth upon implantation (Schultheiss et al., 2005; Levenberg et al., 2005; Schauerte et al., 2006). Gastrointestinal (GI) tract is a complex tissue with multiple layers; therefore, thicker tissues are constructed to provide nutrients to every cellular layers. For this, prevascularization is done after anastomosis to the host vasculature that is available at the final site of implantation for ready perfusion (Lovett et al., 2009; Rouwkema et al., 2008). The restructured scaffold is then perfused with angiogenic growth factors such as FGF2, VEGF, transforming growth factor-β and more recently platelet-derived growth factor BB to promote mobilization and recruitment of endothelial cells as well as stabilization of newly formed vessels (Richardson et al, 2001).

The prominent GI-related pathologies for which TE is being considered are short bowel syndrome, fecal incontinence, and gastroesophageal reflux disease among others. Bioengineering of GI tract is definitely a better option to the invasive surgeries and pharmacological approaches. This technique also offers to investigate molecular mechanisms that contribute to pathophysiology of functional GI disorders by de novo generation of 3D neuromuscular structures.

7.11   FUTURE ASPECTS OF REGENERATIVE MEDICINE AND TISSUE ENGINEERING

Regenerative medicine is the next big revolution to treat a number of diseases. 3D-bioprinted constructs or organs enable continuous manipulations of cells and scaffolds for appropriate host's response; thus, this will allow constructing tailor-made grafts which are more patient specific. Also, it will help to position the cells within specific regions of the scaffold and possibly mimic native tissues. New knowledge on graft vascularization and innervation will help us understand the graft integration with host tissue. Additional improvement with regard to controlled release of growth factors within 3D-bioprinted constructs and organs will allow effective healing and regeneration process. Care should be taken to minimize the immunological rejection by modulating desirable immune responses in the 3D-bioprinted tissues and organs. This helps in alleviating fears of their safety and rejection as an increased knowledge on stem cell behavior and controlled differentiation is achieved. 3D-bioprinted constructs and organs provide right niche for the transplanted cells allowing them to grow under normal conditions with minimized immune rejection for improved regenerative medicine strategies. The onus completely lies on the shoulders of scientists and clinicians to mimic nature or work in parallel to nature to develop innovative biomaterials and technologies such as nanotechnology to advance this field.

KEYWORDS

- tissue engineering
- reconstructive surgery
- visceral organs
- stem cells
- scaffolds
- bioreactors

REFERENCES

Abou Neel, E. A. and Young, A. M. Antibacterial adhesives for bone and tooth repair. In: Joining and Assembly of Medical Materials and Devices. **2013**, pp. 491–513. Woodhead Publishing.

Allen, J. W. and Bhatia, S. N. Improving the next generation of bioartificial liver devices. *Semin Cell Dev Biol.* **2002**, 13: 447–454.

Andrade, C. F., Wong, A. P., Waddell, T. K., Keshavjee, S. and Liu, M. Cell-based tissue engineering for lung regeneration. *Am J Physiol Lung Cell Mol Physiol.* **2007**, 292: L510–L518.

Arnal-Pastor, M., Chachques, J. C., Pradas, M. M. and Vallés-Lluch, A. Biomaterials for cardiac tissue engineering. In: Regenerative Medicine and Tissue Engineering. **2013**. Intech Open.

Aronson, N. Making personalized medicine more affordable. *Ann N Y Acad Sci.* **2015**, 1346(1): 81–89.

Atala, A., Bauer, S. B., Soker, S., Yoo, J. J. and Retik, A. B. Tissue-engineered autologous bladders for patients needing cystoplasty. *Lancet.* **2006**, 367(9518): 1241–1246.

Atala, A., Kasper, F. K. and Mikos, A. G. Engineering complex tissues. *Sci Transl Med.* **2012**, 4(160): 160rv12.

Bara, H. and Sambanis, A. Development and characterization of a tissue engineered pancreatic substitute based on recombinant intestinal endocrine L-cells. *Biotech Bioeng.* **2009**, 103(4): 828–834.

Basile, D. P., Friedrich, J. L., Spahic, J., Knipe, N., Mang, H., Leonard, E. C. et al.. Impaired endothelial proliferation and mesenchymal transition contribute to vascular rarefaction following acute kidney injury. *Am J Physiol.* **2011**, 300: F721.

Basile, D. P. Rarefaction of peritubular capillaries following ischemic acute renal failure: a potential factor predisposing to progressive nephropathy. *Curr Opin Nephrol Hypertens.* **2004**, 13: 1.

Basile, D. P. The endothelial cell in ischemic acute kidney injury: implications for acute and chronic function. *Kidney Int.* **2007**, 72: 151.

Benhardt, H. A. and Cosgriff-Hernandez, E. M. The role of mechanical loading in ligament tissue engineering. *Tissue Eng Part B Rev.* **2009**, 15(4): 467–475.

Berry, M. F., Engler, A. J., Woo, Y. J., Pirolli, T. J., Bish, L. T., Jayasankar, V. et al. Mesenchymal stem cell injection after myocardial infarction improves myocardial compliance. *Am J Physiol Heart Circ Physiol.* **2006,** 290(6): H2196–H2203.

Bianchi, F., Vassalle, C., Simonetti, M., Vozzi, G. I., Domenici, C. and Ahluwalia, A. Endothelial cell function on 2D and 3D micro-fabricated polymer scaffolds: applications in cardiovascular tissue engineering. *J Biomat Sci Polym Ed.* **2006,** 17(1-2): 37–51.

Bilzer, M., Roggel, F. and Gerbes, A. L. Role of Kupffer cells in host defense and liver disease. *Liver Int.* **2006,** 26: 1175–1186.

Blake, J. and Rosenblum, N. D. Renal branching morphogenesis: morphogenetic and signaling mechanisms. *Semin Cell Dev Biol.* **2014,** 36: 2–12.

Brittberg, M. and Lindahl, A. Tissue engineering of cartilage. In: Tissue Engineering. Academic Press. **2008,** 533–557.

Buckberg, G., Hoffman, J. I. E., Mahajan, A., Saleh, S. and Coghlan, C. Cardiac mechanics revisited: the relationship of cardiac architecture to ventricular function. *Circulation.* **2008,** 118: 2571–2587.

Bulger, R. E. and Dobyan, D. C. Recent structure-function relationships in normal and injured mammalian kidneys. *Anat Rec.* **1983,** 205: 1.

Caddeo, S., Boffito, M. and Sartori, S. Tissue engineering approaches in the design of healthy and pathological *in vitro* tissue models. *Front Bioeng Biotech.* **2017,** 5: 40.

Chachques, J. C. Development of bioartificial myocardium using stem cells and nanobiotech-nology templates. *Cardio Res Pract.* **2011,** 2011: 806795.

Chen, P., Marsilio, E., Goldstein, R. H., Yannas, I. V. and Spector, M. Formation of lung alveolar-like structures in collagen-glycosaminoglycan scaffolds *in vitro. Tissue Eng.* **2005,** 11: 1436–1448.

Chen, Y., Soto-Gutierrez, A., Navarro-Alvarez, N., Rivas-Carrillo, J. D., Yamatsuji, T., Shirakawa, Y. et al. Instant hepatic differentiation of human embryonic stem cells using activin A and a deleted variant of HGF. *Cell Transpl.* **2006,** 15: 865–871.

Cheung, D. Y., Duan, B. and Butcher, J. T. Current progress in tissue engineering of heart valves: multiscale problems, multiscale solutions. *Exp Opin Biol Ther.* **2015,** 15: 1155–1172.

Clark, R. A. Wound repair: basic biology to tissue engineering. In: Principles of Tissue Engineering. Academic Press. **2014,** 1595–1617.

Cooper, D. K. A brief history of cross-species organ transplantation. In: Baylor University Medical Center Proceedings. 2012, Jan 1 (Vol. 25, No. 1, pp. 49–57). Taylor & Francis.

Cortes, P., Méndez, M., Riser, B. L., Guérin, C. J., Rodríguez-Barbero, A., Hassett, C. and Yee, J. F-actin fiber distribution in glomerular cells: structural and functional implications. *Kidney Int.* **2000,** 58: 2452–2461.

Cortiella, J., Nichols, J. E., Kojima, K., Bonassar, L. J., Dargon, P., Roy, A. K. et al. Tissue-engineered lung: an *in vivo* and *in vitro* comparison of polyglycolic acid and pluronic F-127 hydrogel/somatic lung progenitor cell constructs to support tissue growth. *Tissue Eng.* **2006,** 12: 1213–1225.

Crapo, P. M., Gilbert, T. W. and Badylak, S. F. An overview of tissue and whole organ decellularization processes. *Biomaterials.* **2011,** 32: 32–33.

Crawford, J. M. The liver and biliary tract. In: Cotran, R. S., Kumar, V., Collins, T (Eds). Robbins Pathologic Basis of Disease. WB Saunders Company, Philadelphia, PA. **1999,** pp. 845–901.

Crow, B. B. A novel bicomponent, hydrogel-bored, biodegradable polymer fiber for tissue engineering and drug delivery applications. The University of Texas at Arlington; **2004.**

Cuppage, F. E and Tate, A. Repair of the nephron following injury with mercuric chloride. *Am J Pathol.* **1967,** 3(51): 405–429.

De Santis, M. M., Bölükbas, D. A., Lindstedt, S. and Wagner, D. E. How to build a lung: latest advances and emerging themes in lung bioengineering. *Eur Respir J.* **2018,** 52(1): 1601355.

De Ugarte, D. A., Morizono, K., Elbarbary, A., Alfonso, Z., Zuk, P. A., Zhu, M. et al.. Comparison of multi-lineage cells from human adipose tissue and bone marrow. *Cells Tissues Organs.* **2003,** 174(3): 101–109.

Demetriou, A. A., Brown, Jr R. S., Busuttil, R. W., Fair, J., McGuire, B. M., Rosenthal, P. et al. Prospective, randomized, multicenter, controlled trial of a bioartificial liver in treating acute liver failure. *Ann Surg.* **2004,** 239(5): 660–667.

Di Donato, M., Toso, A., Dor, V., Sabatier, M., Barletta, G., Menicanti, L., and the RESTORE Group. Surgical ventricular restoration improves mechanical intraventricular dyssynchrony in ischemic cardiomyopathy. *Circulation.* **2004,** 109: 2536–2543.

DiMasi, J. A., Grabowski, H. G. and Hansen, R. W. Innovation in the pharmaceutical industry: new estimates of R&D costs. *J Health Econ.* **2016,** 47: 20–33.

Dixit, R. and Boelsterli, U. A. Healthy animals and animal models of human disease(s) in safety assessment of human pharmaceuticals, including therapeutic antibodies. *Drug Discov Today.* **2007,** 12: 336–342.

Eberli, D. and Atala, A. Tissue engineering using adult stem cells. *Meth Enzymol.* **2006,** 420: 287–302.

Evans, M. J. and Kaufman, M. H. Establishment in culture of pluripotential cells from mouse embryos. *Nature.* **1981,** 292(5819): 154–156.

Fatehullah, A., Tan, S. H. and Barker, N. Organoids as an *in vitro* model of human development and disease. *Nat Cell Biol.* **2016,** 18: 246–251.

Fehrer, C. and Lepperdinger, G. Mesenchymal stem cell aging. *Exp Geront.* **2005,** 40(12): 926–930.

Festing, M. F. W. Is the use of animals in biomedical research still necessary in 2002? Unfortunately, "yes". *ATLA.* **2004,** 32: 733–740.

Fuchs, E. and Segre, J. A. Stem cells: a new lease on life. *Cell.* **2000,** 100: 143–155.

Gadue, P., Huber, T. L., Paddison, P. J. and Keller, G. M. Wnt and TGF-beta signaling are required for the induction of an *in vitro* model of primitive streak formation using embryonic stem cells. *Proc Natl Acad Sci U S A.* **2006,** 103(45): 16806–16811.

Grainger, D. W. Cell-based drug testing; this world is not flat. *Adv Drug Deliv Rev.* **2014,** 3: 69–70.

Grund, S., Bauer, M. and Fischer, D. Polymers in drug delivery—state of the art and future trends. *Adv Eng Mat.* **2011,** 13(3): B61–B87.

Guvendiren, M. and Burdick, J. A. Stiffening hydrogels to probe short- and long-term cellular responses to dynamic mechanics. *Nat Commun.* **2012,** 3(1): 1–9.

Haagsma, B. H. and Pound, A. W. Mercuric chloride-induced tubulonecrosis in the rat kidney: the recovery phase. *Br J Exp Path.* **1980,** 619(3): 229–241.

Hasan, A., Paul, A., Vrana, N. E., Zhao, X., Memic, A., Hwang, Y. S., t al. Microfluidic techniques for development of 3D vascularized tissue. *Biomaterials.* **2014,** 35: 7308–7325.

Hay, M., Thomas, D. W., Craighead, J. L., Economides, C. and Rosenthal, J. Clinical development success rates for investigational drugs. *Nat Biotech.* **2014,** 32(1): 40–51.

Helen, W. H. Bridging the translational gap: collaborative drug development and dispelling the stigma of commercialization. *Drug Discov Today.* **2016,** 21(2): 299–305.

Hellman, B. The frequency distribution of the number and volume of the islets of Langerhans in man. *Acta Soc Med Up.* **1959**, *6:* 432–460.

Hellman, B. Actual distribution of the number and volume of the islets of Langerhans in different size classes in non-diabetic humans of varying ages. *Nature.* **1959**, *184(19)*: 1498–1499.

Hengstler, J. G., Brulport, M., Schormann, W., Bauer, A., Hermes, M., Nussler, A. K. et al.. Generation of human hepatocytes by stem cell technology: definition of the hepatocyte. *Exp Opin Drug Metab Toxicol.* **2005**, 1: 61–74.

Heyde, M., Partridge, K. A., Oreffo, R. O., Howdle, S. M., Shakesheff, K. M. and Garnett, M. C. Gene therapy used for tissue engineering applications. *J Pharm Pharmacol.* **2007**, 59(3): 329–350.

Hoganson, D. M., Pryor, H. I. and Vacanti, J. P. Tissue engineering and organ structure: a vascularized approach to liver and lung. *Pediatr Res.* **2008**, 63(5): 520–526.

Hosseini, V., Maroufi, N. F., Saghati, S., Asadi, N., Darabi, M., Ahmad, S. N. et al. Current progress in hepatic tissue regeneration by tissue engineering. *J Transl Med.* **2019**, 17(1): 383–387.

Howard, D., Buttery, L. D., Shakesheff, K. M. and Roberts, S. J. Tissue engineering: strategies, stem cells, and scaffolds. *J Anatomy.* **2008**, 213(1): 66–72.

Hsia, C. C. W., Hyde, D. M. and Weibel, E. R. Lung structure and the intrinsic challenges of gas exchange. *Comp Physiol.* **2016**, 6: 827–830.

Huang, S. X. L., Islam, M. N., O'Neill, J., Hu, Z., Yang, Y. G., Chen, Y. W. et al. Efficient generation of lung and airway epithelial cells from human pluripotent stem cells. *Nat Biotechnol.* **2013**, 32: 84–87.

Hubbell, J. A. Biomaterials in tissue engineering. *Biotechnology (N Y).* **1995**, 13(6): 565–576.

Huebsch, N., Arany, P. R., Mao, A. S. et al. Harnessing traction-mediated manipulation of the cell/matrix interface to control stem cell fate. *Nat Mater.* **2010**, 9: 518–526.

Hwang, J. H., Yuk, S. H., Lee, J. H., Lyoo, W. S., Ghil, S. H., Lee, S. S. et al. Isolation of muscle-derived stem cells from rat and its smooth muscle differentiation. *Mol Cells.* **2004**, 17(1): 57–61.

Ichai, P. and Samuel, D. Treatment of patients with hepatic failure: the difficult place of liver support systems. *J Hepatol.* **2004**, 41: 694–695.

Ikada, Y. Challenges in tissue engineering. *J Royal Soc Interface.* **2006**, 3(10): 589–601.

Inanç, B., Elcin, A. E. and Elcin, Y. M. Human embryonic stem cell differentiation on tissue engineering scaffolds: effects of NGF and retinoic acid induction. *Tissue Eng Part A.* **2008**, 14(6): 955–964.

Inoue, Y., Tsuda, S., Nakagawa, K., Hojo, M. and Adachi, T. Modeling myosin-dependent rearrangement and force generation in an actomyosin network. *J Theor Biol.* **2011**, 281: 65–73.

Itoh, H., Nishino, M. and Hatabu, H. Architecture of the lung: morphology and function. *J Thorac Imaging.* **2004**, 19: 221–224.

Jawad, H., Lyon, A. R., Harding, S. E., Ali, N. N. and Boccaccini, A. R. Myocardial tissue engineering. *Br Med Bull.* **2008**, 87: 31–47.

Jen, K. Y., Haragsim, L. and Laszik, Z. G. Kidney microvasculature in health and disease. *Exp Model Ren Dis Pathog Diagn.* **2011**, 169: 51–57.

Jungermann, K. and Katz, N. Functional hepatocellular heterogeneity. *Hepatology.* **1982**, 2: 385–395.

Jungermann, K. and Katz, N. Functional specialization of different hepatocyte populations. *Physiol Rev.* **1989**, 69: 708–764.

Kanczler, J. M., Barry, J., Ginty, P., Howdle, S. M., Shakesheff, K. M. and Oreffo, R. O. Supercritical carbon dioxide generated vascular endothelial growth factor encapsulated poly(D-L-lactic acid) scaffolds induce angiogenesis *in vitro*. *Biochem Biophys Res Commun.* **2007**, 352(1): 135–141.

Kaushik, G., Leijten, J. and Khademhosseini, A. Concise review: organ engineering: design, technology, and integration. *Stem Cells.* **2017**, 35(1): 51–60.

Keane, T. J., Swinehart, I. T. and Badylak, S. F. Methods of tissue decellularization used for preparation of biologic scaffolds and *in vivo* relevance. *Methods.* **2015**, 84: 25–31.

Kellar, C. A. Solid organ transplantation overview and deletion criteria. *Am J Manag Care.* **2015**, 21: S4–S11.

Kelly, J. H. and Sussman, N. L. The hepatic extracorporeal liver assist device in the treatment of fulminant hepatic failure. *ASAIO J.* **1994**, 40: 83–85.

Kerckhofs, G., Sainz, J., Wevers, M., Van de Putte, T. and Schrooten, J. Contrast-enhanced nanofocus computed tomography images the cartilage subtissue architecture in three dimensions. *Eur Cell Mater.* **2013**, 25: 179–189.

Kern, S., Eichler, H., Stoeve, J., Kluter, H. and Bieback, K. Comparative analysis of mesenchymal stem cells from bone marrow, umbilical cord blood, or adipose tissue. *Stem Cells.* **2006**, 24: 1294–1301.

Keung, A. J., Healy, K. E., Kumar, S. and Schaffer, D. V. Biophysics and dynamics of natural and engineered stem cell microenvironments. *Wiley Interdiscip Rev Syst Biol Med.* **2010**, 2(1): 49–64.

Kim, B. S. and Mooney, D. J. Development of biocompatible synthetic extracellular matrices for tissue engineering. *Trend Biotech.* **1998**, 16(5): 224–230.

Knackstedt, C., Gramley, F., Schimpf, T., Mischke, K., Zarse, M., Plisiene, J. et al. Association of echocardiographic atrial size and atrial fibrosis in a sequential model of congestive heart failure and atrial fibrillation. *Cardiovasc Pathol.* **2008**, 17(5): 318–324.

Kocica, M. J., Corno, A. F., Carreras-Costa, F., Ballester-Rodes, M., Moghbel, M. C., Cueva, C. N. C. et al. The helical ventricular myocardial band: global, three-dimensional, functional architecture of the ventricular myocardium. *Eur J Cardiothorac Surg.* **2006**, 29: S21–S27.

Korecky, B., Hai, C. M. and Rakusan, K. Functional capillary density in normal and transplanted rat hearts. *Can J Physiol Pharmacol.* **1982**, 60: 23–29.

Korossis, S., Bolland, F., Ingham, E., Fisher, J., Kearney, J. and Southgate, J. Tissue engineering of the urinary bladder: considering structure-function relationships and the role of mechanotransduction. *Tissue Eng.* **2006**, 12(4): 635–644.

Krebs, N., Neville, C. and Vacanti, J. Cellular transplantation for liver diseases. In: Halberstadt, C., Emerich, D. (Eds). Cellular Transplantation from Laboratory to Clinic. Academic Press, Burlington, MA. **2007**, 215–240.

Krishna, M. Microscopic anatomy of the liver. *Clin Liver Dis.* **2013**, 2: S4.

Kruger, G. M., Mosher, J. T., Bixby, S., Joseph, N., Iwashita, T. and Morrison, S. J. Neural crest stem cells persist in the adult gut but undergo changes in self-renewal, neuronal subtype potential, and factor responsiveness. *Neuron.* **2002**, 35(4): 657–669.

Kulig, K. M. and Vacanti, J. P. Hepatic tissue engineering. *Transpl Immunol.* **2004**, 12: 303–310.

Kumar, A. H., Metharom, P., Schmeckpeper, J., Weiss, S., Martin, K. and Caplice, N. M. Bone marrow-derived CX3CR1 progenitors contribute to neointimal smooth muscle cells via fractalkine CX3CR1 interaction. *FASEB J.* **2010**, 24(1): 81–92.

Lalwani, G., Henslee, A. M., Farshid, B., Lin, L., Kasper, F. K., Qin, Y. X. et al. Two-dimensional nanostructure-reinforced biodegradable polymeric nanocomposites for bone tissue engineering. *Biomacromolecules.* **2013,** 14(3): 900–909.

Lam, Q., Freedman, B. S., Morizane, R., Lerou, P. H., Valerius, M. T. and Bonventre. J. V. Rapid and efficient differentiation of human pluripotent stem cells into intermediate mesoderm that forms tubules expressing kidney proximal tubular markers. *J Am Soc Nephrol.* **2014,** 25(6): 1211–1225.

Langer, R. and Vacanti, J. P. Tissue Engineering. Science, New York, NY. **1993,** 260(5110): 920–926.

Le Visage, C., Yang, S. H., Kadakia, L., Sieber, A. N., Kostuik, J. P. and Leong, K. W. Small intestinal submucosa as a potential bioscaffold for intervertebral disc regeneration. *Spine.* **2006,** 31(21): 2423–2430.

Lee, K. D., Kuo, T. K., Whang-Peng, J., Chung, Y. F., Lin, C. T., Chou, S. H., Chen, J. R., Chen. Y. P. and Lee, O. K. *In vitro* hepatic differentiation of human mesenchymal stem cells. *Hepatology.* **2004,** 40: 1275–1284.

Lee, S. H. and Shin, H. Matrices and scaffolds for delivery of bioactive molecules in bone and cartilage tissue engineering. *Adv Drug Deliv Rev.* **2007,** 59(4-5): 339–359.

Lelongt, B. and Ronco, P. Role of extracellular matrix in kidney development and repair. *Pediatr Nephrol.* **2003,** 18(8): 731–742.

Levenberg, S., Rouwkema, J., Macdonald, M., Garfein, E. S., Kohane, D. S., Darland, D. C. et al. Engineering vascularized skeletal muscle tissue. *Nat Biotech.* **2005,** 23(7): 879–884.

Loh, Q. L. and Choong, C. Three-dimensional scaffolds for tissue engineering applications: role of porosity and pore size. *Tissue Eng Part B Rev.* **2013,** 19(6): 485–502.

Longnecker, D. S. Anatomy and Histology of the Pancreas. Pancreapedia: The Exocrine Pancreas Knowledge Base. **2014** Mar 20.

Lopez, P. P., Gogna, S. and Khorasani-Zadeh, A. Anatomy, abdomen and pelvis, duodenum. In: StatPearls. StatPearls Publishing. **2019.**

Lovett, M., Lee, K., Edwards, A. and Kaplan, D. L. Vascularization strategies for tissue engineering. *Tissue Eng Part B Rev.* **2009,** 15(3): 353–370.

Lu, T. Y., Lin, B., Kim, J., Sullivan, M., Tobita, K., Salama, G. and Yang, L. Repopulation of decellularized mouse heart with human-induced pluripotent stem cell-derived cardiovascular progenitor cells. *Nat Commun.* **2013,** 4: 2307–2318.

MacNeil, S. Biomaterials for tissue engineering of skin. *Mater Today.* **2008,** 11(5): 26–35.

Mae, S. I., Shono, A., Shiota, F. et al. Monitoring and robust induction of nephrogenic intermediate mesoderm from human pluripotent stem cells. *Nat Commun.* **2013,** 4: 1367.

Magee, J. C., Barr, M. L., Basadonna, G. P., Johnson, M. R., Mahadevan, S., McBride, M. A. et al. Repeat organ transplantation in the United States, 1996–2005. *Am J Transplant.* **2007,** 7: 1424.

Makadia, H. K. and Siegel, S. J. Polylactic-co-glycolic acid (PLGA) as biodegradable controlled drug delivery carrier. *Polymers.* **2011,** 3(3): 1377–1397.

Malik, N. and Rao, M. S. A review of the methods for human iPSC derivation. *Methods Mol Biol.* **2013,** 997: 23.

Martin, G. R. Isolation of a pluripotent cell line from early mouse embryos cultured in medium conditioned by teratocarcinoma stem cells. *Proc Natl Acad Sci U S A.* **1981,** 78: 7634–7638.

Martino, M. M., Tortelli, F., Mochizuki, M., Traub, S., Ben-David, D., Kuhn, G. A. et al. Engineering the growth factor microenvironment with fibronectin domains to promote wound and bone tissue healing. *Sci Transl Med.* **2011,** 3(100): 100ra89.

Marx, U., Andersson, T. B., Bahinski, A., Beilmann, M., Beken, S., Cassee, F. R. et al. Biology-inspired microphysiological system approaches to solve the prediction dilemma of substance testing. *ALTEX.* **2016,** 33: 272–321.

Mathur, A., Loskill, P., Shao, K., Huebsch, N., Hong, S., Marcus, S. G. et al. Human iPSC-based cardiac microphysiological system for drug screening applications. *Sci Rep.* **2015,** 5: 8883.

Mercer, R. R., Russell, M. L. and Crapo, J. D. Alveolar septal structure in different species. *J Appl Physiol.* **1994,** 77: 1060.

Metharom, P., Kumar, A. H., Weiss, S. and Caplice, N. M. A specific subset of mouse bone marrow cells has smooth muscle cell differentiation capacity—brief report. *Arterioscler Thromb Vasc Biol.* **2010,** 30(3): 533–535.

Mikos, A. G., Herring, S. W., Ochareon, P., Elisseeff, J., Lu, H. H., Kandel, R. et al. Engineering complex tissues. *Tissue Eng.* **2006,** 12: 3307.

Miller, P. G. and Shuler, M. L. Design and demonstration of a pumpless 14 compartment microphysiological system. *Biotechnol Bioeng.* **2016,** 113: 2213.

Mohand-Said, S., Hicks, D., Dreyfus, H. and Sahel, J. A. Selective transplantation of rods delays cone loss in a retinitis pigmentosa model. *Arch Ophthalmol.* **2000,** 118(6): 807–811.

Mosig, A. S. Organ-on-chip models: new opportunities for biomedical research. *Future Sci OA.* **2016,** 3: FSO130.

Nagy, A., Gocza, E., Diaz, E. M., Prideaux, V. R., Iványi, E., Markkula, M. et al. Embryonic stem cells alone are able to support fetal development in the mouse. *Development.* **1990,** 110(3): 815–821.

Nakayama, K. H., Batchelder, C. A., Lee, C. I. and Tarantal, A. F. Decellularized rhesus monkey kidney as a Three-Dimensional Scaffold for Renal Tissue Engineering. *Tissue Eng A.* **2010,** 16: 2207.

Narine, K., Wever, O. D., Valckenborgh, D. V., Francois, K., Bracke, M., Desmet, S. et al. Growth factor modulation of fibroblast proliferation, differentiation, and invasion: implications for tissue valve engineering. *Tissue Eng.* **2006,** 12(10): 2707–2716.

Nayyer, L., Patel, K. H., Esmaeili, A., Rippel, R. A., Birchall, M., O'Toole, G. et al. Tissue engineering: revolution and challenge in auricular cartilage reconstruction. *Plast Reconstr Surg.* **2012,** 129(5): 1123–1137.

Nerem, R. M. The challenge of imitating nature. In: Lanza, R., Langer, R., Vacanti, J. Principles of tissue engineering. San Diego (CA) USA: Academic Press; **1997**: 9–15.

Noor, N., Shapira, A., Edri, R., Gal, I., Wertheim, L. and Dvir, T. 3D printing of personalized thick and perfusable cardiac patches and hearts. *Adv Sci.* **2019,** 6(11): 1900344.

Oh, S. H., Witek, R. P., Bae, S. H., Zheng, D., Jung, Y., Piscaglia, A. C. and Petersen, B. E. Bone marrow-derived hepatic oval cells differentiate into hepatocytes in 2-acetylaminofluorene/ partial hepatectomy-induced liver regeneration. *Gastroenterology.* **2007,** 132: 1077–1087.

Oliver, J. Correlations of structure and function and mechanisms of recovery in acute tubular necrosis. *Am J Med.* **1953,** 15(4): 535–557.

Opitz, F. M., Schenke-Layland, K., Cohnert, T. U., Starcher, B., Halbhuber, K. J., Martin, D. P. and Stock, U. A. Tissue engineering of aortic tissue: direct consequence of suboptimal elastic fiber synthesis *in vivo. Cardiovasc Res.* **2004,** 63(4): 719–730.

Ott, H. C., Clippinger, B., Conrad, C., Schuetz, C., Pomerantseva, I., Ikonomou, L., Kotton, D. and Vacanti, J. P. Regeneration and orthotopic transplantation of a bioartificial lung. *Nat Med.* **2010,** 16: 927.

Ott, H. C., Matthiesen, T. S., Goh, S. K., Black, L. D., Kren, S. M., Netoff, T. I. and Taylor, D. A. Perfusion-decellularized matrix: using nature's platform to engineer a bioartificial heart. *Nat Med.* **2008,** 14: 213.

Parker, K. K. and Ingber, D. E. Extracellular matrix, mechanotransduction and structural hierarchies in heart tissue engineering. *Philos Trans R Soc Lond B Biol Sci.* **2007,** 362(1484): 1267–1279.

Paul S. M., Mytelka, D. S., Dunwiddie, C. T., Persinger, C. C., Munos, B. H., Lindborg, S. R. and Schacht, A. L. How to improve R&D productivity: the pharmaceutical industry's grand challenge. *Nat Rev Drug Discov.* **2010,** 9(3): 203–214.

Petersen, B. E., Bowen, W. C., Patrene, K. D., Mars, W. M., Sullivan, A. K., Murase, N. et al. Bone marrow as a potential source of hepatic oval cells. *Science.* **1999,** 284: 1168–1170.

Petersen, T. H., Calle, E. A., Zhao, L., Lee, E. J., Gui, L., Raredon, M. B. et al. Tissue-engineered lungs for *in vivo* implantation. *Science.* **2010,** 329: 538.

Pocock, G., Richards, C. D. and Richards, D. A. Human Physiology. Oxford University Press; **2013**.

Poornejad, N., Schaumann, L. B., Buckmiller, E. M., Roeder, B. L. and Cook, A. D. Current cell-based strategies for whole kidney regeneration. *Tissue Eng Part B Rev.* **2016,** 22(5): 358–370.

Pound, P. and Bracken, M. B. Is animal research sufficiently evidence based to be a cornerstone of biomedical research. *BMJ.* **2014,** 348: g3387.

Poveda, F., Gil, D., Martí, E., Andaluz, A., Ballester, M. and Carreras, F. Helical structure of the cardiac ventricular anatomy assessed by diffusion tensor magnetic resonance imaging with multiresolution tractography. *Rev Española Cardiol Engl Ed.* **2013,** 66: 782.

Pryor, H. I. and Vacanti, J. P. The promise of artificial liver replacement. *Front Biosci.* **2008,** 13: 2140–2159.

Puche, J. E., Saiman, Y. and Friedman, S. L. Hepatic stellate cells and liver fibrosis. *Compr Physiol.* **2013,** 3: 1473.

Radisic, M. Biomaterials for cardiac tissue engineering. *Biomed Mater (Bristol, England).* **2015,** 10(3): 030301.

Ramkisoensing, A. A., de Vries, A. A., Atsma, D. E., Schalij, M. J. and Pijnappels, D. A. Interaction between myofibroblasts and stem cells in the fibrotic heart: balancing between deterioration and regeneration. *Cardiovasc Res.* **2014,** 102(2): 224–231.

Rappaport, A. M., Borowy, Z. J., Lougheed, W. M. and Lotto, W. N. Subdivision of hexagonal liver lobules into a structural and functional unit. Role in hepatic physiology and pathology. *Anatom Rec.* **1954,** 119(1): 11–33.

Ren, G., Chen, X., Dong, F., Li, W., Ren, X., Zhang, Y. and Shi, Y. Concise review: mesenchymal stem cells and translational medicine: emerging issues. *Stem Cells Transl Med.* **2012,** 1(1): 51–58.

Ren, X., Moser, P. T., Gilpin, S. E., Okamoto, T., Wu, T., Tapias, L. F. et al. Engineering pulmonary vasculature in decellularized rat and human lungs. *Nat Biotechnol.* **2015,** 33: 1097.

Richardson, S. M., Hoyland, J. A., Mobasheri, R., Csaki, C., Shakibaei, M. and Mobasheri, A. Mesenchymal stem cells in regenerative medicine: opportunities and challenges for articular cartilage and intervertebral disc tissue engineering. *J Cell Physiol.* **2010,** 222(1): 23–32.

Richardson, T. P., Peters, M. C., Ennett, A. B. and Mooney, D. J. Polymeric system for dual growth factor delivery. *Nat Biotechnol*. **2001**, 19(11): 1029–1034.

Ripamonti, U. and Duneas, N. Tissue engineering of bone by osteoinductive biomaterials. *MRS Bull*. **1996**, 21(11): 36–39.

Ross, E. A., Williams, M. J., Hamazaki, T. et al. Embryonic stem cells proliferate and differentiate when seeded into kidney scaffolds. *J Am Soc Nephrol*. **2009**, 20(11): 2338–2347.

Salmon, A. H. J., Neal, C. R. and Harper, S. J. New aspects of glomerular filtration barrier structure and function: five layers (at least) not three. *Curr Opin Nephrol Hypertens*. **2009**, 18: 197.

Salvatori, M., Peloso, A., Katari, R. and Orlando, G. Regeneration and bioengineering of the kidney: current status and future challenges. *Curr Urol Rep*. **2014**, 15(1): 379.

Samadikuchaksaraei, A., Cohen, S., Isaac, K., Rippon, H. J., Polak, J. M., Bielby, R. C. et al. Derivation of distal airway epithelium from human embryonic stem cells. *Tissue Eng*. **2006**, 12: 867–875.

Schäfer, K. H., Micci, M. A. and Pasricha, P. J. Neural stem cell transplantation in the enteric nervous system: roadmaps and roadblocks. *Neurogastroenterol Mot*. **2009**, 21(2): 103–112.

Schauerte, P., Schimpf, T., Mischke, K., Zarse, M., Schmid, M., Plisiene, J. et al. Morphology and function of the intrinsic cardiac nervous system. *Herz*. **2006**, 31(2): 96–100.

Schoen, F. J. and Levy, R. J. Founder's Award, 25th Annual Meeting of the Society for Biomaterials, perspectives. Providence, RI, April 28–May 2, 1999. Tissue heart valves: current challenges and future research perspectives. *J Biomed Mater Res*. **1999**, 47(4): 439–465.

Schultheiss, D., Gabouev, A. I., Cebotari, S., Tudorache, I., Walles, T., Schlote, N. et al. Biological vascularized matrix for bladder tissue engineering: matrix preparation, reseeding technique and short-term implantation in a porcine model. *J Urol*. **2005**, 173(1): 276–280.

Seglen, P. O. Preparation of rat liver cells. I. Effect of Ca^{2+} on enzymatic dispersion of isolated, perfused liver. *Exp Cell Res*. **1972**, 74: 450–454.

Shen, X., Tanaka, K. and Takamori, A. Coronary arteries angiogenesis in ischemic myocardium: biocompatibility and biodegradability of various hydrogels. *Artif Organs*. **2009**, 33(10): 781–787.

Shi, Y., Inoue, H., Wu, J. C. and Yamanaka, S. Induced pluripotent stem cell technology: a decade of progress. *Nat Rev Drug Discov*. **2016**, 16: 115.

Shirato, I., Tomino, Y., Koide, H. and Sakai, T. Fine structure of the glomerular basement membrane of the rat kidney visualized by high-resolution scanning electron microscopy. *Cell Tissue Res*. **1991**, 266: 1.

Song, H. Y., Jeon, E. S., Kim, J. I., Jung, J. S. and Kim, J. H. Oncostatin M promotes osteogenesis and suppresses adipogenic differentiation of human adipose tissue-derived mesenchymal stem cells. *J Cell Biochem*. **2007**, 101: 1238–1251.

Song, J. J. and Ott, H. C. Organ engineering based on decellularized matrix scaffolds. *Trends Mol Med*. **2011**, 17(8): 424–432.

Song, J. J., Guyette, J. P., Gilpin, S. E., Gonzalez, G., Vacanti, J. P. and Ott, H. C. Regeneration and experimental orthotopic transplantation of a bioengineered kidney. *Nat Med*. **2013**, 19: 646.

Soto-Gutierrez, A., Navarro-Alvarez, N., Zhao, D., Rivas-Carrillo, J. D., Lebkowski, J., Tanaka, N. Differentiation of mouse embryonic stem cells to hepatocyte-like cells by co-culture with human liver nonparenchymal cell lines. *Nat Protoc.* **2007,** 2: 347–356.

Spanjaard, E. and de Rooij, J. Mechanotransduction: Vinculin provides stability when tension rises. *Curr Biol.* **2013,** 23: R159–R161.

Spoerri, R. Histological studies on nerve elements and their endings at the epithelial cells of the gastric mucosa. *J Comp Neurol.* **1949,** 90(2): 151–171.

Stokes, C. L., Cirit, M. and Lauffenburger, D. A. Physiome-on-a-chip: the challenge of 'scaling' in design, operation, and translation of microphysiological systems. *CPT Pharm Syst Pharmacol.* **2015,** 4: 559.

Suciati, T., Howard, D., Barry, J., Everitt, N. M., Shakesheff, K. M. and Rose, F. R. Zonal release of proteins within tissue engineering scaffolds. *J Mater Sci Mater Med.* **2006,** 17(11): 1049–1056.

Sullivan, D. C., Mirmalek-Sani, S. H., Deegan, D. B. et al. Decellularization methods of porcine kidneys for whole organ engineering using a high-throughput system. *Biomaterials.* **2012,** 33(31): 7756–7764.

Sun, J. and Tan, H. Alginate-based biomaterials for regenerative medicine applications. *Materials.* **2013,** 6(4): 1285–1309.

Sutherland, M. L., Fabre, K. M. and Tagle, D. A. The National Institutes of Health Microphysiological Systems Program focuses on a critical challenge in the drug discovery pipeline. *Stem Cell Res Ther.* **2013,** 4(Suppl 1): I1.

Taguchi, A., Kaku, Y., Ohmori, T. et al. Redefining the *in vivo* origin of metanephric nephron progenitors enables generation of complex kidney structures from pluripotent stem cells. *Cell Stem Cell.* **2014,** 14(1): 53–67.

Takahashi, K. and Yamanaka, S. Induction of pluripotent stem cells from mouse embryonic and adult fibroblast cultures by defined factors. *Cell.* **2006,** 126(4): 663–676.

Takahashi, K., Tanabe, K., Ohnuki, M. et al. Induction of pluripotent stem cells from adult human fibroblasts by defined factors. *Cell.* **2007,** 131(5): 861–872.

Takasato, M. and Wymeersch, F. J. Challenges to future regenerative applications using kidney organoids. *Curr Opin Biomed Eng.* **2020,** 13: 144–151.

Takasato, M., Er, P. X., Becroft, M. et al., Directing human embryonic stem cell differentiation towards a renal lineage generates a self-organizing kidney. *Nat Cell Biol.* **2014,** 16(1): 118–126.

Talens-Visconti, R., Bonora, A., Jover, R., Mirabet, V., Carbonell, F., Castell, J. V. et al. Hepatogenic differentiation of human mesenchymal stem cells from adipose tissue in comparison with bone marrow mesenchymal stem cells. *World J Gastroenterol.* **2006,** 12: 5834–5845.

Taylor-Weiner, H., Ravi, N. and Engler, A. J. Traction forces mediated by integrin signaling are necessary for definitive endoderm specification. *J Cell Sci.* **2015,** 128: 1961–1968.

Tian, H., Bharadwaj, S., Liu, Y., Ma, P. X., Atala, A. and Zhang, Y. Differentiation of human bone marrow mesenchymal stem cells into bladder cells: potential for urological tissue engineering. *Tissue Eng Part A.* **2010,** 16(5): 1769–1779.

Vacanti, J. P. Beyond transplantation: third annual Samuel Jason Mixter lecture. *Arch Surg.* **1988,** 123(5): 545–549.

Vaquette, C., Pilipchuk, S. P., Bartold, P. M., Hutmacher, D. W., Giannobile, W. V. and Ivanovski, S. Tissue engineered constructs for periodontal regeneration: Current status and future perspectives. *Adv Healthc Mater.* **2018,** 7(21): 1800457.

Vashist, A. and Ahmad, S. Hydrogels in tissue engineering: scope and applications. *Curr Pharm Biotechnol.* **2015**, 16(7): 606–620.

Vernetti, L., Gough, A., Baetz, N., Blutt, S., Broughman, J. R., Brown, J. A. et al. Functional coupling of human microphysiology systems: intestine, liver, kidney, proximal tubule, blood-brain barrier, and skeletal muscle. *Sci Rep.* **2017**, 7: 42296.

Vining, K. H, and Mooney, D. J. Mechanical forces direct stem cell behaviour in development and regeneration. *Nat Rev Mol Cell Biol.* **2017**, 18(12): 728–742.

Vunjak-Novakovic, G., Lui, K. O., Tandon, N. and Chien, K. R. Bioengineering heart muscle: a paradigm for regenerative medicine. *Ann Rev Biomed Eng.* **2011**, 13: 245–267.

Weibel, E. R. and Knight, B. W. A morphometric study on the thickness of the pulmonary air-blood barrier. *J Cell Biol.* **1964**, 21: 367.

Wen, J. H., Vincent, L. G., Fuhrmann, A. et al. Interplay of matrix stiffness and protein tethering in stem cell differentiation. *Nat Mater.* **2014**, 13: 979–987.

West, J. B. Comparative physiology of the pulmonary blood-gas barrier: the unique avian solution. *Am J Physiol Regul Integr Comp Physiol.* **2009**, 297: R1625.

Wu, J., Zeng, F., Weisel, R. D. and Li, R. K. Stem cells for cardiac regeneration by cell therapy and myocardial tissue engineering. *Adv Biochem Eng Biotechnol.* **2009**, 114: 107–128.

Wu, Q., Bao, J., Zhou, Y., Wang, Y., Du, Z., Shi, Y., Li, L. and Bu, H. Optimizing perfusion-decellularization methods of porcine livers for clinical-scale whole-organ bioengineering. *Biomed Res Int.* **2015**, 2015: 785474.

Xia, Y., Nivet, E., Sancho-Martinez, I. et al. Directed differentiation of human pluripotent cells to ureteric bud kidney progenitor-like cells. *Nat Cell Biol.* **2013**, 15(12): 1507–1515.

Xu, H., Othman, S. F. and Magin, R. L. Monitoring tissue engineering using magnetic resonance imaging. *J Biosci Bioeng.* **2008**, 106(6): 515–527.

Xu, J. J., Diaz, D. and O'Brien, P. J. Applications of cytotoxicity assays and pre-lethal mechanistic assays for assessment of human hepatotoxicity potential. *Chem Biol Interact.* **2004**, 150: 115–128.

Yamanaka, S. and Yokoo, T. Current bioengineering methods for whole kidney regeneration. *Stem Cells Int.* **2015**, 2015: 724047.

Yao, C., Markowicz, M., Pallua, N., Noah, E. M. and Steffens, G. The effect of cross-linking of collagen matrices on their angiogenic capability. *Biomaterials.* **2008**, 29(1): 66–74.

Young, A. A. and Cowan, B. R. Evaluation of left ventricular torsion by cardiovascular magnetic resonance. *J Cardiovasc Magn Reson.* **2012**, 14: 49.

Young, H. M. Neural stem cell therapy and gastrointestinal biology. *Gastroenterology.* **2005**, 129(6): 2092–2095.

Yue, K., Trujillo-de Santiago, G., Alvarez, M. M., Tamayol, A., Annabi, N. and Khademhosseini, A. Synthesis, properties, and biomedical applications of gelatinmethacryloyl (GelMA) hydrogels. *Biomaterials.* **2015**, 73: 254–271.

Zhou, R., Acton, P. D. and Ferrari, V. A. Imaging stem cells implanted in infarcted myocardium. *J Am Coll Cardiol.* **2006**, 48(10): 2094–2106.

CHAPTER 8

Polysaccharides and Proteins-based Hydrogels for Tissue Engineering Applications

ROBERTA CASSANO, FEDERICA CURCIO, MARIA LUISA DI GIOIA, DEBORA PROCOPIO, and SONIA TROMBINO*

Department of Pharmacy, Health and Nutritional Sciences, University of Calabria, Arcavacata di Rende, Cosenza, Italy

Corresponding author. E-mail: sonia.trombino@unical.it

ABSTRACT

Tissue engineering is a branch of science that studies the possibility of repairing organs and tissues of the human body, such as muscles, bones, cartilage, and skin, damaged by a disease, accident, or aging, restoring its integrity and functionality without resorting to transplants or prostheses, thus ensuring a better quality of life for patients. To achieve this, it is necessary to integrate biological components, such as cells and growth factors, with biomaterials. In particular, implants made up of living cells are designed to proliferate on biocompatible and bioabsorbable materials. Among these, materials of natural origin are more interesting because they are characterized by several very important properties to create a favorable microenvironment for the healing process. This chapter fits into this context and aims to describe the polysaccharides- and protein-based biomaterials particularly useful for tissue engineering and their major applications.

8.1 INTRODUCTION

In recent years, the need for biomaterials useful for the promotion, regeneration, or replacement of damaged tissues has increased considerably.

Tissue engineering represents a new frontier for the biomedical field and its primary purpose is to repair or even replace damaged tissues and organs such as muscles, bones, and cartilages (Langer and Vacanti, 1993; Saunders and Ma, 2019) from diseases, trauma, or aging, restoring their integrity and functionality, thus permitting a better quality of life. The purpose of tissue engineering is to use scaffold matrices to fill the tissues and/or cells and, therefore, treat the tissues after a transplant (Howard et al., 2008). Tissue scaffolds cannot only cover the wound and provide a physical barrier, but can also offer a cellular skin with excretive biological components to stimulate re-epithelialization and formation of granulation tissue (Yadav and Chauhan, 2017). Various materials can be used as scaffolds for distinct tissue. Among them, natural polymers are most attractive; thanks to their bioactive properties such as antimicrobial, immunomodulatory, cell proliferative, and angiogenic for their similarieties with the extracellular matrix (ECM), biodegradability, and good biological performance (Mano et al., 2007). All these factors are very important to create a favorable microenvironment for the healing process (Velema and Kaplan, 2006; Sahana and Rekha, 2018). In this context, polysaccharides and proteins are natural biomaterials, which have found many applications in tissue regeneration. In particular, polysaccharides are characterized by functional groups that are essential for the development of materials applicable in tissue regeneration as well as exhibiting a high biocompatibility and biodegradability. Biomaterials, based on proteins, have also been explored for tissue engineering. Although proteins are highly biocompatible, they are also characterized by rapid degradation and low mechanical resistance that cause a lack of structural support during the formation of the new tissue (Khan and Ahmad, 2013). Among the most promising biomaterials used in biomedical field are hydrogels, a class of materials with three-dimensional (3D) network of hydrophilic polymers chains capable of retaining a significant amount of water (Peppas and Hoffman, 2020). Hydrogels have good biocompatibility, production flexibility, variable composition, and physical properties (Lee and Kim, 2018) that enable to mimic the highly hydrated ECM and to facilitate nutrients and oxygen transport due to their porous structure (Lee and Mooney, 2012; Caló and Khutoryanskiy, 2015; Saunders and Ma, 2019).

The present chapter aims to describe hydrogels based on polysaccharides such as chitosan, cellulose, alginate, hyaluronic acid, and proteins such as collagen, gelatin, elastin, and their various applications in the field of tissue engineering will be highlighted (Figure 8.1).

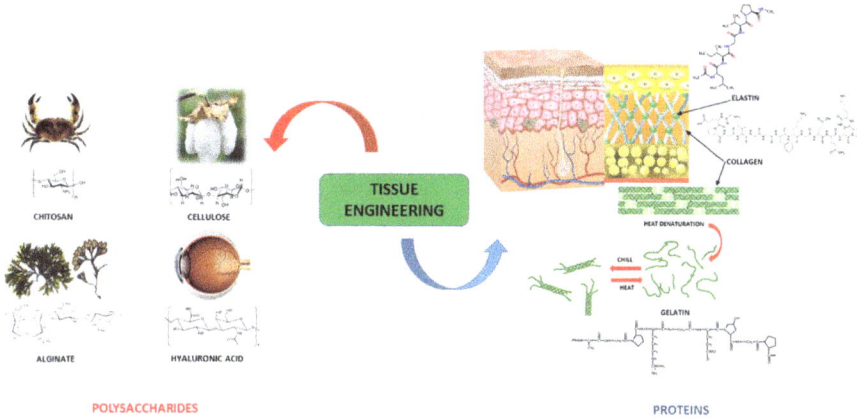

FIGURE 8.1   Natural sources of biomaterials for tissue engineering.

8.2   POLYSACCHARIDE-BASED BIOMATERIALS

Polysaccharides are macromolecules with excellent properties including biodegradability and biocompatibility that are the precious features of polymers application for biomaterial applications (Zhu at al., 2019). For this reason, polysaccharides have recently gained increasing attention from numerous researchers owing to their applications in pharmaceuticals and biomedical field. In this section, the principal polysaccharides used in tissue engineering will be described.

8.2.1   CHITOSAN

Chitosan is a linear polysaccharide composed of (1–4)-2-acetamido-2-deoxy-b-D-glucan (*N*-acetyl-D-glucosamine) and (1–4)-2-amino-2-deoxy-*b*-D-glucan (D-glucosamine) units (Figure 8.2) that can be easily derived from the partial deacetylation of chitin (Rinaudo, 2006).

Chitosan has drawn considerably more attention due to its environmentally friendly nature, biocompatibility, biodegradability, and availability (Baranwal et al., 2018). It is also particularly interesting in bone regeneration because it facilitates the attachment and proliferation of osteoblasts as well as the process of bone mineralization (Sheehy et al., 2013). Furthermore, this polysaccharide can be enzymatically degraded by lysozyme (Varum et al., 1997; Pangburn et al., 1982), a polycationic protein present in the ECM of human cartilage (Moss et al., 1997; Greenwald et al., 1972) and, for this reason, it is able to modulate chondrocyte morphology, differentiation, and stimulating chondrogenesis. Furthermore, compared to many synthetic polymers, chitosan degradation products are nontoxic (Levengood and Zhang, 2014). Therefore, various methodologies have been developed to obtain chitosan hydrogels and foams as 3D scaffolds particularly useful for tissue engineering (Croisier and Jérôme, 2013).

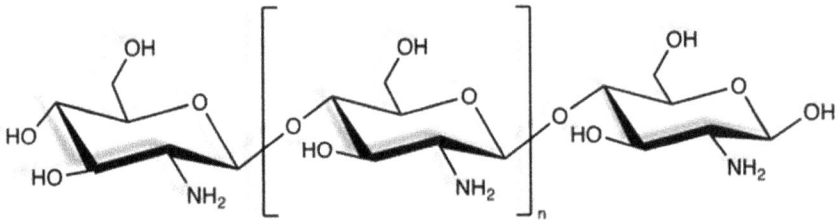

FIGURE 8.2   Chitosan chemical structure.

Several injectable chitosan-based hydrogels have been developed for cartilage repair (Choa et al., 2004; Hong et al., 2007; Chena and Chen, 2006). These hydrogels can be prepared by both physical and chemical cross-linking methods. In particular, reversible physical interactions in poly(N-isopropylacrylamide) (PNIPAM)- or polyethylene glycol (PEG)-grafted chitosan derivatives have been used to obtain physically cross-linked hydrogels (Bhattarai et al., 2005; Berger et al., 2004). These physical gels are generally characterized by a low stability, low mechanical strength, and rapid degradation. Chemically cross-linked injectable chitosan hydrogels are prepared using redox-initiated cross-linking (Hong et al., 2006) and photo-initiated cross-linking (Amsden et al., 2006). Furthermore, the properties of these chemically cross-linked hydrogels such as gelation time, gel modulus, and hydrogel degradability can be tuned by changing the molecular weight of polymers and the cross-linking densities. In fact, Hong et al. (2007) reported the preparation of methacrylated chitosan-based hydrogels using ammonium persulfate and N,N,N',N'-tetramethylethylenediamine with increased concentration of the initiator. Consequently, the gelation time could be reduced and the enzymatic degradation of the resulting hydrogels could be decreased.

Naderi-Meshkin et al. (2014) proposed the synthesis of a chitosan-beta glycerophosphate-hydroxyethyl cellulose (CH-GP-HEC) scaffold with a sol–gel transition at 37 °C. Chondrogenic factors or mesenchymal stem cells

(MSCs) were included in the hydrogel. Subsequently, in order to correct the defects of the cartilage tissue, the CH-GP-HEC hydrogel was injected into the lesion site and the viability of the encapsulated MSCs was assessed by coloring with iodide-fluorescein diacetate and propidium. After inducing a differentiation process with the growth factor tβ3, the chondrogenic differentiation capacity of the encapsulated human MSC (hMSC) was determined. These cells, inserted inside the CH-GP-HEC hydrogel, showed excellent survival and proliferation rates during the 28 days of observation. The CH-GP-HEC hydrogel also provided suitable conditions for chondrogenic differentiation of the encapsulated hMSCs.

Another interesting study was proposed in 2014 by Choi et al. They investigated the incorporation of type II collagen (Col II) and chondroitin sulfate (CS) in chitosan-based injectable hydrogels gelled after exposure, in the presence of riboflavin, to visible blue light (VBL). Infact, Col II and CS are components of the cartilage ECM that play a crucial role in chondrogenesis. Unfortunately, the direct use of scaffolds for cartilage regeneration is limited due to their instability and rapid enzymatic degradation. For this reason, Choi and collaborators thought of incorporating Col II and CS into a chitosan hydrogel. Since the unmodified hydrogel was able to promote the multiplication and placement of cartilaginous ECMs allowed by encapsulated chondrocytes and MSCs, the idea of incorporating Col II or CS into the chitosan hydrogels has contributed to increasing the process of chondrogenesis, especially by Col II. This is attributable to the binding of integrin α10 to Col II, which promoted an increased cell-matrix adhesion, thus favoring the cartilage regeneration.

In 2018, Wu et al. obtained PNIPAM-g-chitosan injectable and thermosensitive hydrogel characterized by the absence of toxicity. They are characterized by high biocompatibility, biodegradability and, after injection, show a rapid phase transition, therefore are ideal candidates as vectors of cells or implanted scaffolding. In order to strengthen its mechanical properties, Wu and collaborators have thought of covalently bonding thiol side chains in chitosan through the conjugation of *N*-acetylcysteine by carbodiimide. After oxidation of the thiols in disulfide bonds, the hydrogels showed a better compression modulus.

Through *in vitro* proliferation studies, a great biocompatibility of hydrogels toward MSCs, fibroblasts, and osteoblasts has been shown allowing the encapsulation of cells without toxicity. These results suggested the potentiality of the thiol-modified thermosensitive polysaccharide hydrogels as cell-laden biomaterial for tissue regeneration.

An interesting work was also proposed by Xu and collaborators in 2018. They made a biodegradable composite carboxymethyl chitosan (CMCS) hydrogel conductive by in situ chemical polymerization using poly(3,4-ethylendioxythiophene) (PEDOT) as a conductive polymer layer. This hydrogel has proven to be potentially useful for nerve tissue engineering. In dependence of the different contents of PEDOT, the physicochemical and electrochemical properties of the conductive hydrogels (PEDOT/CMCS) were analyzed. In addition, *in vitro* studies have shown the lack of toxicity of the PEDOT/CMCS hydrogels, the adhesive capacity, the viability, and cell proliferation. In particular, after a culture for 9 days, the PEDOT layer of the conductive hydrogels improved the diffusion and proliferation of pheochromocytoma cells in rat-like neurons even in the absence of electrical stimulation. Furthermore, the inclusion of PEDOT in the CMCS hydrogels allowed the hydrogel to have both greater mechanical strength and conductivity and to preserve their biocompatibility. These results suggested the use of these conductive hydrogels (PEDOT/CMCS) as nerve regeneration scaffold materials. An injectable chitosan-based hydrogel, useful for bone tissue engineering, was developed by Saekhor and colleagues. In particular, they wanted to obtain a water-soluble and thixotropic chitosan particularly useful as an injectable liquid with the ability to form a hydrogel under physiological conditions. For this reason, chitosan was reacted with carboxymethyl chloride to obtain CMCS. The latter was conjugated with α-cyclodextrin (α-CD) to produce CMCSCD. This conjugation improved the solubility, in knowledge, of the hydrophobic cavity to produce as cross-linking points by forming an inclusion complex with PEG. The sol–gel transition was formed within 450 ± 10 min to obtain a complete (yellow) soft gel. Through the scanning electron microscope, both the surface and cross-section were observed, showing an interconnected porous structure of the gel, making it suitable for transport of extracellular fluid and nutrients and hormones to cells and waste removal. Moreover, *in vitro* experiment with sarcoma osteogenic (SaOS-2) cell line indicated that this injectable hydrogel was potentially compatible, nontoxic to the SaOS-2 cells, and capable to promote cell proliferation. On the basis of all obtained results, the CMCSCD/PEG demonstrated to be a promising scaffold for bone tissue engineering. Very recently also, Nezhad-Mokhtari et al. have developed a new injectable hydrogel based on collagen, aldehyde modified-nanocrystalline cellulose, and chitosan loaded with gold nanoparticles (collagen/ADH-CNCs/CS-Au) for tissue engineering applications (Nezhad-Mokhtari et al., 2020). In particular, solutions of collagen/CS-Au and ADH-CNCs were mixed resulting in an intermacromolecular Schiff base cross-linking reaction, obtaining a rapid formation of the hydrogel. With the aim to control the microscopic morphology, swelling degree, gelation time, and degradation rate, various molar blending ratio of collagen/CNCs/CS-Au were used. The MTT assay, performed with mouse fibroblast cells (NIH 3T3), highlighted the effectiveness and nontoxicity of the obtained hydrogel. In addition, the reinforcing with the addition of CNCs and CS-Au, to form the hydrogel, was an interesting approach to improve the mechanical strength and degradation resistance of the scaffold. It could be concluded that also this hydrogel may be a good candidate as a new biomaterial for tissue engineering applications.

8.2.2   CELLULOSE

Cellulose (Figure 8.3) is a glucose polysaccharide that has a straight chain consisting of several (1–4) linked D-glucose units. It is the most plentiful biopolymer on earth and found in the cell wall of green plants, many algae, and other microorganisms such as oomycetes or bacteria (Novotna et al., 2013).

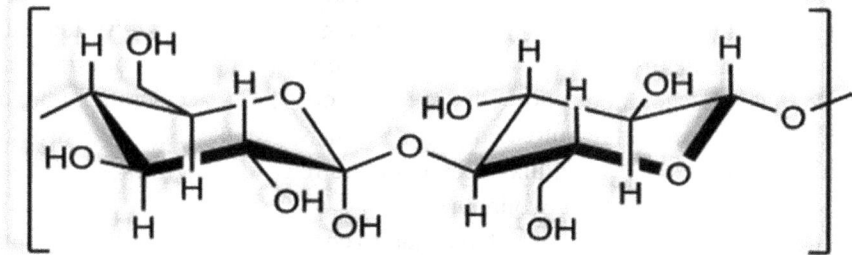

FIGURE 8.3   Cellulose chemical structure.

Bacterial cellulose (BC) is an interesting material as implant and scaffold in tissue engineering (Peterson and Gatenholm, 2011). In fact, it is notable for biocompatibility, mechanical resistance, and ability to be structurally and chemically engineered at nano-, micro-, and macroscales. BC hydrogels are promising materials for making dressings thanks to its properties such as purity, maintaining adequate humidity, and flexibility in adapting to any wound, forming a tight barrier between the wound itself and the external environment, thus avoiding bacterial infections (Valle et al., 2017).

Cellulose (CB) hydrogels can be obtained from pure and native cellulose by dissolving with LiCl/dimethylacetamide (DMAc), *N*-methylmorpholine-*N*-oxide (NMMO), ionic liquids (ILs), alkalis/urea (or thiourea), or producing them from BC (Shen et al., 2016). Cellulose derivatives usually include esters such as cellulose acetate phthalate (CAP) [e.g., cellulose acetate (CA), cellulose acetate trimellitate], hydroxypropyl methylcellulose phthalate, cellulose acetate butyrate (CAB), or ethers [e.g., methyl cellulose (MC), ethyl cellulose (EC), hydroxyethyl cellulose (HEC), carboxymethyl cellulose (CMC), sodium carboxymethyl cellulose (NaCMC), hydroxypropyl cellulose, and hydroxypropyl methylcellulose (HPMC)]. Other types of hydrogel are constituted from mixtures of natural polymers, polyvinyl alcohol, polyelectrolyte complexes, interpenetrating polymer network, and inorganic hybrid cellulose hydrogels (Chang and Zhang, 2011; Onofrei and Filimon, 2016; Sannino et al., 2009). These hydrogels are being studied for possible biomedical applications and, in particular, in tissue engineering (Kabir et al., 2018).

The capacity of a hydrogel made of BC/acrylic acid (AA) to release human epidermal keratinocytes and dermal fibroblasts (DFs), useful for the full-thickness skin lesions treatment, was evaluated by Loh and collaborators (Loh et al., 2018). Through *in vitro* studies, they proved the excellent cell attachment of the BC/AA hydrogel, the maintaining of cell viability with a narrow migration, and allowing a cell transfer. *In vivo* studies, histological, immunohistochemistry, and transmission electron microscopy analysis indicated that hydrogel alone and hydrogel with cells (HCs) accelerated wound healing compared to the untreated controls. Therefore, the BC/AA hydrogel could be an interesting cellular vector for the release of keratinocytes and fibroblasts, thus promoting wound healing.

In the same year, Boyer et al. have made a composite hydrogel containing a small amount of nanoreinforced clay, called laponite, which can stick within the hydroxypropyl methylcellulose (Si-HPMC) silicate hydrogel structure. Therefore, composite hydrogels were made by mixing laponites with Si-HPMC thus, developing a hybrid interpenetrating network that increased their mechanical properties. The *in vitro* investigations showed no side effects from the laponites. Furthermore, through *in vivo* studies, conducted for 6 weeks using nude mice, the capacity of the hybrid scaffold, made with composite hydrogel and chondrogenic cells, to form cartilage tissue was evaluated. Histological studies showed that the new cartilage-like tissue was characterized by an ECM including glycosaminoglycans (GAGs) and collagens. These results indicated the possibility of using the composite hydrogel for the treatment of cartilage defects. With the aim to obtain a biomaterial to treat tissue defects, Ghorbani and Roshangar have prepared and characterized injectable hydrogels based on collagen and modified nanocrystalline cellulose [cellulose nanocrystals (CNCs)] (Ghorbani and Roshangar, 2019). The surface of CNCs was functionalized with aldehyde groups using an oxidation manner of nanocrystalline cellulose in water with sodium periodate. The surface morphology of hydrogels with different ratios of CNCs has been analyzed evaluating the macroscopic physical properties and microscopic internal structure. Swelling tests showed that the hydrogels maintain their structure over the course of 60 days and were, thus, suitable for longer term applications. The results of toxicity studies for CNCs, aldehyde-modified CNCs, and the CNC-reinforced hydrogels support the potential application of these materials for biomedical applications.

Recently, Li et al. have proposed a green and simple method to prepare a series of all-natural chitosan-dialdehyde bacterial cellulose (CS-DABC) hydrogels. In particular, for the first time, to prepare these hydrogels, was used ascorbic acid as solvent to dissolve chitosan and the natural fiber DABC as reinforcing and cross-linking agent (Li et al., 2020). The disadvantage of the use of acetic acid and other toxic cross-linking agents was bypassed making these hydrogels biocompatible. Moreover, due to the supporting of DABC nanofibers and introduction of dynamic balance of the Schiff base structure in the cross-linked network, these hydrogels exhibited good mechanical properties, self-healing ability, and injectability. Consequently, these hydrogels can be used as good sustained release systems of drugs to promote wound healing indicating great potential in the field of wound dressings or tissue engineering. Among the latest interesting research on cellulose-based hydrogels for tissue engineering applications, there is the work of Gupta and his collaborators (2020). They proposed a green synthesis to prepare nanoparticles using eco-friendly chemicals such as silver, a broad spectrum natural antimicrobial substance, and curcumin a natural polyphenol with healing properties. The hydrophobicity of curcumin was bypassed by its microencapsulation in hydroxypropyl-cyclodextrins, which, in turn, were then loaded into BC hydrogels. These hydrogels demonstrated broad-spectrum antimicrobial activity against three common pathogenic microbes that infect wounds such as *Staphylococcus aureus*, *Pseudomonas aeruginosa*, and *Candida auris*. They showed also with antioxidant properties, high cytocompatibility, with the tested cell lines. In addition, the high moisture content and the good level of transparency of the hydrogels indicated a possible application in the management of chronic wounds with high microbial bioburden.

8.2.3 ALGINATE

Alginate (Figure 8.4) is a natural anionic and hydrophilic polysaccharide typically obtained from brown seaweed and bacteria. It contains blocks of β-(1→4)-linked-D-mannuronic acid (M) and α-(1→4)-linked-L-guluronic acid (G) monomers (Figure 8.4). Alginate is interesting for many biomedical applications due to its excellent biocompatibility, low toxicity, low cost, and for its ability to gel in the presence of bivalent cations such as Ca^{2+} (Langer and Vacanti, 1993; Lee and Mooney, 2012). In particular, alginate hydrogels have a structural resemblance to the extracellular matrices of living tissues. In fact, alginate-based treatments could maintain a physiologically moist microenvironment, minimize bacterial infection at the wound site, and facilitate healing.

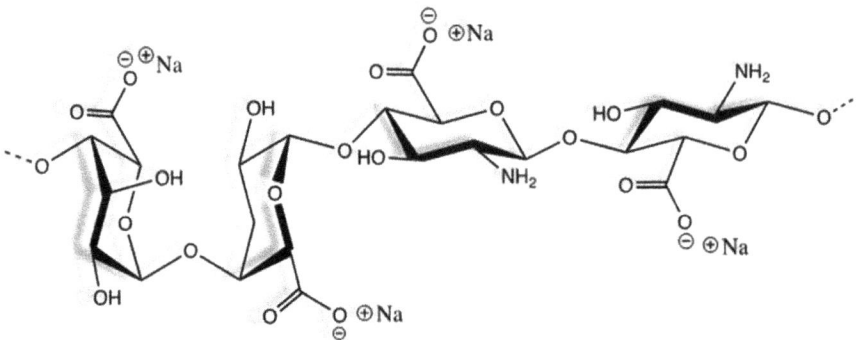

FIGURE 8.4   Alginate chemical structure.

Furthermore, alginate is an appropriate material for several tissue engineering applications such as cell encapsulations and biofabrications (Li et al., 2006; Song at al., 2011). Nevertheless, alginate is not able to promote cell attachment due to poor cell–material interactions, causing slow degradation with unfavorable degradation kinetics (Gao et al., 2009). To overcome these drawbacks, specific proteins have been considered for their similarity to the ECM to enhance cellular interaction and to improve degradability, biocompatibility, and the availability of alginate hydrogel (Wang and Shansky, 2012).

To this aim, Silva et al. (2014) developed a hybrid hydrogel based on alginate and keratin extracted from wool. This hydrogel was made in 2D and 3D conformations and was characterized by chemical–physical analyses. Studies on primary human umbilical vein endothelial cells have also been performed to highlight the ability of these hybrid hydrogels to promote cell attachment, proliferation, diffusion, and viability. It has been shown that the cells seeded on the 2D hydrogel surface remained viable for up to 10 days of culture, forming a monolayer and showing the typical endothelial morphology, instead the encapsulated cells remained viable for up to 4 weeks. During this culture time, the number and mitochondrial activity of the cells increased and the cells started to propagate. Hence, hybrid alginate/keratin hydrogels could be promising biomaterial for regenerative medicine applications.

In 2017, Chen et al. developed a drug-loaded hydrogel, produced using ion cross-linking, for use in oral bone tissue regeneration (Chen et al., 2017). This hydrogel was made of calcium alginate at different concentrations (12.5, 25, and 50 mg/mL) and displayed a high plastic behavior and biological properties suitable for promoting the regeneration of oral bone tissue. The swelling degree, degradation time, and release rate of bovine serum albumin were also assessed. Human periodontal ligament cells and bone marrow stromal cells were maintained in culture together with calcium alginate hydrogen and polylactic acid as control and then the cellular proliferation was examined. Inflammatory-related factor gene expressions of human periodontal ligament cells and osteogenesis-related gene expressions of bone marrow stromal cells were observed. The materials, implanted in the subcutaneous tissue of the rabbits, showed a favorable biocompatibility. The results of the studies demonstrated that calcium alginate hydrogels caused less inflammation than the polylactic acid and had superior osteoinductive bone ability to the polylactic acid. The drug-loadable calcium alginate hydrogel system could represent an interesting approach for bone defect reparation and, thus, useful in clinical dental applications.

With the aim to verify the mineralization and differentiation potential of human dental pulp stem cells (DPSCs) seeded onto scaffolds based on alginate and nanohydroxyapatite, it has been previously described and evaluated by Turco et al (2009). Sancilio and collaborators (2018), in their work, made use of hydroxyapatite (HAp) as inorganic strengthening and osteoconductive element of alginate/HAp composite scaffolds. These scaffolds are actually valued as possible strategy in bone tissue engineering because they can efficiently support the adhesion, colonization, and matrix deposition of osteoblast-like cells without any supplementary chemical alginate modification.

In particular, Sancilio and collaborators inserted the HAp in an alginate solution and the internal gelation was generated by the addition of delta-lactone of the D-gluconic acid which induced the slow hydrolysis of the acid with consequent direct calcium ion release from HAp. Human DPSCs are clonogenic cells capable of differentiating in multiple lineages. To this end, the components of the ECM, the vitality parameters, and oxidative stress, as well as the gene expression profile of the markers related to both early and late mineralization process, were assessed and analyzed.

So, Sancilio et al. have demonstrated that DPSCs expressed osteogenic differentiation-related markers and promoted calcium deposition and biomineralization when growing onto alginate/HAp scaffolds. Therefore, these alginate/HAp scaffolds have proven to be composite materials suitable for tissue engineering, as they are able to promote specific tissue regeneration as well as the formation of mineralized matrices and the regeneration of natural bone.

More recently, Reakasame and Boccaccini described, in their review, the possibility of using oxidized alginate (OA)-based hydrogels that have drawn considerable importance as a biodegradable material for tissue engineering applications due to the higher degradation rate and the presence in OA of more reactive groups than native alginate (Reakasame and Boccaccini, 2018). So, the OA-based hydrogel could be successfully used in various engineering tissue applications such as repair of bone, cartilage, cornea, blood vessel, and other soft tissues. With the aim to mimic the complex inorganic/organic structure of bone, Diaz-Roriguez et al. synthesized new biomimetic hydrogels based on mineralized calcium alginate following the addition of biomineral calcium carbonate microparticles obtained from mussels or oysters (OYs) shells. This innovative strategy also has the advantage of exploiting natural components, since alginate would have the function of forming the biodegradable polymer matrix while the calcium carbonate stimulating cell differentiation by mimicking the nanostructure of the tissue. Alginate hydrogels containing 7 mg/mL of OY particles promoted the osteogenic differentiation of hMSCs. Thus, the incorporation of calcium carbonate particles in alginate networks was able to modulate cell differentiation. Furthermore, the presence of calcium carbonate in alginate matrix could improve long-term stability of alginate hydrogels. So, Roriguez et al. highlighted the importance of the type of alginate and the origin of calcium carbonate to obtain valid systems for the engineering of bone tissue capable of modulating both mechanical properties and cell differentiation.

In 2019, Homaeigohar et al. functionalized graphite nanofilaments to get better, mechanical, electrical, and biological properties of an alginate hydrogel and accelerated nerve regeneration. CA functionalization by a green and simple approach permitted to induce the formation of oxygen containing functional groups on the surface of graphite nanofilaments, thereby ensuring their uniform distribution within the alginate matrix. Its biocompatibility has even been enhanced as shown by the use of *in vitro* MSCs. The uniformly distributed nanofilaments increased the mechanical stability of the nanocomposite hydrogel compared to pure one by up to three times. Furthermore, the nanofilaments were able to give electrical contact and intercellular signaling stimulating their biological activity. *In vivo* tests highlighted the applicability of the nanocomposite hydrogel for implantation within body showing no adverse reaction and no inflammatory responses after 2 weeks after its implant. The obtained results demonstrated that the electroactive nanocomposite hydrogel, stimulating nerve generation, could be potentially useful for neural tissue engineering applications.

In 2020, Shafei and coworkers designed and realized an alginate-based hydrogel loaded with exosomes (EXOs), nano-size membrane vesicles isolated from cultured adipose-derived stem cells that could promote migration, proliferation, and angiogenesis process in skin wound through modulation of the secretory activity of DFs and could improve the synthesis and secretion of collagen/elastin with a better re-epithelialization (Shafei et al., 2020). The degradability evaluation of EXOs-loaded hydrogel and cell viability studies confirmed the favorable properties of hydrogel for *in vitro* and *in vivo* applications. Moreover, the release of EXO from alginate hydrogel indicated that this structure was suitable for controlled release of small bioactive molecules including secreted EXO derivatives and growth factors. Consequently, alginate hydrogel could enhance wound closure, collagen synthesis, and vessel formation in the wound area and it could represent a good therapeutic strategy for skin wounds healing. Recently, Ehterami and collaborators also developed a vitamin D3-loaded alginate hydrogel for wounds healing. Various vitamin D3 concentrations were added to sodium alginate and cross-linked by calcium carbonate in combination with D-gluconolactone. The swelling behavior, weight loss, microstructure, and cyto- and hemocompatibility of obtained hydrogels were assessed. Furthermore, the therapeutic efficacy of prepared materials was evaluated in the full-thickness dermal wound model. The hydrogels study through scanning electron microscopy (SEM) showed their highly porosity and the presence of interconnected pores. In addition, the hydrogels resulted in biodegradable (being its weight loss percentage of about 89% in 14 days) hemo- and cytocompatible. In particular, *in vivo* studies indicated that the alginate hydrogel/3,000 IU vitamin D3 exhibited more highest capacity of wound closure, best performance, and induced highest re-epithelialization and granular tissue formation. These results indicated that alginate hydrogels with 3000 IU of vitamin D3 could be useful as a dressing to treat skin wounds (Ehterami et al., 2020).

8.2.4   HYALURONIC ACID

Hyaluronic acid (HA) (Figure 8.5) is a GAG, composed by repeating disaccharide units of *N*-acetyl-D-glucosamine and D-glucuronic acid, and synthesized in bacteria, birds, and mammals.

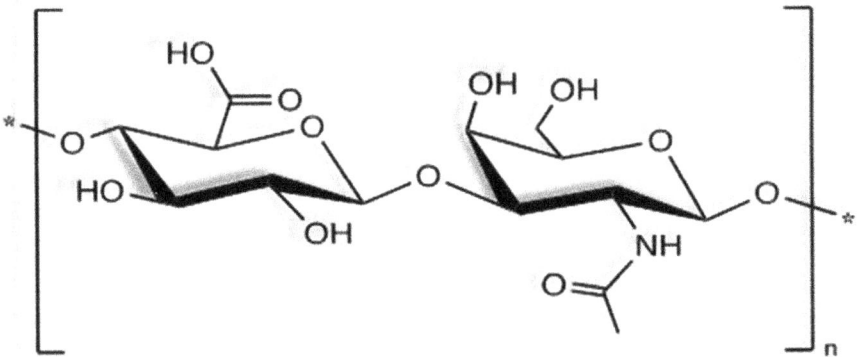

FIGURE 8.5   Hyaluronic acid chemical structure.

It is found in the body in pericellular matrices, various body fluids, and in specialized tissues such as the vitreous humor of the eye and cartilage. Its physical properties and viscoelastic behavior make HA a precious biomaterial thanks also to the ability of assembly into extracellular and pericellular matrices and its effects on cell signaling (Falcone et al., 2006). HA is characterized by physicochemical properties such as the solubility and the presence of reactive functional groups that allow chemical changes on HA, which makes it attractive for tissue regeneration. Furthermore, these materials do not cause allergies or inflammations and their hydrophilicity which make them particularly interesting also as injectable fillers via the skin and soft tissues (Hemshekhar et al., 2016; Trombino et al., 2019).

Tan et al. reported a new biodegradable and biocompatible hydrogels and composites derived from oxidized HA and water-soluble chitosan after mixing, without the addition, of a chemical cross-linking agent (Tan et al., 2011). Furthermore, the gelation was obtained by the Schiff base reaction between amino and aldehyde groups of polysaccharide derivatives. In particular, N-succinyl chitosan and aldehyde hyaluronic acid were synthesized to prepare composite hydrogel and its potential as an injectable scaffold was shown encapsulating the bovine articular chondrocyte. Therefore, the composite hydrogel promoted cell survival and cells were able to preserve the morphology of the chondrocytes. These characteristics suggested the possibility of using injectable composite hydrogels in tissue engineering.

In 2018, Sani et al. made a elastic, antimicrobial, and adhesive hydrogel composed of methacrylated HA (MeHA) and an elastin-like polypeptide (ELP), which can be rapidly photoreticulated in situ for the purpose of regenerating and repairing different tissues. Therefore, hydrogel hybrids with various physical properties have been designed and modifying the concentrations of MeHA and ELP. In addition, adhesion tests have shown that the MeHA/ELP hydrogels have a greater adhesive force toward the tissue than the commercial tissue adhesives. The incorporation of zinc oxide (ZnO) nanoparticles conferred antimicrobial properties to the hydrogel that inhibited the growth of methicillin-resistant *S. aureus* (MRSA) compared to controls. Furthermore, the MeHA/ELP hydrogels did not induce any significant inflammatory response. They could also be efficiently biodegraded by promoting the integration of new autologous tissue. In a recent paper, Rezaeeyazdi et al. described the preparation of several injectable cryogels based on HA and gelatin. Their idea was to combine both physicochemical characteristics of HA and intrinsic cell adhesion characteristics of gelatin, providing sufficient physical support for attachment, survival, and diffusion of cells. The physical characteristics of gelatin cryogels, such as mechanics and injection, have also improved after copolymerization with HA. The adhesion of mouse fibroblast cell lines (3T3), grown in HA cryogels, was increased when expressed with gelatin. In addition, the cryogels had a minimal effect on the activation of dendritic cells in the bone marrow, underlining their cytocompatibility. *In vitro* studies have shown that HA-copolymerized gelatin has not significantly changed their intrinsic biological characteristics, so the HA-cogelatin cryogels combine the favorable capacity of single biopolymer giving a strong system from the point of mechanical view, susceptible to cells, with macroporous and injectable structure and, therefore, interesting for tissue engineering applications.

Han et al. proposed a biocompatible and in situ cross-linkable hydrogel arised from HA. The hydrogel was obtained through a bioorthogonal reaction and tested for the regeneration of cartilage *in vivo*. The gelling reaction is attributable to copper-free click reactions between an azide and a dibenzyl cyclooctyne (DBCO). In particular, the HA-PEG4-DBCO hydrogel was synthesized and cross-linked through 4-arm PEG azide and the effects of the relationship between HA-PEG4-DBCO and PEG 4-arm azide on gelation time, microstructure, morphology superficial, balance swelling, and compression module were also evaluated. In order to evaluate the *in vitro* and *in vivo* capacity of the obtained hydrogel as injectable scaffold, chondrocytes were encapsulated inside it. The obtained results underlined how the hydrogel is capable of supporting cell survival and the cells able to regenerate cartilage tissue confirming the ability of the injectable hydrogel to be used in tissue engineering applications. In 2019, Luo et al. preapared two in situ injectable hydrogels made of gelatin (sc-G) and HA/gelatin (HA/G) for hemorrhage control. In particular, these materials were prepared by cross-linking gelatin and HA with N-(3-dimethylaminopropyl)-N'-ethylcarbodiimide hydrochloride (EDC) and N-hydroxysuccinimide on the surface of the tissue in situ and analyzed by rheological, stability, cytotoxicity, and burst resistance tests. Their hemostatic capacity was assessed in a bleeding rat model of the liver. The sc-G and HA/G hydrogels that were able to gel in the 90s and 50s, respectively, have been shown to be suitable for cell attachment and proliferation. Bursting forces was even greater than that of fibrin glue. The hemostatic power of the HA/G hydrogel was found to be better than that of the sc-G hydrogel and was comparable to that of fibrin. These results indicated a possible use in particular of HA/G hydrogel as tissue sealant for hemorrhage control in clinic. A remarkable study undertaken by Makvandi and coworkers reported the synthesis of thermosensitive and injectable hydrogels synthesis, containing tricalcium phosphate, HA, and corn silk extract-nanosilver (CSE-Ag NPs) for potential use in bone tissue regeneration applications. In particular, spherical silver nanoparticles were synthesized through a microwave-assisted green approach using corn silk extract without using toxic chemical reagents thus, making them more suitable for clinical and biomedical applications. Rheological experiments indicated that the thermosensitive hydrogels had gelification temperature (T_{gel}) close to body one. The samples containing silver had an antibacterial activity against several gram-positive and gram-negative bacterial strains without cytotoxicity after 24 h. In addition, MSCs inserted in the nanocomposite exhibited high bone differentiation indicating the use of this material as a potential scaffold for bone tissue regeneration. In the same period, Wang et al. developed and characterized a new injectable HA hydrogel functionalized with tyramine through dual-enzymatically cross-linked by horseradish peroxidase and galactose oxidase (GalOX). They evaluated the gelation time, swelling behavior, water content, mechanical strength, degradation rate, cytotoxicity *in vitro*, and immune response *in vivo*. The results of these analyses highlighted that the properties of hydrogel (HT) such as good injectability, favorable cytocompatibility to mice bone marrow mesenchymal stem cells, and low inflammatory response verified by cytotoxicity test *in vitro* and after *in vivo* subcutaneous injection *in vivo*. The authors suggested the possibility of adjusting gelation time, swelling behavior, and degradation rate of the HT hydrogel varying the concentrations of HT and GalOX in a determined range. These interesting results supported the use of these hydrogel for application in 3D stem cell culture and in tissue engineering.

8.3 PROTEIN-BASED BIOMATERIALS

Like polysaccharides, proteins are versatile macromolecules that perform essential functions in living systems in almost all biological processes. They are characterized by several interesting properties such as large-scale availability, low cost, biocompatibility, biodegradability, and chemical reactivity. Given their unique properties, proteins have been thoroughly used for the development of innovative materials for biomedical applications (Silva et al., 2018). Moreover, the mechanical and modifiable structural properties of protein-based hydrogels make these scaffolds interesting for tissue engineering and regeneration. With the use of protein structures, it is also possible to insert sequences that facilitate cell adhesion to the substrate and overall cell growth (Schloss et al., 2016). In this section, the most promising proteins-based materials, their properties, and applications in tissue engineeering are described.

8.3.1 COLLAGEN

Collagen (Figure 8.6) is the most abundant protein in animals. This fibrous protein consists of a right-handed bundle of three parallel and left-handed polyproline II helices. Twenty-eight different types of collagen composed of at least 46 distinct polypeptide chains that have been found in vertebrates and many other proteins also contain collagen domains (Shoulders and Raines, 2009).

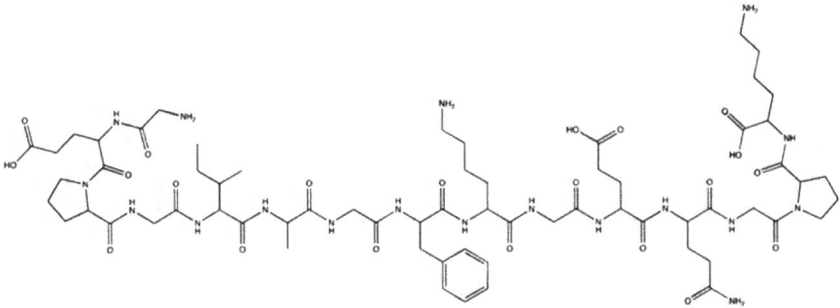

FIGURE 8.6   Collagen chemical structure.

This protein appealing in medical applications thanks to its presence in all connective tissue and its various properties such as: excellent biocompatibility and safety, biodegradability, and weak antigenicity. The protein contains specific cell adhesion domains including arginine-glycine-aspartic acid. After the integrin receptor on the cell surface binds to the RDG domain on the collagen molecule, cell adhesion is actively induced. The latter interaction allows the progression of cell growth as well as the differentiation and regulation of various cellular functions (Yamada et al., 2014). The main applications of collagen for tissue engineering concern bone substitutes, skin replacement, and artificial blood vessels and valves (Lee at al., 2001). Cahn et al. described a porous 3D collagen scaffold material with uniform pore size of 80 m to support capillary formation *in vitro* and favor the vascularization when implanted *in vivo* (Saunders and Ma, 2019). For the synthesis of the scaffolds, type I bovine collagen was utilized. *In vitro* scaffolds seeded with primary human microvascular endothelial cells suspended in human fibrin gel were able to form CD31-positive capillary-like structures. *In vivo*, following subcutaneous implantation in mice, the cell-free collagen scaffolds were vascularized by the host neovessels; in the meantime, there was a gradual degradation of the scaffold material for 8 weeks. Moreover, collagen scaffolds, filled with human fibrinogen gel, were implanted in the subcutaneous tissue inside a chamber that enclosed the femoral vessels of the rats. Subsequently, the angiogenic sprouts of the femoral vessels entered the scaffolds and these, after 4 weeks, entirely degraded. In the same model, collagen scaffolds seeded with stem cells derived from human adipose (ASC) produced greater increase in vascular volume compared to cell-free collagen scaffolds. In addition, the collagen scaffolds, obtained by Chan and collaborators, being also biocompatible, could be used to promote the growth of more strong vascularized tissue engineered grafts with a consequent better survival of the implanted cells.

In 2008, Nocera et al. proposed a collagen isolated printable from the bovine Achilles tendon and evaluated the purity of the collagen isolated by means of electrophoresis on sodium dodecyl sulfate gel and polyacrylamide. They discovered that the bands corresponded to α1, α2, and β chains possessed a little contamination from other small proteins. Collagen gels and solutions have been used to obtain scaffold by means of 3D printing. First, the researchers designed and manufactured an inexpensive 3D printer, then tested collagen printing, and made 3D-printed collagen scaffolds at pH 7. The scaffold porosity was excellent. After observation of the scaffolds microstructure, using SEM, a porous mesh of fibrillar collagen was observed. Moreover, the 3D-printed collagen scaffold was not cytotoxic with cell viability higher than 70% using Vero cell lines (derived from the kidney of an African green monkey) and fibrobalst NIH 3T3. *In vitro* tests with both cells lines showed that the collagen scaffolds had the capacity to favor the cell attachment and proliferation. Also, a new fibrillar collagen mesh was seen after 2 weeks of culture at 37°C. With the aim to treat patients with renal failure, Lee et al. investigated the possibility to inject collagen hydrogel in renal tissue. The collagen hydrogel was then injected into the kidneys of normal mice and rat kidneys with ischemia/reperfusion injury. Subsequently, the kidneys of both animal models were studied for up to 4 weeks to check for tissue response. The infiltrating host cells present in the injection regions expressed renal stem/progenitor cell markers as well as MSC markers. After this treatment, both glomeruli, significantly higher, were found in the injected regions compared to the normal regions of the renal cortex in both normal- and ischemic-injured kidneys. Furthermore, after the injection of collagen hydrogel, renal activity, after the ischemia/reperfusion injury, was regained. Therefore, the insertion of biomaterials into the kidney can be an excellent strategy to facilitate the regeneration of glomerular and tubular structures in normal and injured kidneys (Lee et al., 2018).

In 2019, Samadian and collaborators prepared and characterized a collagen hydrogel loaded with naringin as scaffold for peripheral nerve damage treatment. The microstructure, biodegradation, swelling behavior, and cyto-/hemocompatibility of the hydrogel were evaluated. Finally, the efficacy of the obtained hydrogel on the sciatic nerve crush injury was studied in the animal model. The characterization tests showed a porous structure of the hydrogel with the presence of interconnected pores and pore average size of 90 μm. The degradation tests proved that a loss of about 70% of the primary weight of the hydrogel after 4 weeks of storage. *In vitro* studies revealed a high cell proliferation on collagen/naringin hydrogel higher than the control group (tissue culture plate) at both 48 and 72 h after cell seeding and even significantly higher than pure collagen at 72 h.

Moreover, the animal study confirmed the positive effect of the proposed hydrogels on the healing of the induced nerve injury. All results showed that the prepared collagen/naringin hydrogel could be used as a sophisticated alternative to healing peripheral nerve damages.

In their study, Zhang et al. hypothesized that the use of an ECM collagen I hydrogel loaded with histone deacetylase 7 peptide 7-amino-acid-phosphorylated (7Ap) could hold back ventricular remodeling and improving heart function after heart attack and myocardial infarction (MI) (Zhang et al., 2019). In fact, the phosphorylated form of 7A (7Ap) was reported to promote in situ tissue repair via the mobilization and recruitment of endogenous stem cell antigen-1 positive (Sca-1) stem cells. In this study, an MI model was established through ligation of the left anterior descending coronary artery of C57/B6 mice. In particular, collagen I hydrogel loaded with 7Ap was injected intramyocardially into the infarcted region of the left heart wall. After local delivery, 7Ap collagen increased the formation of neomicrovessels, improved the recruitment and differentiation of antigen-1-positive stem cells, decreasing cell apoptosis, and promoting the progression of the cardiomyocyte cycle. Moreover, 7Ap collagen limited fibrosis in the left ventricle wall, reducing thinning of the infarcted area, and significantly improving cardiac efficiency 2 weeks after heart infart. These results indicated the positive impact of implanting 7Ap-collagen hydrogel as a novel constituent for the myocardial infarction treatment.

Recently, Nabavi et al. proposed an interesting strategy to stimulate bone regeneration, employing a type I collagen hydrogel entrapping tacrolimus, an immunosuppressant drug useful after organ transplantation to reduce the activity of the patient's immune system and, therefore, avoid the risk of organ rejection. For this reason, various amounts of tacrolimus (10 g/mL, 100 g/mL, and 1000 g/mL, respectively) were added to the hydrogel. The drug-loaded hydrogels were characterized. In particular, swelling capacity, porosity, weight loss, blood compatibility, cell proliferation, and drug release were evaluated. The obtained hydrogel, enclosed in a gelatin and polycaprolactone film, was put on the injured part of Wistar rats showing a high porosity and a sufficient degree of swelling, good drug release capacity, and fine hemocompatibility behavior. Also, *in vivo* studies enhanced the importance of the developed hydrogel for bone healing. Very interesting is also the study proposed by Nilforoushzadeh et al. that fabricated and characterized engineered collagen-fibrin-based scaffold to generate intrinsic microvasculature in a dermal and epidermal skin substitute to use in patients with hard to heal diabetic wounds. In particular, they characterized hydrogel evaluating the biological compatibility and cell proliferation, migration, and vitality in skin organotypic cell culture. The performance of the prevascularized hydrogel transplanted on five human subjects as an intervention group with diabetic wounds was analyzed and compared with nonvascularized skin grafts as a control on five patients. There was an important increase in skin thickness and density in the vascular beds of the hypodermis assessed by skin scanner respect to that in the control group. These preliminary data indicated that the hydrogel collagen-fibrin could be a good candidate for accelerating the healing process in patients with hard to heal diabetic wounds.

8.3.2   GELATIN

Gelatin (Figure 8.7) is a protein-based material derived from the hydrolysis of collagen. It is very useful in biomedical and pharmaceutical fields (Jain and Kumar, 2013; Tonsomboon et al., 2013) due to its biodegradable, biocompatible nature, low immunogenicity, and its commercial availability at low cost. The advantages include its solubility in aqueous systems, a sol–gel transition at 30 °C (Bohidar and Jena, 1994), and the possibilty to be cross-linked or modified with the inclusion of other materials to significantly alter its mechanical and biochemical properties (Jain and Kumar, 2013).

In their review, Soman et al. described the possibility to use gelatin methacrylamide as a gel-based system with tunable stiffness, which could be controlled without significantly changing its chemical composition. Generation of gelatin methacrylamide gels of different elastic moduli has been previously demonstrated (Nichol et al., 2010). These materials would be an effective tool for applications in ocular tissue engineering also on the basis of the result shown in other biomedical application such as cartilage repair (Medvedeva et al., 2018) generating blood vessels (Chen et al., 2012) and also cardiac tissue development. With the aim to find inexpensive skin substitutes useful in patients with burn injuries and chronic wounds, Nicholas et al. developed a hydrogel cellularized (PG-1) by using two polymers, pullulan, an economic antioxidant polysaccharide and gelatin. After inserting human fibroblasts and keratinocytes onto PG-1, a cellularized bilayer skin substitute was gained. This new cellularized PG-1 was compared *in vivo* to one acellular and no hydrogel (control) by means of a mouse excisional skin biopsy

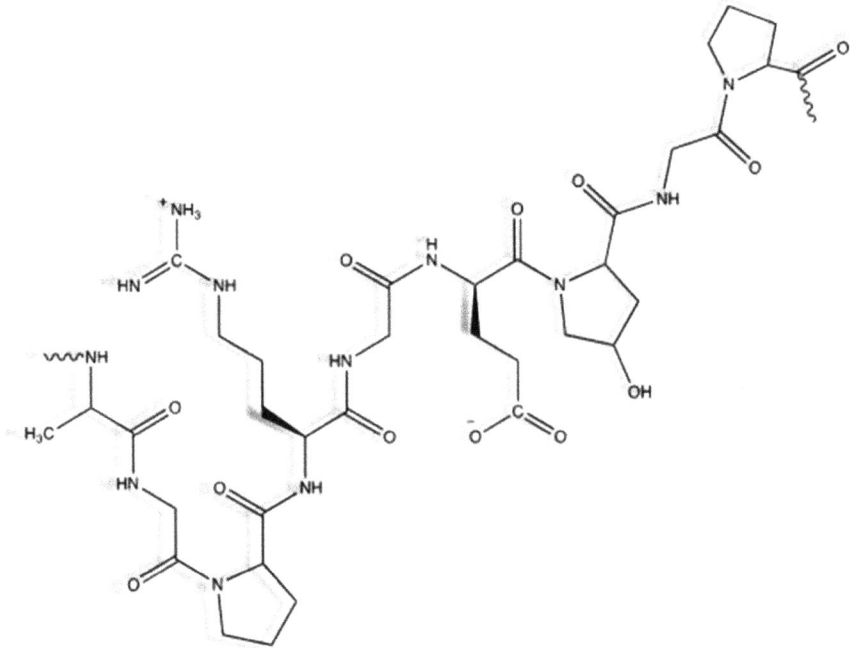

FIGURE 8.7   Gelatin chemical structure.

template. PG-1 showed an average pore size of 61.69 μm with an ideal elastic modulus, swelling behavior, and biodegradability. In addition, the excellent viability, proliferation, differentiation, and morphology of skin cells were evaluated by means of *in vivo*/dead assays, 5-bromo-2′-deoxyuridine proliferation assays, and confocal microscopy. Immunohistochemical analyses of excisional wounds treated with cellularized PG-1 showed the formation of a thicker newly formed skin with a higher presence of actively proliferating cells and incorporation of human cells than acellular or control PG-1. Excisional wounds treated with acellular or cellular hydrogels showed significantly less macrophage infiltration and increased angiogenesis 14 days after skin biopsy respect to control. All obtained results suggested that cellularized PG-1 could promote skin regeneration and wound healing. Dong et al. have designed an injectable PEG gelatin hydrogel with highly tunable properties to enhance stem cell retention useful for wound healing. The hydrogel was obtained from a multifunctional PEG-based hyperbranched polymer and a commercially available thiolated gelatin. This material showed a spontaneous gelation within about 2 min under the physiological condition. In addition, with the aim to support murine adipose-derived stem cells (ASCs) growth and maintain their stemness, Dong and coworkers incapsulated them into the PEG-gelatin hydrogel. Moreover, they tuned hydrogel mechanical properties, biodegradability, and cellular responses by changing the formulation and cell seeding densities. *In vivo* studies, with old female FVB mice, showed that in situ hydrogel improved significantly cell retention, enhances angiogenesis, and accelerates wound closure. The obtained results suggested that injectable PEG-gelatin hydrogel can be used for regulating stem cell behaviors in 3D culture, delivering cells for wound healing to overcome all the limitation of conventional nerve suturing methods such as scar tissue formation, the limited adhesive, and mechanical strength of fibrin-based adhesives. Soucy et al. have engineered composite neuro-supportive hydrogels with strong tissue adhesion. These composites were obtained by photocross-linking two natural polymers, gelatin-methacryloyl (GelMA) and methacryloyl-substituted tropoelastin (MeTro). These lasts are characterized by modifiable mechanical properties by varying the GelMA/MeTro ratio. Furthermore, GelMA/MeTro hydrogels showed 15-fold higher adhesive strength to nerve tissue ex vivo respect to fibrin control. Moreover, the composites were shown to support Schwann cell viability and proliferation as well as neurite extension and glial cell participation *in vitro*, which are essential cellular components for nerve regeneration. Therefore, subcutaneously implanted GelMA/MeTro hydrogels showed slower degradation *in vivo* respect to pure GelMA, suggesting its potential to support the growth of slowly regenerating nerves. Thus, GelMA/MeTro composites can be useful as clinically important biomaterials to regenerate nerves and reduce the need for microsurgical suturing during nerve reconstruction.

Recently, Contessi Negrini et al. obtained a 3D-printed hydrogel potentially useful for the regeneration of damaged or missing adipose tissue (AT). 3D-printed hydrogel scaffolds are characterized by macroscopic shape, microarchitecture, extracellular matrix-mimicking structure, degradability, and soft-tissue biomimetic mechanical properties that give them very interesting materials for AT reparation. The authors presented a simple and cost-effective 3D-printing strategy using gelatin-based ink to fabricate scaffolds idoneous for AT engineering. In particular, the ink was prepared by mixing gelatin and N,N'-methylenebisacrylamide as cross-linker to initiate the reaction. Subsequently, the solution was loaded in the cartridge, at 35 °C, of a pneumatic extrusion-based 3D printer and after printed on a cooled surface with a temperature of 4 °C, in an appropriate time for ink printability, as verified by rheological tests. The printed gelatin hydrogels were successively cross-linked at different temperatures to optimize their stability and fix the printed structure. The gelatin scaffolds remained stable for 21 days at physiological temperature, with compressive mechanical properties mimicking those of AT and they showed no indirect cytotoxic effects on a 3T3-L1 preadipocyte cell line. In addition, the printed scaffolds successfully promoted adhesion and proliferation of primary human preadipocytes. Moreover, *in vitro* tests showed no cytotoxic effects and the ability of the gelatin hydrogels to support adhesion, proliferation, and differentiation of primary human preadipocytes toward the adipogenic phenotype thus, demonstrating the potential of the 3D-printed gelatin hydrogels as scaffolds for AT engineering.

Ardhani et al. have developed a gelatin hydrogel membrane mimicking the physicochemical structure of the nerve and furnishing calcium ions in an axonal environment and useful for the regeneration of the nerves. This gelatin membrane has been modified with carbonated hydroxyapatite (CHA), similar in composition to human bone (Eliaz and Metoki, 2017). CHA has been incorporated for improving both the mechanical and scaffolding properties of the gelatin membrane that its stability in physiological conditions. In addition, this scaffold provided an intracellular controlled release to ensure a better axonal environment and promote nerve regeneration. The obtained gelatin membrane showed an ideal microstructure fundamental to prevent the regrowth of the fibrous tissue at the lesion site, allowing an adequate diffusion of glucose and specific proteins. Furthermore, the calcium release into the environment has favored neuronal growth, without suppressing the release of acetylcholine esterase and also the lengthening of neuritis was dramatically higher in the gelatin membrane incorporated with CHA. The preliminary obtained results encourage the use of this CHA-gelatin membrane as a medical device for nerve reconstruction.

8.3.3 ELASTIN

Elastin (Figure 8.8) is a key ECM protein that is fundamental for the elasticity and resilience of many vertebrate tissues including large arteries, lungs, ligaments, tendons, skin, and elastic cartilage (Daamen et al., 2007). This protein possesses a hydrophobic structure and is characterized by many interesting properties such as good elasticity, long-term stability, self-assembly, biocompatibility, and biodegradability. This can be applied in biomaterials in different forms such as insoluble fibers, hydrolyzed soluble form, recombinant tropoelastin (fragments), repeats of synthetic peptide sequences, and as block copolymers of elastin, possibly in combination with other biopolymers. It has recently gained attention in the field of biomedical materials and in particular as tissue engineering scaffolds, dermal substitutes, and other biomedical materials (Annabi et al., 2009).

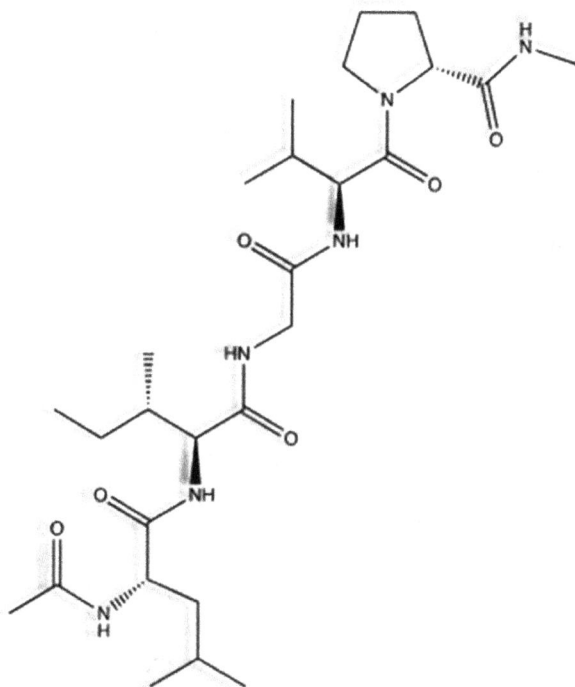

FIGURE 8.8   Elastin chemical structure.

Annabi et al. have proposed the possibility to make porous α-elastin hydrogels through high pressure CO_2 (Yamada et al., 2014). In particular, α-elastin was chemically cross-linked with hexamethylene diisocyanate that reacts with various functional groups in elastin such as lysine, cysteine, and histidine. High pressure CO_2 affected fabricated hydrogels properties. In fact, the pore size of the hydrogels was enhanced 20-fold when, for example, the pressure was increased from 1 to 60 bar. The swelling ratio of the samples fabricated by high pressure CO_2 resulted also higher compared to that the gels produced under atmospheric pressure. The compression modulus of α-elastin hydrogels was increased as the applied strain magnitude was modified from

40% to 80%. The compression modulus of hydrogels produced under high pressure CO_2 was threefold lower than the gels formed at atmospheric conditions due to the increased porosity of the gels produced by high pressure CO_2. The results obtained by Annabi and coworkers demontrated that the large pores within the 3D structures of these elastin-based hydrogels considerably promoted cellular penetration and growth throughout the matrices. Therefore, these hydrogels could be potentially useful for applications in tissue engineering. Although generally used collagen scaffolds have good biochemical properties, they are not beneficial due to their weak mechanical and physical properties. Several studies reported the realization of combined elastin scaffolds with other natural polymers such as HA, alginate, and collagen. Very recent is the work of Saniet et al. that realized an elastic, antimicrobial, and adhesive hydrogel composed of MeHA and an ELP as an adhesive and antimicrobial biomaterial characterized by a possibility to be rapidly photocross-linked in situ for the regeneration and repair of different tissues. So, hybrid hydrogels with a wide range of physical properties were engineered by modifying MeHA and ELP concentrations. Adhesion studies demonstrated that the MeHA/ELP hydrogels exhibited higher adhesive strength with respect to commercially tissue adhesives. Furthermore, through the incorporation of ZnO nanoparticles, MeHA/ELP hydrogels were also rendered antimicrobial and capable to significantly inhibit the growth of MRSA with respect to controls. Moreover, the composite adhesive hydrogels promoted *in vitro* mammalian cellular growth, spreading, and proliferation. *In vivo* subcutaneous implantation demonstrated that MeHA/ELP hydrogels did not elicit any significant inflammatory response and could be also biodegraded while promoting the integration of new autologous tissue.

With the aim to reinforce the collagen matrix, characterized by poor mechanical and physical properties, the collagen was linked with ELP to optimize the composite composition using a novel statistical method of response surface methodology (RSM) (Gurumurthy et al., 2018). In particular, a composite prepared using 6 mg/mL collagen and 18 mg/mL ELP showed an optimal combination of all three tensile properties. Physical properties of 6:18 mg/mL composite were compared to 6:0 mg/mL collagen-only hydrogel with a swelling ratio of differential scanning calorimetry and Fourier-transform infrared spectroscopy showed that ELP reduced the amount of residual water in the composites and highlighted the presence of collagen–ELP interactions. SEM images of the collagen-only hydrogel showed a porous and dense fibrillar in the collagen fibrillar microstructure, while the collagen-ELP composite showed a dense collagen microstructure with characteristic ELP aggregates. Therefore, due to the low water content and dense microstructure, the 6:18 mg/mL collagen-ELP composite exhibited advanced mechanical properties. These composites, prepared by Gurumurthy et al., have formed good quality rigid porous structures that are very useful in the field of tissue engineering.

Silva et al., in their study, produced and characterizated novel hybrid hydrogels based on alginate combined with elastin extracted from bovine neck ligament without the use of cross-linking agents. The properties of elastin were combined with the excellent chemical and mechanical stability of alginate. Two hybrid hydrogels were produced: 2D films obtained using sonication method and 3D microcapsules produced by pressure-driven extrusion. The complete physicochemical characterization demonstrated the positive effect of elastin on the key properties of the alginate-based hydrogels to obtain fibroblast attachment, proliferation, spreading, and viability. The alginate/E hybrid hydrogel can be promising biomaterial for soft-tissue regeneration and suitable for the production of engineering more complex scaffolds, for example, by 3D printing approaches.

Cipriani and collaborators evaluated injectable in situ cross-linkable elastin-like recombinamers (ELRs) to improve cartilage regeneration. ELRs are class of proteinaceous polymers bioinspired by natural elastin and designed using recombinant technologies. They realized both ELR-based hydrogel and ELR-based hydrogel incorporated with rabbit mesenchymal stromal cells (rMSCs) for the regeneration of subchondral defects. The performance of these hydrogel was evaluated *in vivo* in New Zealand rabbits. In particular, the cylindrical osteochondral defects were filled with an aqueous ELR solution and the rabbits were sacrificed after 4 months in order to make a histological evaluation of the biomaterial performance such as cell infiltration, the quality of the surrounding matrix, and the new matrix in defects. Both strategies favored cartilage regeneration, but in particular the hydrogel containing rMSC allowed adequate bone regeneration, while the ELR-based HA induced excellent regeneration of hyaline cartilage. These data suggested that the ELR-based bioactive hydrogel could improve cartilage regeneration both with and without rMSCs embedded supports infiltration and de novo matrix synthesis. In a very recent and interesting review, Sarangthem et al. have highlighted the advantageous role of ELPs for regeneration of skin injuries. Elastin derivatives, in particular, when applied to chronic wounds, can promote wound closure and improve the strength and flexibility of the healed area. They also can improve the healing process essential for restoration of skin's barrier function in short period after injury. Furthermore, the sol–gel transition of elastin derivatives allows complete coverage of wound area, protecting from external pathogens and incorporation of antibacterial components further accelerate the healing process.

8.4   FUTURE PROSPECTS

In the last year, the increase in the field of tissue engineering, especially in the production of biocompatible and biodegradable scaffolds, has allowed the regeneration of tissues with similar characteristics to their corresponding natural ones. However, despite the promising results obtained, much remains to be done so that materials with appropriate structure can be produced that allow the cells to spread in all its parts and to grow thanks to the right nutritional contribution. The production of a tissue ex novo requires significantly longer times compared to those for implanting a prosthesis or a traditional implant. Nevertheless, given the premises and the first results, investing in regenerative engineering, as demonstrated by the various literature data, here explained, represent the starting point for possible future applications and for the development of new technologies.

8.5   CONCLUSION

The design and application of biomaterials in tissue engineering have made great strides in the last years with extraordinary impact in various clinical applications. In particular, the development of new materials, of natural origin, has made it possible to improve the performance of the scaffolds, positively conditioning both the biological response, and the speed and quality of a new tissue proliferation. Therefore, in this chapter, various and interesting approaches, based on protein and carbohydrate hydrogels, are described, suggesting a very promising future for their application in tissue engineering.

KEYWORDS

- **biomaterials**
- **polysaccharides hydrogels**
- **proteins hydrogels**
- **tissue engineering applications**

REFERENCES

Amdsen, B. G., Sukarto, A., Knight, D. K. and Shapka, S. N. Methacrylated glycol chitosan as a photopolymerizable biomaterial. *Biomacromolecules*. **2007**, 8: 3758–3766.

Annabi, M., Mithieux, S. M., Boughton, E. A., Ruys, A. J., Weiss, A. S. and Dehghani, F. Synthesis of highly porous cross-linked elastin hydrogels and their interaction with fibroblasts *in vitro*. *Biomaterials*. **2009**, 8: 4550–4557.

Annabi, N., Mithieux, S. M., Weiss, A. S. and Dehghani, F. The fabrication of elastin-based hydrogels using high pressure CO$_2$. *Biomaterials*. **2009**, 2: 1–7.

Ardhani, R., Ana, I. D. and Tabata, Y. Gelatin hydrogel membrane containing carbonate hydroxyapatite for nerve regeneration scaffold. *J Biomed Mater Res*. **2020**, 3: 1–13.

Baranwal, A., Kumara, A., Priyadharshinib, A., Oggub, G. S., Bhatnagar, I., Srivastava, A. and Chandra, P. Chitosan: An undisputed biofabrication material for tissue engineering and biosensing applications. *Int J Biol Macromols*. **2018**, 110: 110–123.

Berger, J., Reist, M., Mayer, J. M., Felt, O. and Gurny, R. Structure and interactions in chitosan hydrogels formed by complexation or aggregation for biomedical applications. *Eur J Pharm Biopharm*. **2004**, 51: 35–52.

Bhattarai, N., Ramay, H. R., Gunn, J., Matsen, F. A. and Zhang, M. PEG-grafted chitosan as an injectable thermosensitive hydrogel for sustained protein release. *J Control Release*. **2005**, 103: 609–624.

Bohidar, H. B. and Jena, S. S. Study of sol-state properties of aqueous gelatin solutions. *J Chem Phys*. **1994**, 100: 6888–6895.

Boyer, C., Figueiredo, L., Pace, R., Lesoeur, J., Rouillon, T., LeVisage, C. et al. Laponite nanoparticle-associated silated hydroxypropylmethyl cellulose as an injectable reinforced interpenetrating network hydrogel for cartilage tissue engineering. *Acta Biomater*. **2018**, 65: 112–122.

Caló, E. and Khutoryanskiy, V. V. Biomedical applications of hydrogels: a review of patents and commercial products. *Eur Polym J*. **2015**, 65: 252–267.

Chan, E. C., Kuo, S. M., Kong, A. M., Morrison, W. A., Dusting, G. J., Mitchell, G. M. et al. Three-dimensional collagen scaffold promotes intrinsic vascularisation for tissue engineering applications. *PLoS One*. **2016**, 22: 1–22.

Chang, C. and Zhang, L. Cellulose-based hydrogels: present status and application prospects. *Carbohydr Polym*. **2011**, 84: 40–53.

Chen, F., Rousche, K. and Tuan, R. Technology insight: adult stem cells in cartilage regeneration and tissue engineering. *Nat Rev Rheumatol*. **2006**, 2: 373–382.

Chen, L., Shen, R., Komasa, S., Xue, Y., Jin, B., Hou, Y. et al. Drug-loadable calcium alginate hydrogel system for use in oral bone tissue repair. *Int J Mol Sci*. **2017**, 18: 989–1006.

Chen, Y. C., Lin, R. Z., Qi, H., Yang, Y., Bae, H., Melero-Martin, J. M. et al. Functional human vascular network generated in photocross-linkable gelatin methacrylate hydrogels. *Adv Funct Mater*. **2012**, 22: 2027–2039.

Choa, J. H., Kim, K. D., Park, K. D., Jung, M. C., Yang, W. I., Han, S. W. et al., Chondrogenic differentiation of human mesenchymal stem cells using a thermosensitive poly(*N*-isopropylacrylamide) and water-soluble chitosan copolymer. *Biomaterials*. **2004**, 25: 5743–5751.

Choi, B., Kim, S., Lin, B., Wu, B. M. and Lee, M. Cartilaginous extracellular matrix-modified chitosan hydrogels for cartilage tissue engineering. *ACS Appl Mater Interfaces*. **2014**, 6: 20110–20121.

Cipriani, F., Ariño Palao, B., Gonzalez de Torre, I., Vega Castrillo, A., Aguado Hernández, H. J., Alonso Rodrigo, M. et al. An elastin-like recombinamer-based bioactive hydrogel embedded with mesenchymal stromal cells as an injectable scaffold for osteochondral repair. *Regen Biomater.* **2016,** 6: 335–347.

Negrini, N. C., Celikkin, N., Tarsini, P., Farè, S. and Święszkowski, W. Three-dimensional printing of chemically cross-linked gelatin hydrogels for adipose tissue engineering. *Biofabrication.* **2020,** 12: 025001–025017.

Croisier, F. and Jérôme, C. Chitosan-based materials for tissue engineering. *Eur Polym J.* **2013,** 49: 780–792.

Daamen, W. F., Veerkamp, J. H., Van Hest, J. C. and Van Kuppevelt, T. H. Elastin as a biomaterial for tissue engineering. *Biomaterials.* **2007,** 28: 4378–4398.

Diaz-Rodriguez, P., Garcia-Triñanes, P., Echezarret Lópezd M. M., Santoveña, A. and Landina, M. Mineralized alginate hydrogels using marine carbonates for bone tissue engineering applications. *Carbohydr Polym.* **2018,** 195: 235–242.

Dong, Y., Sigen A., Rodrigues, M., Li, X., Kwon, S. H., Kosaric, N. et al. Injectable and tunable gelatin hydrogels enhance stem cell retention and improve cutaneous wound healing. *Adv Funct Mater.* **2017,** 27: 1606619–1606631.

Ehterami, A., Salehi, M., Farzamfar, S., Samadian, H., Vaez, A., Sahrapeyma, H. et al. A promising wound dressing based on alginate hydrogels containing vitamin D3 cross-linked by calcium carbonate/D-glucono-δ-lactone. *Biomed Eng Lett.* **2020,** 3: 309–319.

Eliaz, N. and Metoki, N. Calcium phosphate bioceramics: a review of their history, structure, properties, coating technologies, and biomedical applications. *Materials.* **2017,** 10: 1–104.

Falcone, S. J., Palmeri, D. and Berg, R. A. Biomedical applications of hyaluronic acid. In: Polysaccharides for Drug Delivery and Pharmaceutical Applications. 2006, 8: 155–174.

Gao, C., Liu, M., Chen, J. and Zhang, X. Preparation and controlled degradation of oxidized sodium alginate hydrogel. *Polym Degrad Stability.* **2009,** 94: 1405–1410.

Ghorbani, M. and Roshangar, L. Construction of collagen/nanocrystalline cellulose-based hydrogel scaffolds: synthesis, characterization, and mechanical properties evaluation. *Int J Polym Mater Biomat.* **2019,** 3: 1563–1535.

Greenwald, C. R. A. A., Josephson, S., Diamond, H. S. and Tsang, A. Human cartilage lysozyme. *J Clin Invest.* **1972,** 51: 2261–2270.

Gupta, A., Briffa, S. M., Swingler, S., Gibson, H., Kannappan, V., Adamus, G. et al. Synthesis of silver nanoparticles using curcumin-cyclodextrins loaded into bacterial cellulose-based hydrogels for wound dressing applications. *Biomacromolecules.* **2020,** 21: 1802–1811.

Gurumurthy, B., Griggs, J. A. and Janorkar, A. V. Optimization of collagen-elastin-like polypeptide composite tissue engineering scaffolds using response surface methodology. *J Mech Behav Biomed Mater.* **2018,** 84: 116–125.

Han, S. S., Yoon, H. Y., Yhee, J. Y., Cho, M. O., Shim, H. E., Jeong, J. E. et al. In situ cross-linkable hyaluronic acid hydrogels using copper-free click chemistry for cartilage tissue engineering. *Polym Chem.* **2018,** 9: 20–27.

Hemshekhar, M., Thushara, R. M., Chandranayaka, S., Sherman, L. S., Kemparaju, K. and Girish, K. S. Emerging roles of hyaluronic acid bioscaffolds in tissue engineering and regenerative medicine. *Int J Biol Macromol.* **2016,** 86: 917–928.

Homaeigohar, S., Tsai, T. Y., Young, T. H., Yang, H. Y. and Ji, Y. R. An electroactive alginate hydrogel nanocomposite reinforced by functionalized graphite nanofilaments for neural tissue engineering. *Carbohydr Polym.* **2019,** 224: 115112–115123.

Hong, Y., Mao, Z., Wang, H., Gao, G. and Shen, J. Covalently cross-linked chitosan hydrogel formed at neutral pH and body temperature. *J Biomed Mater Res Part A*. **2006,** 79: 913–922.

Hong, Y., Song, H., Gong, Y., Mao, Z., Gao, C. and Shen, J. Covalently cross-linked chitosan hydrogel: properties of *in vitro* degradation and chondrocyte encapsulation. *Acta Biomater.* **2007,** 3: 23–31.

Howard, D., Lee Buttery, D., Shakesheff, K. M. and Roberts, S. J. Tissue engineering: strategies, stem cells, and scaffolds. *J Anat.* **2008,** 213: 66–72.

Jain, E. and Kumar, A. Disposable polymeric cryogel bioreactor matrix for therapeutic protein production. *Nat Protoc.* **2013,** 8: 821–835.

Kabir, S. M. F., Sikdar, P. P., Haque, B., Bhuiyan, M. A. R., Ali, A. and Islam, M. N. Cellulose-based hydrogel materials: chemistry, properties, and their prospective applications. *Prog Biomater.* **2018,** 7: 153–174.

Saekhor, K., Udomsinprasert, W., Honsawek, S. and Tachaboonyakia, W. Preparation of an injectable modified chitosan-based hydrogel approaching for bone tissue engineering. *Int J Biol Macromol.* **2019,** 123: 167–173.

Khan, F. and Ahmad, S. R. Polysaccharides and their derivatives for versatile tissue engineering application. *Macromol Biosci.* **2013,** 13: 395–421.

Langer, R. and Vacanti, J. P. Tissue engineering. *Science.* **1993,** 260: 920–926.

Lee, J. H. and Kim, H. W. Emerging properties of hydrogels in tissue engineering. *J Tissue Eng.* **2018,** 9: 1–4.

Lee, K. Y. and Mooney, D. J. Hydrogels for tissue engineering. *Chem Rev.* **2001,** 101: 1869–1880.

Lee, K. Y. and Mooney, D. J. Alginate: properties and biomedical applications. *Prog Polym Sci.* **2012,** 37: 106–126.

Lee, S. J., Wang, H. J., Kim, T. H., Choi, J. S., Kulkarni, G., Jackson, J. D. et al. In situ tissue regeneration of renal tissue induced by collagen hydrogel injection. *Stem Cells Transl Med.* **2018,** 7: 241–250.

Levengood, S. K. L. and Zhang, M. Chitosan-based scaffolds for bone tissue engineering. *J Mater Chem B.* **2014,** 2: 3161–3184.

Li, H. B., Jiang, H., Wang, C. H., Duan, C. M., Ye, Y., Su, X. P. et al. Comparison of two types of alginate microcapsules on stability and biocompatibility *in vitro* and *in vivo*. *Biomed Mater.* **2006,** 1: 42–47.

Li, W., Wang, B., Zhang, M., Wu, Z., Wei, J., Jiang, Y. et al. All natural injectable hydrogel with self-healing and antibacterial properties for wound dressing. *Cellulose.* **2020,** 27: 2637–2650.

Loh, E. Y. X., Mohamad, N., Fauzi, M. B., Ng, M. H., Ng, S. F. and Amin, M. C. I. M. Development of a bacterial cellulose-based hydrogel cell carrier containing keratinocytes and fibroblasts for full-thickness wound healing. *Sci Rep.* **2018,** 8: 2875.

Luo, J. W., Liua, C., Wu, J. H., Lin, L. X., Fan, H. M., Zhao, D. H. et al. In situ injectable hyaluronic acid/gelatin hydrogel for hemorrhage control. *Mater Sci Eng.* **2019,** 3: 628–634.

Makvandi, P., Ali, G. W., Della Sala, F., Abdel-Fattah, W. I. and Borzacchiello, A. Hyaluronic acid-/corn silk extract-based injectable nanocomposite: a biomimetic antibacterial scaffold for bone tissue regeneration. *Mater Sci Eng.* **2020,** 8: 110195–110205.

Mano, J. F., Silva, G. A., Azevedo, H. S., Malafaya, P. B., Sousa, R. A., Silva, S. S. et al. Natural origin biodegradable systems in tissue engineering and regenerative medicine: present status and some moving trends. *J Royal Soc Interf.* **2007,** 17: 999–1030.

Medvedeva, E. V., Grebenik, E. A., Gornostaeva, S. N., Telpuhov, V. I., Lychagin, A. V., Timashev, P. S. et al. Repair of damaged articular cartilage: current approaches and future directions. *Int J Mol Sci.* **2018,** 19: 2366–2389.

Moss, J. M., Van Damme, M. P. I., Murphy, W. H., Stanton, P. G., Thomas, P. and Preston, B. N. Purification, characterization, and biosynthesis of bovine cartilage lysozyme isoforms. *Arch Biochem Biophys.* **1997,** 339: 172–182.

Nabavi, M. H., Salehi, M., Ehterami, A., Bastami, F., Semyari, H., Tehranchi, M. et al. A collagen-based hydrogel containing tacrolimus for bone tissue engineering. *Drug Deliv Transl Res.* **2020,** 10: 108–121.

Naderi-Meshkin, H., Andreas, K., Matin, M. M., Sittinger, M., Bidkhori, H. R., Ahmadiankia, N. et al. Chitosan-based injectable hydrogel as a promising in situ forming scaffold for cartilage tissue engineering. *Cell Biol Int.* **2014,** 38: 72–84.

Nezhad-Mokhtari, P., Akrami-Hasan-Kohal, M. and Marjan Ghorbani, M. An injectable chitosan-based hydrogel scaffold containing gold nanoparticles for tissue engineering applications. *Int J Biol Macromol.* **2020,** 154: 198–205.

Nichol, J. W., Koshy, S., Bae, H., Hwang, C. M. and Khademhosseini, A. Cell-laden microengineered gelatin methacrylate hydrogels Jason. *Biomaterials.* **2011,** 31: 5536–5544.

Nicholas, M. N., Jeschke, M. G. and Amini-Nik, S. Cellularized bilayer pullulan-gelatin hydrogel for skin regeneration. *Tissue Eng.* **2016,** 22: 9–10.

Nilforoushzadeh, M. A., Sisakht, M. M., Amirkhani, M. A., Seifalian, A. M., Banafshe, H. R., Verdi, J. et al. Engineered skin graft with stromal vascular fraction cells encapsulated in fibrin–collagen hydrogel: A clinical study for diabetic wound healing. *J Tissue Eng Regen Med.* **2020,** 14: 424–440.

Nocera, A. D., Comín, R., Salvatierra, N. A. and Cid, M. P. Development of 3D printed fibrillar collagen scaffold for tissue engineering. *Biomed Microdevices.* **2018,** 20: 26–39.

Novotna, K., Havelka, P., Sopuch, T., Kolarova, K., Vosmanska, V., Lisa, V. et al. Cellulose-based materials as scaffolds for tissue engineering. *Cellulose.* **2013,** 20: 2263–2278.

Onofrei, M. and Filimon, A. Cellulose-based hydrogels: Designing concepts, properties, and perspectives for biomedical and environmental applications. *Polym Sci Res Adv Pract Appl Edu Aspects.* **2016,** 3: 108–120.

Pangburn, S., Trescony, P. and Heller, J. Lysozyme degradation of partially deacetylated chitin, its films and hydrogels. *Biomaterials.* **1982,** 3: 105–108.

Peppas, A. N. and Hoffman, A. S. Hydrogels. In: *Biomaterials Science: An Introduction to Materials in Medicine* (4th edition). Wagner, W. R., Sakiyama-Elbert, S. E., Yaszemski, M. J. (Eds). **2020,** 1.3.2 E153–166.

Petersen, N. and Gatenholm, P. Bacterial cellulose-based materials and medical devices: current state and perspectives. *Appl Microbiol Biotechnol.* **2011,** 91: 1277–1286.

Reakasame, S. and Boccaccini, A. R. Oxidized alginate-based hydrogels for tissue engineering applications: a review. *Biomacromolecules.* **2018,** 19: 3–21.

Rezaeeyazdi, M., Colombani, T., Memic, A. and Bencherif, S. A. Injectable hyaluronic acid-co-gelatin cryogels for tissue engineering. *Appl Mater.* **2018,** 11: 1374–1388.

Rinaudo, M. Chitin and chitosan: properties and applications. *Prog Polym Sci.* **2006,** 31: 603–613.

Sahana, T. G. and Rekha, P. D. Biopolymers: applications in wound healing and skin tissue engineering. *Mol Biol Rep.* **2018,** 45: 2857–2867.

Samadian, H., Vaez, A., Ehterami, A., Salehi, M., Farzamfar, S., Sahrapeyma, H. Sciatic nerve regeneration by using collagen type I hydrogel containing naringin. *J Mater Sci Mater Med.* **2019,** 30: 107–117.

Sancilio, S., Gallorini, M., Di Nisio, C., Marsich, E., Di Pietro, R., Schweikl, H. alginate/hydroxyapatite-based nanocomposite scaffolds for bone tissue engineering improve dental pulp biomineralization and differentiation. *Stem Cells Int.* **2018,** 2018: 1–13.

Sani, E. S., Portillo-Lara, R., Spencer, A., Yu, W., Geilich, B. M., Noshadi, I. et al. Engineering adhesive and antimicrobial hyaluronic acid/elastin-like polypeptide hybrid hydrogels for tissue engineering applications. *ACS Biomater Sci Eng.* **2018,** 4: 2528–2540.

Sannino, A., Demitri, C. and Madaghiele, M. Biodegradable cellulose-based hydrogels: design and applications. *Materials.* **2009,** 2: 353–373.

Sarangthem, V., Singh, T. D. and Dinda, A. K. Emerging role of elastin-like polypeptides (ELPs) in regenerative medicine. *Adv Wound Care.* **2020,** 1: 1–37.

Saunders, L. and Ma, P. X. Healing supramolecular hydrogels for tissue engineering applications. *Macromol Biosci.* **2019,** 19: 313–324.

Schloss, A. C., Williams, D. M. and Regan, L. J. Protein-based hydrogels for tissue engineering. In: Protein-based Engineered Nanostructures. Cortajarena, A. and Grove, T. (Eds). **2016,** 940: 167–177.

Shafei, S., Khanmohammadi, M., Heidari, R., Ghanbari, H., Nooshabadi, V. T., Farzamfar, S. et al. Exosome-loaded alginate hydrogel promotes tissue regeneration in full-thickness skin wounds: An *in vivo* study. *J Biomed Mater Res.* **2020,** 5: 545–556.

Sheehy, J., Vinardella, T., Buckley, C. T. and Kelly, D. J. Engineering osteochondral constructs through spatial regulation of endochondral ossification. *Acta Biomater.* **2013,** 9: 5484–5492.

Shen, X., Shamshina, J. L., Berton, P., Gurau, G. and Rogers, R. D. Hydrogels based on cellulose and chitin: fabrication, properties, and applications. *Green Chem.* **2016,** 18: 53–75.

Shoulders, M. D. and Raines, R. T. Collagen structure and stability. *Ann Rev Biochem.* **2009,** 78: 929–958.

Silva, R., Singh, R., Sarker, B., Papageorgiou, D. G., Juhasz, J. A., Roether, J. A. et al. Hybrid hydrogels based on keratin and alginate for tissue engineering. *J Mater Chem.* **2014,** 2: 5441–5451.

Silva, S. S., Fernandes, E. M., Pina, S., Silva-Correia, J., Vieira, S., Oliveira, J. M. et al. Natural-origin materials for tissue engineering and regenerative medicine. *Comp Biomater II.* **2018,** 2: 228–252.

Soman, P., Chung, P. H., Zhang, A. P. and Chen, S. Digital microfabrication of user-defined 3D microstructures in cell-laden hydrogels. *Biotechnol Bioeng.* **2013,** 110: 1–11.

Song, S. J., Choi, J., Park, Y. D., Hong, S., Lee, J. J., Ahn, C. B. et al. Sodium alginate hydrogel-based bioprinting using a novel multinozzle bioprinting system. *Artif Organs.* **2011,** 35: 1132–1136.

Soucy, J. R., Sani, E. S., Portillo Lara, R., Diaz, D., Dias, F., Weiss, A. S. et al. Photocross-linkable gelatin/tropoelastin hydrogel adhesives for peripheral nerve repair. *Tissue Eng Part A.* **2018,** 24: 17–18.

Tan, H., Chu, C. R., Payne, K. A. and Marra, K. G. Injectable in situ forming biodegradable chitosan–hyaluronic acid-based hydrogels for cartilage tissue engineering. *Biomaterials.* **2009,** 30: 2499–2506.

Tonsomboon, K., Strange, D. G. T. and Oyen, M. L. Gelatin nanofiber-reinforced alginate gel scaffolds for corneal tissue engineering. *Proc Eng Med Biol Soc.* **2010,** 2013: 6671–6674.

Trombino, S., Servidio, C., Curcio, F. and Cassano, R. Strategies for hyaluronic acid-based hydrogel design in drug delivery. *Pharmaceutics.* **2019,** 11: 407–424.

Turco, G., Marsich, E. and Bellomo, F. Alginate/hydroxyapatite biocomposite for bone ingrowth: a trabecular structure with high and isotropic connectivity. *Biomacromolecules.* **2009,** 10: 1575–1583.

Valle, L. J. D., Diaz, A. and Puiggali, J. Hydrogels for biomedical applications: cellulose, chitosan, and protein/peptide derivatives. *Gels*. **2017,** 27: 1–28.

Varum, K. M., Myhr, M. M., Hjerde, R. J. N. and Smidsrød, O. *In vitro* degradation rates of partially *N*-acetylated chitosans in human serum. *Carbohyd Res*. **1997,** 299: 99–101.

Velema, J. and Kaplan, D. Biopolymer-based biomaterials as scaffolds for tissue engineering. *Adv Biochem Eng Biotechnol*. **2006,** 102: 187–238.

Wang, L., Li, J., Zhang, D., Ma, S., Zhang, J., Gao, F. et al. Dual-enzymatically cross-linked and injectable hyaluronic acid hydrogels for potential application in tissue engineering. *RSC Adv*. **2020,** 10: 2870–2876.

Wang, L. and Shansky, J. Design and fabrication of a biodegradable, covalently cross-linked shape-memory alginate scaffold for cell and growth factor delivery. *Tissue Eng Part A*. **2012,** 18: 2000–2007.

Wu, S. W., Liua, X., Miller, A. L., Cheng, Y. S., Yeh, M. L. and Lu, L. Strengthening injectable thermosensitive NIPAAm-g-chitosan hydrogels using chemical cross-linking of disulfide bonds as scaffolds for tissue engineering. *Carbohyd Polym*. **2018,** 192: 308–316.

Xu, C., Guan, S., Wang, S., Gong, W., Liu, T., Ma, X. et al. Biodegradable and electroconductive poly(3,4-ethylenedioxythiophene)/carboxymethyl chitosan hydrogels for neural tissue engineering. *Mater Sci Eng C*. **2018,** 84: 32–43.

Yadav, R. B. and Chauhan, M. K. A review: chitosan as 3D matrix for tissue engineering. *Int J Res Pharm Sci*. **2017,** 3: 66–69.

Yamada, S., Yamamoto, K., Ikeda, T., Yanagiguchi, K. and Hayashi, Y. Potency of fish collagen as a scaffold for regenerative medicine. *Biomed Res Int*. **2014,** 2014: 1–8.

Zhang, J., Sisley, A. M. G., Anderson, A. J., Taberner, A. J., McGhee, C. N. J. and Dipika, V. Characterization of a novel collagen scaffold for corneal tissue engineering. *Tissue Eng Part C Methods*. **2015,** 22: 1–15.

Zhu, T., Mao, J., Cheng, Y., Liu, H., Lv, L., Ge, M. et al. Recent progress of polysaccharide-based hydrogel interfaces for wound healing and tissue engineering. *Adv Mater Interfaces*. **2019,** 6: 1–23.

Index

For Product Safety Concerns and Information please contact our EU
representative GPSR@taylorandfrancis.com
Taylor & Francis Verlag GmbH, Kaufingerstraße 24, 80331 München, Germany

www.ingramcontent.com/pod-product-compliance
Lightning Source LLC
Chambersburg PA
CBHW060810220326
41598CB00022B/2585